PRACTICAL GASTROENTEROLOGY

PRACTICAL GASTROENTEROLOGY

Edited by Ronald L. Koretz, M.D.

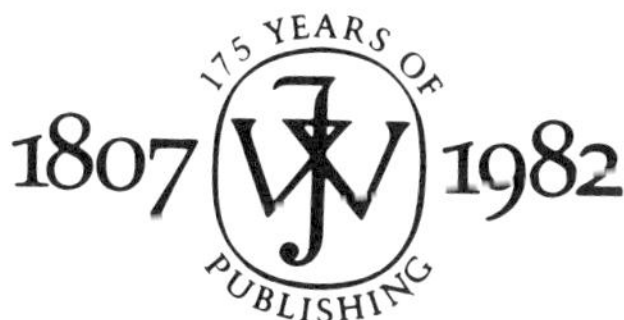

A WILEY MEDICAL PUBLICATION

JOHN WILEY & SONS / **New York · Chichester · Brisbane · Toronto**

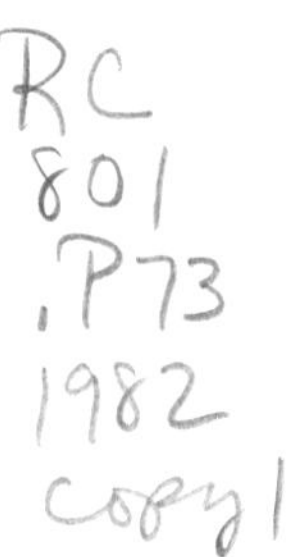

Library of Congress Cataloging in Publication Data:

Main entry under title:

Practical gastroenterology.

(Postgraduate medicine for the primary care
physician)
   Bibliography: p.
   Includes index.
   1. Digestive organs—Diseases.   2. Gastroenterology.   I. Koretz, Ronald.   II. Series.   [DNLM:
1. Gastrointestinal diseases. WI 100 P895]
RC801.P73   616.3'3   81–3373
ISBN 0–471–09513–3   AACR2

Printed in the United States of America

10 9 8 7 6 5 4 3 2 1

To Grace, Brandon, Sherilyn, and Justin
for all those lost weekends

Contributors

Marvin Derezin, M.D., Associate Clinical Professor, Department of Medicine, Division of Gastroenterology, UCLA School of Medicine, Los Angeles, California

Neil Kaplowitz, M.D., Associate Professor, Department of Medicine, UCLA School of Medicine; Chief, Division of Gastroenterology, Wadsworth Veterans Administration Hospital; Director, Combined UCLA–Wadsworth Gastroenterology Training Program, Los Angeles, California

Ronald L. Koretz, M.D., Associate Professor, Department of Medicine, UCLA School of Medicine, Los Angeles, California; Chief, Division of Gastroenterology, Department of Medicine, Olive View Medical Center, Van Nuys, California

Martin A. Pops, M.D., Professor, Department of Medicine, Division of Gastroenterology, UCLA School of Medicine, Los Angeles, California

Arthur D. Schwabe, M.D., Professor, Department of Medicine; Chief, Division of Gastroenterology, UCLA School of Medicine, Los Angeles, California

Wilfred M. Weinstein, M.D., Professor, Department of Medicine, Division of Gastroenterology, UCLA School of Medicine, Los Angeles, California

UCLA Department of Medicine Committee on Continuing Education

Sanford Bloom, M.D., Adjunct Associate Professor of Medicine, Division of Family Practice

Glenn Braunstein, M.D., Associate Professor of Medicine, Division of Endocrinology

Robert Brook, M.D., Associate Professor of Medicine and Public Health, Division of General Internal Medicine and Health Services Research

William Cabeen, M.D., Assistant Clinical Professor of Medicine, Division of Cardiology

Harold Carlson, M.D., Associate Professor of Medicine, Division of Endocrinology

Sheryl Crowley, Program Representative, Division of Medicine, UCLA Extension

Arlene Fink, Ph.D., Associate Social Sciences Researcher, Department of Medicine

Stanley S. Franklin, M.D., Clinical Professor of Medicine, Division of Nephrology

Robert Gale, M.D., Associate Professor of Medicine and Microbiology and Immunology, Division of Hematology/Oncology

Jeffrey Galpin, M.D., Assistant Professor of Medicine, Division of Infectious Disease

Gary L. Gitnick, M.D., Professor of Medicine, Division of Gastroenterology

Ralph Gold, M.D., Clinical Instructor of Medicine, Division of Family Practice

Harvey C. Gonick, M.D., Adjunct Professor of Medicine, Division of Nephrology

Arnold Gurevitch, M.D., Adjunct Associate Professor of Medicine, Division of Dermatology

Jackie Kosecoff, Ph.D., Associate Social Sciences Researcher, Department of Medicine

Richard Meyer, M.D., Associate Professor of Medicine, Division of Infectious Disease

Linda Olt, M.A., Editor, Department of Medicine

Harold Paulus, M.D., Professor of Medicine, Division of Rheumatology

Michael Reza, M.D., Assistant Clinical Professor of Medicine, Division of Rheumatology

William Rodney, M.D., Assistant Professor of Medicine, Division of Family Practice

Gregory Sarna, M.D., Assistant Professor of Medicine, Division of Hematology/Oncology

Andrew Saxon, M.D., Associate Professor of Medicine; Chief, Division of Clinical Immunology and Allergy

     COMMITTEE ON CONTINUING EDUCATION

Martin Shickman, M.D., Clinical Professor of Medicine; Director, Department of Continuing Education in Health Sciences, UCLA Extension; Assistant Dean for Postgraduate Medical Education, UCLA School of Medicine

Vasant Udhoji, M.D., Adjunct Professor of Medicine, Division of Cardiology

Stuart Vener, M.D., Assistant Clinical Professor of Medicine, Division of Endocrinology

Irwin Weinstein, M.D., Clinical Professor of Medicine, Division of Hematology

Thomas Yoshikawa, M.D., Associate Professor of Medicine, Division of Infectious Disease

Roy Young, M.D., Vice Chairman for Clinical Services and Training, Department of Medicine

This publication was developed in association with a course sponsored by UCLA Extension, Health Sciences Division.

Preface

Gastroenterologic problems confront the practicing physician every day. At the same time, the literature in this field is growing at a seemingly exponential rate. (There are currently nine major clinical journals that deal solely with diseases of the gastrointestinal tract and liver in addition to the general medicine, surgery, and pediatric publications.) We are being continuously bombarded with new tests, new therapies, and, occasionally, even new diseases.

The intent of this book is to synthesize some of the accepted recent inroads with the older avenues and present a unified approach to particular gastrointestinal problems. It is not our purpose to review the recent literature in a "what's new" format; such works become outdated rapidly. Rather, the information in each chapter should provide a basis (for attacking these various disorders) that will remain appropriate for many years to come.

Emphasis has been placed on practicality. This is not a textbook of gastroenterology. As you will see, pathophysiologic concepts have not been covered except where they have direct bearing on patient management. Similarly, obscure or sophisticated gastroenterologic disorders or decisions have been omitted or only covered to provide insight as to why particular steps might be taken. This book will not substitute for specialist consultation in patients with particularly complex problems. On the other hand the recommendations in the various chapters will direct primary physicians to reasonable steps that they can take themselves in common problems.

The authors have been selected because of their past proven ability to communicate effectively with audiences of clinicians. Although they have different particular fields of special interest, they all share the common background of a great deal of clinical experience. When they write of a particular method of handling a problem, they will be telling you what has worked for them in countless individual experiences. Sometimes a method is well established scientifically; at other times it is only supported by their "uncontrolled" observations.

The book has been divided into two sections, one dealing with common symptoms and the other with common disease entities. This reflects the situation in the real world, where patients have either isolated symptoms (and a diagnosis needs to be made) or identified disease complexes (where management considerations are the first priority).

The authors of the chapters in Part I were asked to construct their discussions around the answers to the following questions, aimed at establishing a diagnosis or providing nonspecific therapy:

1. What are the important aspects of history?
2. What are the important physical findings to seek?
3. What laboratory tests or procedures should be ordered?
4. What are the major diagnostic considerations?
5. What symptomatic therapy can be given in the absence of a specific diagnosis?

The chapters in Part II will pick up the story after a diagnosis has been established. Again the authors were requested to respond to a set of questions, this time dealing more with therapy and prognosis:

1. How do I make the diagnosis?
2. What additional workup does the patient require?
3. How should I treat the patient?
4. What should I expect from successful therapy?
5. What might cause a failure of treatment?
6. What are the side effects of treatment?
7. How should the patient be followed?
8. What complications of the disease can occur?
9. How should these complications be managed?

Although a few of the chapters (Chapters 12, 16, 20, and 22) could not be so structured, the remainder will follow these formats.

We hope this volume will find its major use in the day-to-day care of your patients. If the book finds its way to the more accessible area of your bookshelf, our efforts will have been justified.

R. L. K.

Contents

PRACTICAL
GASTROENTEROLOGY

SYMPTOMS

1

ARTHUR D. SCHWABE

Abdominal Pain

One of the most common complaints associated with disorders of the gastrointestinal tract is abdominal discomfort or pain. It may emanate from any segment of the digestive tube, from any of the solid viscera in the abdomen, or from any of the tissues lining, surrounding, or suspending these viscera, such as the visceral or parietal peritoneum, the mesentery, or the omentum. Pain in these structures may be caused by distention or stretching, inflammation, ischemia or, in the case of hollow viscera, by spasm.

WHAT ARE THE IMPORTANT ASPECTS OF HISTORY?

The history is of primary importance in arriving at a rapid diagnosis. Clinicians who are most proficient in eliciting the origin of the pain from a barrage of descriptive material rely on the answers to the following eight questions:

1. What is the exact location of the pain? (location)
2. How quickly did the pain arise? (onset)
3. How long did the pain last? (duration)
4. How does the pain feel? (character)
5. To what other areas does the pain radiate? (radiation)
6. What may aggravate or precipitate the pain? (aggravating or precipitating factors)
7. What measures relieve or stop the pain? (relief)
8. What other symptoms accompany the pain? (accompanying symptoms)

Let us now examine how the information elicited from these simple questions may help us to focus on the most likely cause of the pain.

Location

Pain from structures within the abdominal cavity is perceived in more superficial areas of the abdominal wall. Since a number of viscera are innervated by the same spinal segment, pain emanating from several viscera may be localized in one area. Patients should be asked to point to the area of discomfort.

In general, pain that arises from the stomach, duodenum, pancreas, liver, or biliary tree is felt in the upper part of the abdomen. Pain from the small bowel is appreciated in the periumbilical area, and pain from the colon is felt in the lower abdomen (Table 1). The discomfort is sometimes sharply localized to a small area of the abdomen. For example, many patients with duodenal ulcers can point to a half-dollar–sized area in the epigastrium, and those with sigmoid diverticulitis may have discomfort confined to the left lower quadrant. The localization of pain emanating from a hollow viscus also depends on the character and severity of the pathologic process and the involvement of adjacent structures. Distention and spasm are referred to the midline; inflammation with peritonitis localizes wherever the process lies.

Onset

The rate of onset of pain may indicate the pathologic process and may also help the physician to localize the pain. An abrupt or

Table 1 Location of Pain from Abdominal Structures

Area of Pain	Affected Structure	Clinical Examples
Substernal area	Esophagus	Esophagitis Esophageal cancer
Shoulder	Diaphragm	Subphrenic abscess
Epigastrium	Stomach	Gastric ulcer
	Duodenum	Duodenal ulcer
	Gall bladder	Biliary colic
	Liver	Hepatitis
	Bile ducts	Cholangitis
	Pancreas	Pancreatitis
Right scapula	Biliary tract	Biliary colic
Midback	Pancreas	Pancreatic cancer
	Aorta	Aortic aneurysm
Periumbilical area	Small intestine	Obstruction, intussusception, intestinal angina
Hypogastrium	Colon	Diverticulitis, ulcerative colitis
Sacral area	Rectum	Proctitis, perirectal abscess

explosive onset is characteristic of rupture (of a hollow viscus or aneurysm) or of stones (biliary or renal) that suddenly impact a narrow orifice. An inflammatory process, such as appendicitis or pancreatitis, usually has a gradual onset.

Duration

Pain that lasts only a few seconds or minutes is usually due to distention or spasm of a hollow viscus. Epigastric discomfort that lasts 15 to 45 minutes or until it is relieved by food or antacids is characteristic of peptic ulcer disease. In other abdominal conditions pain is often of much longer duration. Biliary colic reaches a level of maximum intensity that persists for several hours. In pancreatitis the pain usually continues for several days. Patients who complain of chronic or unremitting pain for several weeks may have a retroperitoneal tumor, such as a lymphoma or carcinoma of the pancreas. Persistent pain that lasts for months or years is most likely due to a chronic motility disorder or to addiction to narcotics.

Character

It is often difficult for patients to describe their pains in terms that can be interpreted by a physician. However, a number of adjectives can usually be elicited and may be characteristic of a specific disorder. These include: aching, burning, dull, gnawing (peptic ulcer); squeezing, steady, vise-like (biliary colic); cramping, intermittent, knife-like, pulsating, sharp (irritable colon, inflammatory bowel disease). If patients continue to describe their pain as "indigestion" or an "upset stomach," the physician may have to draw diagrams or provide examples of sensations that most patients can understand.

Radiation

Disorders of certain abdominal structures give rise to pain that may radiate or is referred to specific areas. Irritation of the diaphragm, for instance, is referred to the shoulder, usually on the same side. Biliary colic may radiate to the right scapula or the midthoracic spine. A posterior, penetrating duodenal ulcer or pancreatitis usually produces pain that radiates to the back. Ureteral colic tends to radiate downward into the groin or testicles, or both. A knowledge of the areas to which pain from abdominal viscera are referred may greatly facilitate the diagnosis.

Aggravating or Precipitating Factors

Bending forward or lying flat in bed often aggravates or initiates the discomfort of reflux esophagitis. Ingestion of a meal rich in fat may precipitate an attack of biliary colic. Motion, including coughing, exacerbates the pain of peritonitis. Patients with generalized peritonitis are most comfortable lying quietly in bed, avoiding any movement whatsoever. Passage of stool will tend to aggravate the symptoms of proctitis and perianal disease.

Relief

Once the abdominal pain has become manifest, patients can usually identify a number of positions, maneuvers, or activities that

Maneuver or Activity	Structure(s) Involved	Clinical Examples
Belching	Stomach	Gastric distention
Eating	Stomach, duodenum	Peptic ulcer
Vomiting	Stomach, duodenum	Pyloric obstruction
Leaning foward	Retroperitoneal	Carcinoma of the pancreas
Sitting position	structures	Chronic pancreatitis
		Retroperitoneal lymphoma
Flexion of both knees	Peritoneum	Peritonitis
Flexion of right thigh	Right psoas muscle	Appendiceal abscess
Flexion of left thigh	Left psoas muscle	Diverticular abscess
Passage of stool or flatus	Colon	Irritable colon

tend to ameliorate or obliterate the pain (Table 2). These observations by the patients may be important clues to the nature of the underlying process. Equally important are those factors that have no effect on the pain. For example, vomiting will provide relief in the presence of pyloric or duodenal obstruction, but it will have no effect on the pain associated with acute cholecystitis, pancreatitis, or renal colic.

Accompanying Symptoms

The coexistence of fever with or without chills and diaphoresis indicates an inflammatory process in the abdomen. Hematemesis or melena, or both, with pain in the epigastrium is most likely due to hemorrhagic gastritis or peptic ulcer. The simultaneous occurrence of diarrhea suggests an infectious or inflammatory process of the bowel. Frequent urination may indicate an inflammatory process adjacent to the bladder, such as appendicitis, diverticulitis, or pelvic inflammatory disease. Epigastric pain followed by jaundice should suggest disease of the biliary tract.

Other Significant Historical Information

Certain population groups are at risk for particular diseases associated with abdominal pain. For example, American Indians have a high risk of developing gallstones at an early age. Intestinal vascular disease is more likely to develop in elderly patients, particularly those with hypercoagulable states or extensive atherosclerosis, or both. Diverticulitis and gastrointestinal cancer are also more likely to develop in elderly patients.

WHAT ARE THE IMPORTANT PHYSICAL FINDINGS TO SEEK?

The origin of abdominal pain may be surmised from abnormalities in the skin, neck, eyegrounds, breasts, chest, heart, or skeleton as well as the abdomen. The scrotum and inguinal canals should be examined carefully for the presence of hernias. Thorough rectal and pelvic examinations may support the diagnosis of acute appendicitis, pelvic abscess, or pelvic inflammatory disease. A detailed description of all the physical findings associated with abdominal pain is beyond the scope of this chapter. Emphasis is therefore given to highly significant abdominal signs, which are important in establishing a diagnosis.

Gastric Peristalsis

Visible waves that move from the left upper quadrant across the upper abdomen toward the right upper quadrant represent gastric peristalsis and indicate gastric outlet obstruction. A gastric succussion splash four or more hours after the patient eats is frequently present as well.

Abdominal Distention

Visible distention of the abdomen may be due to partial bowel obstruction, accumulation of gas, or ascites. Partial obstruction is usually accompanied by nausea, cramping abdominal pain, hyperperistalsis, succussion splashes, and, occasionally, by visible peristalsis. In gaseous distention the abdomen is tympanitic and bowel sounds are either normal or decreased. Ascites can be demonstrated by percussion, the observation of shifting dullness, or a fluid wave.

Bowel Sounds

Bowel sounds are noises produced by the movement of gas, fluid, and chyme through the intestine. The absence of bowel sounds indicates a state of intestinal paralysis caused by ileus or peritonitis. Increased bowel sounds may be heard in the presence of intestinal inflammation, infection, or obstruction. Intermittent, high-pitched bowel sounds, which rise to a crescendo and then pass away, are characteristic of bowel obstruction.

Abdominal Bruits, Hums, and Murmurs

Vascular sounds originating in the abdomen may be valuable clues in localizing and interpreting the origin of abdominal pain. A systolic arterial murmur over the liver may be found in hepatoma and a venous hum may accompany portal hypertension. Mesenteric arterial compression or partial occlusion may be accompanied by a bruit in the midline. However, advanced mesenteric vascular disease may exist in the absence of any bruit. A splenic artery aneurysm may cause left upper quadrant pain and may give rise to a palpable and audible bruit. A pulsating abdominal mass accompanied by a bruit near the midline is characteristic of an aortic aneurysm.

Hepatic Friction Rub

A friction rub may be palpated or heard over the liver or over the right lower chest anteriorly or anterolaterally. A hepatic friction rub is usually caused by a malignant tumor, but may also be present in liver abscess, gonococcal perihepatitis, or after a percutaneous liver biopsy.

Absence of Hepatic Dullness

Absence of hepatic dullness on percussion indicates either a small shrunken liver from previous liver disease or the presence of free air in the abdominal cavity.

Palpable Gallbladder

A gallbladder that is visible or palpable in the right upper quadrant is caused most frequently by a carcinoma of the head of the pancreas or ampulla. Occasionally the gallbladder may also be felt when the cystic duct or common bile duct is obstructed by a stone or when the gallbladder is extensively infiltrated and thickened by a primary carcinoma.

Murphy's Sign

Murphy's sign, the sudden termination of inspiratory effort and induction of right upper quadrant pain elicited by pressure in the region of the gallbladder, is useful in supporting the diagnosis of acute cholecystitis. The maneuver is performed with the patient in the supine position. The examiner carefully palpates the liver, fixes his or her fingers below the liver edge under the costal margin, and then asks the patient to take a deep breath. Deep inspiration causes the liver to descend and drives the inflamed gallbladder against the examiner's fingers.

Psoas Sign

An inflammatory process in contact with the psoas muscle may be detected by a simple maneuver. While in the supine position with the legs fully extended, the patient is asked to elevate one leg. Pain in the hypogastrium may indicate acute appendicitis, diverticulitis, or a pelvic abscess.

Obturator Sign

An inflammatory process in contact with the internal obturator muscle may give rise to the obturator sign. With the patient in the supine position with flexed thigh and knee, the examiner rotates the leg 180 degrees. If this rotation induces pain in the hypogastrium, acute appendicitis or a pelvic abscess should be suspected.

Edema of the Flank

A bulge or pitting edema in the flank indicates a retroperitoneal phlegmon, usually a perinephric or pancreatic abscess.

Ecchymoses

Bluish discoloration or frank ecchymoses at the costovertebral angles (Grey-Turner sign) and around the umbilicus (Cullen's sign) indicate retroperitoneal bleeding. Such hemorrhagic phenomena occur in some cases of hemorrhagic pancreatitis and in other disorders associated with retroperitoneal bleeding.

WHAT LABORATORY TESTS OR PROCEDURES SHOULD BE ORDERED?

The selection of laboratory tests is based on the information obtained from the history and physical examination. A complete blood count, urinalysis, chest x-ray, and electrocardiogram should always be obtained if the pain is of recent onset. Occasionally lobar pneumonia or acute myocardial infarction may present as abdominal pain. If a liver, biliary tract, or pancreatic process is suspected, appropriate blood and urine studies are indicated. In acute diarrheal disorders stools should be cultured and examined for ova and parasites. Several studies deserve special emphasis.

Plain Films of the Abdomen

Films of the abdomen taken with the patient in a supine or upright position are often diagnostic in many acute abdominal conditions and may obviate the need for other more time-consuming and complicated procedures (Table 3).

Ultrasonography

Ultrasonography is a simple, safe technique that is an extremely valuable tool in defining a variety of intraabdominal conditions. It

Diagnostic Finding	Clinical Problem(s)
Calcifications	
Rounded or faceted in RUQ	Gall stones
Globular or ring shaped in RUQ	Porcelain gallbladder, echinococcus cyst
Mottled in RUQ	Metastatic tumor
Curvilinear in midline	Aortic aneurysm
Speckled across midline	Chronic pancreatitis
Irregular lateral to L1 or L2	Renal calculi
Kernel shaped lateral to spine	Ureteral calculi
Elongated, worm-like in RLQ	Appendicolith
Dilatation of hollow viscera	
Of the stomach	Gastric outlet obstruction
Of the small bowel	Small-bowel obstruction
Of the cecum	Cecal ileus, volvulus
Of the colon	Obstruction, volvulus, toxic megacolon
Fingerprinting	
Of the small bowel	Ischemia, edema
Of the colon	Ischemic colitis
Gas or air collections	
Free air under diaphragm	Perforated viscus
Extraluminal, mottled	Abscess
In stomach wall	Emphysematous gastritis
In fascial planes	Clostridial abscess of cecum
In wall of colon	Pneumatosis cystoides
Sentinel loop in small bowel	Acute pancreatitis
Colon cutoff sign	Acute pancreatitis
Masses	Tumors, abscesses
Loss of colonic haustrations	Ulcerative colitis

may demonstrate primary or metastatic tumors, abscesses, cysts, aortic aneurysms, gallstones, enlargement of abdominal viscera, and dilated bile ducts and loops of bowel.

Radionuclide Scans

Radionuclide imaging is useful in evaluating the size, shape, and position of the liver and spleen. Tumors, abscesses, cysts, or hematomas in these organs may be detected by this technique.

Analysis of Peritoneal Fluid

A peritoneal tap and subsequent analysis of peritoneal fluid may provide a quick answer to some acute abdominal conditions. Diagnostic paracentesis should be performed in patients with abdominal pain in whom free intraperitoneal fluid can be demonstrated.

The following determinations should be performed on the fluid obtained: specific gravity, cell count, gram stain, cultures for bacteria, total protein, lactic dehydrogenase, amylase, and cytology. A white blood cell count greater than 250/mm^3 in peritoneal fluid is usually associated with intraabdominal infections, inflammation, or tumor. Bloody ascitic fluid is seen with abdominal trauma, acute hemorrhagic pancreatitis, hepatic vein thrombosis, ruptured aneurysm, ruptured spleen, neoplasms, and tuberculous peritonitis. Fluids with specific gravities greater than 1.016 or a protein level greater than 3 gm/100 ml are considered to be exudates. Exudative ascites is found primarily in the presence of bacterial or tuberculous peritonitis, pancreatitis, peritoneal malignancy, and traumatic rupture of major lymphatic channels. An elevated ascitic fluid amylase is characteristic of pancreatitis. An elevated ascitic fluid lactic dehydrogenase is sometimes associated with peritoneal carcinomatosis.

Sigmoidoscopy

Abdominal pain associated with diarrhea or rectal bleeding, or both, warrants a sigmoidoscopic examination. The mucosa should be inspected carefully, direct smears should be made of rectal mucus, and biopsies should be taken from abnormal areas. Ulcerative, granulomatous, and pseudomembranous colitis are usually identified by a combination of inspection and histologic examination. Amoebas may be seen in rectal mucus or in stained histologic specimens.

Contrast Radiography of Hollow Viscera

In most acute abdominal conditions, particularly in the presence of obvious perforation or generalized peritonitis, examination of hollow viscera with radiographic contrast media is avoided. Water-soluble media may be used after adequate decompression to define the nature of gastric retention or to localize the site of intestinal obstruction. However, in chronic abdominal conditions a regular barium study provides better detail of mucosal abnormalities, such as ulceration, inflammation, infiltration, edema, and stricture.

Cholecystography and Cholangiography

Visualization of the gallbladder and biliary tree may aid in the diagnosis of right upper quadrant pain. The objectives, indications, and contraindications are discussed in Chapters 6 and 18.

WHAT ARE THE MAJOR DIAGNOSTIC CONSIDERATIONS?

This material has been covered in previous sections.

WHAT SYMPTOMATIC THERAPY CAN BE GIVEN IN THE ABSENCE OF A SPECIFIC DIAGNOSIS?

In acute abdominal conditions supportive care, including fluid, electrolyte, and blood replacement, should be instituted as soon as appropriate blood and urine specimens have been obtained. However, motility-inhibiting drugs, such as anticholinergics and opiates, should be withheld until the precise nature of the abdominal pain has been established. Nasogastric suction should be initiated when the diagnosis of gastric retention or small-bowel obstruction is made or suspected. Chronic abdominal pain should be treated only with local measures and mild, nonnarcotic analgesics until a diagnosis is established.

The specific modes of treatment for abdominal conditions associated with pain are detailed in subsequent chapters.

Abcarian H, Eftaiha M, Kraft AR, et al: Colonic complications of acute pancreatitis. *Arch Surg* 114:995–1001, 1979.

Gelin LE, Nyhus LM, Condon RE: *Abdominal Pain: A Guide to Rapid Diagnosis.* Philadelphia, JB Lippincott Co, 1969.

Jones CE, Polk HC, Fulton RL: Pancreatic abscess. *Am J Surg* 129:44–47, 1975.

Mellinkoff SM: *The Differential Diagnosis of Abdominal Pain.* New York, McGraw-Hill Book Co, 1959.

Sharpe JC, Marx FW Jr: *Management of Medical Emergencies,* ed 2. New York, McGraw-Hill Book Co, 1969, pp 351–418.

Silen W: *Cope's Early Diagnosis of the Acute Abdomen,* ed 15. London, Oxford University Press, 1979.

CLINICAL PROBLEMS

I. A 22-year-old man has a three-week history of intermittent epigastric pain, usually occurring daily one to two hours after he eats. The pain is described as "burning." It lasts for one to two hours unless he consumes food or antacid. Physical examination is unremarkable except for some mild epigastric tenderness.

   1. What are the likely diagnostic possibilities?
   2. What tests would be appropriately obtained?
   3. What considerations might prompt a hospital admission?

II. A 35-year-old Spanish American woman states that for the past year she had episodes of steady epigastric pain every month or so. These episodes develop to their maximum in five to ten minutes and last up to two hours. During these periods she cannot find a comfortable position and she usually paces the floor until they resolve. She becomes nauseated and occasionally vomits but this does not provide relief. Her most recent episode was last evening and she finally succumbed to family pressure and went to the doctor. Her physical examination is entirely normal.

1. What are the likely diagnostic possibilities?
2. What tests would be appropriately obtained?
3. What considerations might prompt a hospital admission?

III. A 45-year-old man who had been consuming one quart of whiskey a day for six years is seen in the emergency room. He complains of a steady epigastric pain that has been present for the entire day. Although no position or maneuver completely relieves the pain, he is most comfortable sitting still on the gurney with his knees drawn up to his chest. He has had three similar episodes of this pain during the past two years. On each occasion he was seen in an emergency room and treated with analgesics after he refused admission. His physical examination reveals a temperature of 38.4 C, blood pressure of 105/60, pulse rate of 120, epigastric tenderness, and hypoactive bowel sounds. There is a vague sensation of fullness in the epigastrium.

1. What are the likely diagnostic possibilities?
2. What tests would be appropriately obtained?
3. What considerations might prompt a hospital admission?

Discussion

Before discussing the three cases separately, it should be noted that all three patients had certain features in common. All had recurrent epigastric pain that, while present, was described as steady. In spite of this, three different pathologic entities should have been perceived.

I. 1. As is true for the other two cases, the location of the pain should suggest a process in the stomach, duodenum, gallbladder, liver, or biliary tree. The relation to acid (pain arising when free acid is present) and the relief by buffering should suggest an acid-peptic disorder. Thus the likely diagnosis is peptic ulcer disease, gastritis, or esophagitis. Cancer would be very unlikely in a 22-year-old. Hepatic or biliary tract disease would not have this relationship with food.

2. For the immediate care of the patient, one need not order any tests. In order to confirm the diagnosis of an ulcer, if that

is desired, a barium upper gastrointestinal x-ray or endoscopy should be performed (see Chapter 11). The hemoglobin concentration might also be checked to look for evidence of anemia secondary to bleeding.

3. There is no reason to hospitalize this patient. He does not have incapacitating pain and there is no evidence of either an acute intraabdominal catastrophe or a complication of peptic disease, such as bleeding, obstruction, or perforation. (The clinical presentation of the latter would include the findings of peritonitis.)

II. 1. In this case the pain has no relationship to any maneuver, and the patient describes a "restless" behavior during the pain. This is typical of an obstruction of a smooth-muscle–lined cavity without associated clinical inflammation. The organs in which this process often happens clinically are the gallbladder and biliary tree, the small intestine, and the ureter. (Interestingly and for unclear reasons, processes in the gallbladder and biliary tree do not produce "colic," but rather steady pain.) The absence of the findings of intraabdominal inflammation (e.g., fever or peritonitis) argue against a diagnosis of acute cholecystitis, and the likely diagnosis is pain due to a stone impacted in the gallbladder or biliary tree.

2. Again, the history is quite suggestive and one would proceed to specific tests to establish the diagnosis of cholelithiasis (see Chapter 18).

3. The patient has no evidence of active cholecystitis, and, in fact, is asymptomatic. If her presenting symptom complex consisted of continued pain aggravated by motion (especially if it were now localized in the right upper quadrant), fever, right upper quadrant tenderness and rebound, hypoactive bowel sounds, and a positive Murphy's sign, hospitalization for acute cholecystitis would be appropriate. The presence of icterus would also be an indication for admission.

III. 1. We can now appreciate some of the findings of an intraabdominal inflammatory process. In this patient those findings are fever, aggravation of the pain with movement, abdominal tenderness, and hypoactive bowel sounds. Processes to be considered include acute pancreatitis, acute cholecystitis, or an acutely inflamed intrahepatic process such as an abscess. The remainder of the clinical picture is most consistent with acute pancreatitis.

2. An elevated white blood cell count would add further evidence to the suspicion of intraabdominal inflammation. Other tests should be directed at confirming the diagnosis of pancreatitis (see Chapter 19).

3. Patients with evidence of intraabdominal inflammatory processes should, in general, be admitted to the hospital, especially if they are unknown to the physician.

2 MARTIN A. POPS

Nausea and Vomiting

WHAT ARE THE IMPORTANT ASPECTS OF HISTORY?

Nausea and vomiting, although nonspecific complaints, are important symptoms that imply abnormalities in the motility of the gastrointestinal tract. The frequency of these symptoms in many diverse conditions (e.g., motion sickness, pregnancy, drug toxicity, intestinal or pyloric obstruction, myocardial infarction, postsurgical states, intracranial diseases, and psychoneurosis) make them among the most common encountered in clinical practice. Vomiting may or may not indicate the presence of illness. Most often the symptom accompanies some acute problem that is not serious. However, in order to establish the underlying cause, or at least to exclude significant pathology, several important questions should be posed.

What Is the Timing of the Nausea and Vomiting?

Onset of nausea and vomiting during or immediately after a meal is common in patients with psychoneurosis. It is occasionally seen in patients with a peptic ulcer in the pyloric channel, presumably because of antral motor dysfunction caused by secondary spasm.

When the onset of nausea and vomiting is delayed, that is, when it occurs more than 60 to 90 minutes after a meal, gastric retention states should be considered. This retention may be due to obstruction (e.g., peptic ulcer disease with edema, spasm, and/or fibrosis) or to severe motor disorders of the stomach (e.g., diabetic gastric neuropathy or the postvagotomy state). Vomiting in the morning, on arising and before breakfast, is characteristic of pregnancy and is often described in toxic-metabolic disorders, such as Addison's disease, uremia, or alcoholism.

Are the Nausea and Vomiting Repetitious or Cyclical?

Repetitive vomiting is a more serious symptom than occasional vomiting. Its presence is usually associated with a serious pathologic process. Furthermore, no matter what the cause, it is much more likely to lead to fluid and electrolyte abnormalities and demands prompter therapy.

Is the Vomiting Projectile?

Although a clear definition of projectile vomiting is not available, it is usually taken to mean forceful ejection of vomitus from the mouth. Especially forceful or projectile vomiting is said to be characteristic of raised intracranial pressure and often occurs without nausea or retching (dry heaves). However, vomiting secondary to intracranial lesions is sometimes not projectile and it may be accompanied by nausea and retching.

What Is the Content of the Vomitus?

Vomitus that has the appearance of food that has not been ingested recently (within a few hours) implies gastric retention. Undigested food is also vomited from the esophagus in achalasia or because of an esophageal diverticulum. The latter states are rare; patients with these esophageal disorders report the lack of a sour (acid) or bitter (bile) taste to the vomitus.

Vomitus that contains blood, which appears fresh, in clots, or as "coffee grounds," is of obvious importance. It indicates either a discrete bleeding lesion, such as an ulcer or tumor, or some diffuse process such as gastritis or esophagitis.

Bile seen in the vomitus implies an open connection between the proximal duodenum and the stomach. Bilious vomiting is especially common after surgical procedures in which the pylorus has been interrupted. On the other hand, vomitus that never contains bile might suggest pyloric obstruction.

Does the Vomitus Have Any Particular Odor?

Feculent vomiting suggests intestinal obstruction or ileus and is characteristic of gastrocolic fistula. Feces are rarely vomited; rather the odor is due to the by-products of the associated bacterial overgrowth. Thus, feculent vomiting may also accompany bacterial overgrowth in the proximal small bowel, such as jejunal diverticulosis, scleroderma, or other blind loop syndromes. Feculent vomiting is especially common in patients who have had intestinal bypass surgery for the treatment of obesity.

Are There Other Symptoms that Might Point to the Diagnosis?

It is extremely important to ask the patient about weight loss, dysphagia, fever, and abdominal pain. Patients with psychogenic vomiting do not lose much weight; weight loss can be profound in gastric outlet obstruction. If there is accompanying abdominal pain, one should inquire if the vomiting temporarily relieves the pain. Relief often ensues in acid-peptic disease or proximal bowel obstruction but not in biliary tract or pancreatic disease.

WHAT ARE THE IMPORTANT PHYSICAL FINDINGS TO SEEK?

The most important findings in patients with nausea and vomiting are to be elicited during the examination of the abdomen. Patients with gastric retention will often demonstrate a succussion. This is elicited by rocking the supine patient back and forth while listening in the left subcostal region with a stethoscope. Visible gastric peristaltic waves with or without a succussion suggest mechanical obstruction of the distal stomach. The absence of visible waves suggests paralysis of the stomach, often referred to as gastric atony.

Other important findings include abdominal distention and the character of the bowel sounds. If bowel sounds are very high pitched and tinkling and the abdomen is distended, intestinal obstruction should be suspected, and abdominal mass should be sought. Clues to the diagnosis may include evidence of weight loss, jaundice, an inguinal hernia (which may contain incarcerated bowel) or signs of metabolic disorders (such as hypokalemia, uremia, or Addison's disease).

The physical examination should include a careful look at the optic fundi, where papilledema would suggest an increase in intracranial pressure. A complete physical examination should always be performed in a patient with severe or prolonged nausea and vomiting since the causes and complications of these symptoms are almost myriad.

WHAT LABORATORY TESTS OR PROCEDURES SHOULD BE ORDERED?

Under the circumstances in which a self-limited process is thought to be present, it is best for the physician to observe the patient and to determine only if complications due to vomiting, such as metabolic alkalosis or acute dehydration, are present. Ascertaining the cause is of limited value. Thus, if the symptoms are sudden in onset and short in duration (i.e., lasting only for a few hours), laboratory tests are not necessary and symptomatic therapy only will usually suffice.

When vomiting is frequent and protracted or recurrent, some type of workup becomes necessary. Though the history of the illness and the physical examination are the most helpful, some laboratory determinations may be of additional benefit in establishing a diagnosis or in dictating therapy. These two groups of tests are listed in Table 1. The left column of Table 1 lists those tests that will indicate the severity of the vomiting. The tests and procedures in the right column are obtained to determine the cause of vomiting.

Table 1 Laboratory Tests in the Evaluation of Vomiting

Tests That May Dictate Therapy	Diagnostic Tests
Complete blood cell count: determine degree of hemoconcentration; WBC elevation in infection and inflammation	Flat plate of abdomen: may show dilated stomach or small intestine filled with air and fluid, gallstones, sentinal loop, pancreatic calcification, organomegaly
Urine: over 50% of patients have a concentrated alkaline urine	Upper GI series: of limited value; may show dilated stomach with retention of barium for > three hours
Electrolytes: may show metabolic alkalosis	Nasogastric aspiration: > 300 cc of food or fluid three or more hours after a meal signifies gastric retention
Chest film: determine if patient has aspiration pneumonia	Saline load test or Hunt's test (see text)
	Blood tests: serum calcium, creatinine
	Pregnancy test

If gastric retention is suspected as the cause of the nausea and vomiting, it can often be confirmed by a saline load test (Hunt's test). After the stomach is intubated and emptied as completely as possible, 750 cc of normal saline is infused rapidly via the nasogastric tube. The tube is clamped for 30 minutes, after which the stomach is emptied and the volume is measured. If more than 300 cc of saline is recovered, the test is unequivocally positive for gastric retention. Values of 200 to 300 cc are indeterminate and indicate that the test should be repeated after several hours. Values under 200 cc are normal and suggest unimpaired gastric emptying.

WHAT ARE THE MAJOR DIAGNOSTIC CONSIDERATIONS?

There are literally hundreds of causes of nausea and vomiting. The vast majority of patients who develop these symptoms are suffering from some acute and usually self-limited process and are not seriously ill. However, vomiting may be an early indication of an emergency, such as intestinal obstruction, peritonitis, cholecystitis, pancreatitis, hypertensive encephalopathy, or serious drug overdose. Differentiating the serious causes from the nonserious ones is usually obvious based on the material we have just discussed. Some syndromes that are characterized by nausea and vomiting are specifically discussed in the section on special types of vomiting.

WHAT SYMPTOMATIC THERAPY CAN BE GIVEN IN THE ABSENCE OF A SPECIFIC DIAGNOSIS?

Antiemetic drugs are generally more effective when given prophylactically than for treatment. They may be useful because they depress the vomiting center of the brain, the vestibular apparatus, or peripheral sites such as the stomach or intestine. In initiating drug therapy, the choice of agents depends on the cause of nausea and vomiting.

Antihistamines such as dimenhydrinate (Dramamine), cyclizine (Marezine), and meclizine (Bonine) are recommended for motion sickness or vomiting caused by vestibular dysfunction such as Meniere's disease. Anticholinergics such as scopolamine can also be very effective in vestibular disorders, especially motion sickness.

Antihistamines are also used in morning sickness of pregnancy and may be the safest antiemetics. However, a few reports of teratogenicity in animals due to some of these drugs must give pause for reflection and caution. Probably no antiemetic is absolutely safe in early pregnancy so drugs should be withheld if at all possible.

Phenothiazines such as prochlorperazine (Compazine) or chlorpromazine (Thorazine) are usually effective for nausea and vomiting caused by drugs such as opiates or digitalis, anticancer chemotherapy, and radiation. They are also useful for gastroenteritis and for postoperative vomiting. Because of several toxic effects, such as cholestatic jaundice, blood dyscrasias, and extrapyramidal reactions, they should be used with caution.

A new drug, called metoclopramide, is about to be released commercially in the United States. Extensive use in Europe and trials in this country have shown it to be safe and effective in preventing vomiting in many clinical settings because of its stimulating effect on motor activity of the stomach and small intestine.

The formerly widespread practice of using hypnotic drugs in

the treatment of vomiting is to be condemned. Hypnotics such as barbiturates can reduce the severity of vomiting. However, their marked sedating effects can result in aspiration pneumonia, a serious complication of vomiting.

ADDENDUM: SPECIAL TYPES OF VOMITING

Reflux or Regurgitation

Reflux of gastric contents is sometimes so severe as to produce vomiting. Pyrosis (heartburn) and substernal pain are the dominant symptoms. However, some adults regurgitate food, usually one mouthful at a time, and either expectorate the food or chew and reswallow it. This is called rumination and appears to be similar to what occurs in ruminant animals such as cows or sheep; the exact mechanism by which it occurs is unknown. It does not require therapy or surgical correction.

Nausea and Vomiting in Pregnancy

Nausea and vomiting in pregnancy is generally a mild disorder of early pregnancy. It is characterized by morning nausea and sometimes by vomiting. Fluid and electrolyte depletion are not seen. Symptoms usually disappear by the fourth month, though they may occasionally persist into the second half of pregnancy.

Treatment beyond reassurance is usually not necessary; the ingestion of small frequent feedings of dry foods such as crackers may be of symptomatic benefit. As previously noted, antiemetic drugs should be avoided in early pregnancy because of their teratogenic potential. If medication is necessary, such drugs as dimenhydrinate (Dramamine) or meclizine (Bonine) appear to be safest.

Pernicious vomiting or hyperemesis gravidarum develops in a very few pregnant women. Vomiting becomes intractable and malnutrition or fluid and electrolyte disturbances are the rule. Onset of hyperemesis is usually early in pregnancy; it classically disappears by the fourth month although some patients may continue to vomit through the second, and even into the third, trimester. The incidence of hyperemesis is about 3.5 per 1,000 deliveries. The cause of the vomiting is unknown, though some believe that psychic factors are important. Therapy should be prompt and complete since the mortality rate in untreated patients is high. Treatment consists of fluid and electrolytic replacement. Antiemetic drugs appear to be of little value.

Psychogenic Vomiting

Psychogenic vomiting may be recognized by several of its features. It is usually present for years. In fact, a history of recurrent vomiting in childhood under stressful situations is frequently obtained. Often other members of the family are or have been vomiters. The vomiting typically occurs soon after a meal has begun or just after its completion, and it is often self induced by the insertion of a finger into the pharynx. The vomiting can be suppressed, if necessary, so that the patient has time to run to the bathroom. The majority of patients are women.

Workup sometimes reveals a dilated stomach or, more typically, a dilated duodenum. This appears to be secondary to the vomiting and usually reverts toward normal when the symptoms subside. Antiemetic drugs are usually not helpful. Improvement may be spontaneous or follow successful psychotherapy.

Epidemic Vomiting

Epidemic vomiting has many synonyms, including acute nonbacterial (viral?) gastroenteritis, epidemic nausea and vomiting, and intestinal flu, among others. Vomiting is always acute in onset and is often accompanied by abdominal cramps, diarrhea, and headache. Myalgia, sweating, and fever may also occur. For many years a viral etiology has been suspected and in recent years two likely agents (Norwalk agent and a reovirus-like agent) have been detected in the feces of patients. Rapid recovery is the rule; persistence of symptoms for 10 days and even relapses occurring after three weeks have been reported.

Table 2   Important Causes of Gastric Retention

Obstructive	Nonobstructive
Pyloroduodenal ulcer with scarring or spasm	Gastroparesis of diabetes
Carcinoma of the stomach with antral or pyloric obstruction	Postvagotomy
Pyloric stenosis in children and adults	Anticholinergic drugs
Pyloroduodenal webs or diaphragms	Severe electrolyte disturbance (especially hypokalemia)
Bezoars of the stomach (often follow gastric surgery and vagotomy)	Uremic gastritis
Stricture of the gastric antrum by strong alkali or acid	Nonobstructing gastric ulcer or malignancy
Carcinoma of the pancreas	Psychogenic vomiting?
	Hyperemesis gravidarum
	Intracranial tumors

Gastric Retention

Delayed vomiting, a succussion heard for longer than four hours after the last intake of food or water, or the presence of food in the stomach at the time of an upper gastrointestinal x-ray series (assuming no intake for the prior eight hours) indicates gastric retention. Two major categories of gastric retention are recognized; it is important to differentiate between them. In the first, retention is caused by obstruction of the gastric outlet. The second group consists of a wide variety of conditions that cause gastric retention without obstruction of the gastric outlet. The important causes of gastric retention are listed in Table 2.

SELECTED READING

Bogoch A, Wilson R, Fishman S, et al: The stomach and the duodenum, in Bogoch A (ed): *Gastroenterology*. New York, McGraw-Hill Book Co, 1973, p 460.

Goldstein H, Janin M, Schapiro M, et al: Gastric retention associated with gastroduodenal disease. *Am J Dig Dis* 11:887–897, 1966.

Metzger WH, Cano R, Sturdevant RAL: Effect of metoclopramide in chronic gastric retention after gastric surgery. *Gastroenterology* 71:30–32, 1976.

Rimer DG: Gastric retention without mechanical obstruction. *Arch Intern Med* 117:287–299, 1966.

CLINICAL PROBLEMS

I. A 28-year-old woman complains of nausea and vomiting that has persisted for six weeks. The symptoms are especially prominent in the morning. The vomitus usually consists of small amounts of clear fluid. The patient has lost no weight. She denies abdominal pain. Her last period was 10 weeks earlier but she has always had irregular menses. Her physical examination is unremarkable except for her pelvic examination, which demonstrates bluish discoloration of the cervix and a borderline enlarged uterus.

1. What are the possible causes of the nausea and vomiting?
2. What further tests should be performed?
3. How should the patient be managed?

II. A 38-year-old man has had episodes of vomiting off and on for the past two years. For the past two months, the vomiting has become more severe and he has lost 15 pounds during this time. The vomiting tends to occur later in the day; at times the vomitus contains food eaten hours earlier. The patient often has bouts of epigastric pain that usually occur during the same time as the vomiting. These episodic pains have been noted for years; an evaluation eight years earlier revealed duodenal ulcer disease. The only change the patient has appreciated is that antacids no longer relieve the discomfort. The physical examination demonstrates evidence of weight loss. The abdominal examination demonstrates visible gastric peristalsis and a succussion.

1. What are the possible causes of the nausea and vomiting?
2. What further tests should be performed?
3. How should the patient be managed?

III. A 26-year-old woman is seen for vomiting that has been present on and off for "as long as I can remember." Sometimes the vomiting is induced because the patient "feels uncomfortable." Often the vomiting is temporally related to stressful periods in her life. The vomiting usually occurs close to mealtime. The patient denies weight loss or abdominal pain. Further questioning reveals the presence of a number of somatic complaints including constipation, low back pain, headaches, fatigue, and irregular periods. The physical examination is completely normal.

1. What are the possible causes of the nausea and vomiting?
2. What further tests should be performed?
3. How should the patient be managed?

Discussion

I. 1. The most apparent cause for the patient's symptoms is an early pregnancy.
2. A pregnancy test should be ordered to confirm the diagnostic impression.
3. In general antiemetic drugs should be avoided; if absolutely necessary, dimenhydrinate or meclizine should be used. Reassurance and small frequent feedings of dry food provide symptomatic benefit.

II. 1. This patient has characteristic symptoms of gastric retention. The visible peristaltic waves imply the presence of an obstructive process. The remainder of the history makes an obstructing duodenal ulcer the most likely diagnosis.
2. An upper gastrointestinal barium x-ray may demonstrate the retention; endoscopy will identify the etiology more specifically. A saline load test or measurement of the residual gastric contents three or more hours after a meal will also establish the diagnosis of gastric retention.

The patient should also be evaluated for fluid or electrolyte imbalance. In particular the presence of a hypokalemic alkalosis must be excluded.
3. Much of the management of gastric retention is discussed in the chapter on peptic ulcer disease. The patient should be

managed with intravenous fluids and electrolytes, nasogastric suction, and antiulcer therapy. Many of these patients ultimately require surgical procedures.

III. 1. The long history of vomiting without any overt sequelae points to a psychogenic source. Acute causes of vomiting are not compatible with the illness. Similarly, chronic gastric retention should have some of the features of Case II.

   2. A barium upper gastrointestinal x-ray should be taken to make sure no intermittent obstructing process is present. Occasionally a dilated area of the upper gastrointestinal tract (especially the duodenum) may be seen. Interestingly, in patients with obvious psychological problems, the dilated duodenum does not represent an area of obstruction but rather a manifestation of functional bowel disease, which usually improves with supportive psychotherapy. Patients with psychogenic vomiting should also be evaluated for problems in fluid or electrolyte balance.

   3. Treatment usually entails prolonged, emotionally supportive therapy. This can be performed by the primary physician, often with psychiatric consultation. Antiemetic drugs are of no value.

ARTHUR D. SCHWABE

Diarrhea

WHAT ARE THE IMPORTANT ASPECTS OF HISTORY?

The frequency and consistency of the stool vary considerably throughout the world and are influenced by many factors, particularly the composition of the diet and the bacterial flora in the colon. In the United States the frequency of evacuation of feces in the "normal" population ranges from two to three times a day to twice a week. The mean daily fecal weight is less than 200 gm. Diarrhea may be defined as an increase in the frequency of or a decrease in the consistency of the stool, or both. Fecal water is usually increased. Patients may describe their stools as watery, loose, creamy, mushy, or soft. During the past decade four major pathophysiologic mechanisms operative in the development of diarrhea have been identified. Accordingly, we can classify diarrhea as osmotic, secretory, due to damaged mucosa, or due to deranged intestinal motility.

Osmotic Diarrhea

An excess of solutes poorly absorbed in the intestine creates a luminal osmotic pressure greater than that of plasma, resulting in the movement of water into the intestinal lumen and diarrhea. Osmotically active molecules may accumulate because of impaired digestion, as in intestinal lactase deficiency; defective absorption and transport, as in many malabsorptive syndromes; or after the ingestion of certain laxatives or poorly absorbable sugars.

Since in osmotic diarrhea the movement of water depends on the ingestion of solutes that are poorly absorbed, the diarrhea will cease when the patient fasts. This simple observation is extremely helpful in differentiating osmotic diarrhea from other types. For example, patients may not be aware that they have intestinal lactase deficiency until they have fasted or are asked to stop drinking milk. The sorbitol present in certain brands of chewing gum has been shown to cause an osmotic diarrhea in gum addicts.

Secretory Diarrhea

Active secretion of ions and water from the gastrointestinal tract may be due to exogenous agents, such as bacterial enterotoxins and certain drugs, or endogenous substances, such as specific hormones, hydroxylated fatty acids, or bile salts. The most striking feature of secretory diarrhea is the large stool volume, usually exceeding 1 liter and occasionally 5 liters per day. In most instances the diarrhea persists when the patient fasts. However, when the cause is malabsorption of bile acids or fatty acids or orally administered drugs, the diarrhea may substantially diminish or cease on fasting.

Diarrhea Due to Damaged Mucosa

Diarrhea may occur secondary to an inflammatory mucosal process with consequent fluid exudation or defective absorption of water, electrolytes, or ingested nutrients, or both. Impairment of only water and electrolyte absorption is associated with certain enteric infections and congenital diarrheas. In inflammatory disorders of the small bowel, such as celiac sprue, on the other hand, water, electrolytes, and nutrients may all be malabsorbed.

These diarrheal processes may be ameliorated, but usually do not cease, when the patient fasts. Red or white blood cells (microscopic or gross bleeding and/or pus), or both, are often found in the stool. Systemic signs and symptoms of inflammation (e.g., fever) may be present.

Diarrhea Due to Motility Disorders

Increased or disordered intestinal motility may result in abdominal discomfort and diarrhea. Although the precise mechanisms have not been elucidated, it is likely that neurogenic or hormonal factors, or both, are responsible. In those disorders characterized by hypermotility, it is assumed that liquid chyme is passed so rapidly out of the colon that there is insufficient time for normal absorption of water and electrolytes.

With the exception of diarrhea and abdominal discomfort, the signs and symptoms in these disorders are variable, reflecting the basic disease process. Patients with irritable colon syndrome may have symptoms that are exacerbated with emotional stress. In the carcinoid syndrome periodic cutaneous flushing and wheezing are often prominent. Diabetic enteropathy is usually associated with peripheral neuropathy. The presence of glaucoma should arouse the suspicion that long-acting parasympathomimetic eyedrops, which may cause diarrhea, are being used.

WHAT ARE THE IMPORTANT PHYSICAL FINDINGS TO SEEK?

The abdominal examination is an important component of the diagnostic evaluation. The quality and quantity of the bowel sounds and the presence or absence of distention, tenderness, masses, and organomegaly must be observed. The perineum and rectum should be examined for evidence of local disease such as hemorrhoids, fissures, or fistulas.

WHAT LABORATORY TESTS OR PROCEDURES SHOULD BE ORDERED?

Regardless of the cause of the diarrhea, the patient should be evaluated for evidence of volume and blood loss as well as electrolyte disturbances.

The most common form of diarrhea is a short-lived episode without associated systemic toxicity that is often referred to as viral gastroenteritis. Whether this illness is in fact even viral is an unimportant consideration, since it is self limited. Such episodes require no further workup.

For acute diarrheal states associated with systemic signs, sigmoidoscopy and stool examination and culture should be obtained. Sigmoidoscopy should be carried out in the unprepared bowel. Mucosal biopsy at this time is often helpful. The stool examination should include a microscopic search for red or white blood cells and parasites as well as a gram stain identification of any predominant bacterial forms. In general, barium enemas should not be obtained during this acute phase because of the risk of precipitating a toxic megacolon in some inflammatory processes.

Most of the time, the major diagnostic procedures are undertaken for processes that last for more than one to two weeks, so-called "chronic diarrhea." When evaluating patients with this type of disease, a preliminary classification of the process into one of the four major pathophysiologic mechanisms will direct the selection of diagnostic tests. From a practical standpoint, however, more than one mechanism may be responsible. The diarrhea in a patient with long-standing Crohn's disease of the small intestine may be due to bile acid malabsorption, secondary intestinal lactase deficiency, bypassed or blind loops with bacterial overgrowth, rapid transit through fistulas, malabsorption of nutrients, and disordered motility from extensive inflammation and strictures.

In an osmotic process, determinations of serum sodium, stool pH, and stool osmolality may be useful. The loss of body water greater than that of sodium may be reflected in hypernatremia. Carbohydrate malabsorption results in higher than normal concentrations of fecal fatty acids and lactate, which, in turn, may lower the pH of the stool. In most forms of diarrhea, the osmolality of fecal water, which is an ultrafiltrate of plasma, is equal to the sum of the cations and anions [osmolality = $(Na + K) \times 2$]. In osmotic diarrhea, however, the excess amounts of fecal solute and their breakdown products raise the fecal osmolality, which tends to be greater than twice the sum of the sodium and potassium concentrations.

In secretory processes, the diagnosis depends on the identification of the offending agent. Bacterial food poisoning and other infectious agents can be surmised from the history, particularly if the onset has been acute, if other family members have been affected, or if a patient has traveled to a foreign country. The ingestion of all but the most essential drugs should be discontinued. If infectious agents and drugs have been eliminated, and especially if progression of the diarrhea has been gradual, a search for intrinsic bowel disease and excess hormone production should be performed with appropriate studies. Such an evaluation will usually require gastroenterologic consultation and is beyond the scope of this chapter.

If the diarrhea is thought to be due to damaged mucosa, the most important diagnostic step is to visualize that mucosa. This can be accomplished best by proctosigmoidoscopy, barium contrast studies, or intestinal biopsy.

Most patients with motility disorders should have upper and lower gastrointestinal x-rays, although, statistically, irritable colon syndrome is the usual cause. Thyroid function tests are indicated in patients with clinical features of hyperthyroidism. In the carcinoid syndrome, 24-hour urine specimens for 5-hydroxytryptamine (5-hydroxyindoleacetic acid) and 5-hydroxytryptophan should be obtained. Elevated levels of one or both of these substances are usually present.

WHAT ARE THE MAJOR DIAGNOSTIC CONSIDERATIONS?

The differential diagnosis of diarrhea is greatly simplified by approaching it from a mechanistic point of view. Based on history, physical examination, and, sometimes, a few simple laboratory tests, the process can be relegated to one of the four pathophysiologic categories. Tables 1 to 4 list the major diseases that produce diarrhea by each of these mechanisms.

Osmotic Diarrhea

Intestinal Disaccharidase Deficiency

The intestinal brush border is the site for the disaccharidases lactase, sucrase, isomaltase, glucoamylase, and trehalase. Absence or significant decreases in the concentration of these enzymes results in

Table 1   **Causes of Osmotic Diarrhea**

Intestinal disaccharidase deficiency
    Primary (congenital, acquired, genetic)
    Secondary
        Amyloidosis
        Blind loop syndrome
        Crohn's disease
        Infections
        Sprue
        Whipple's disease
Monosaccharide malabsorption
    Primary glucose-galactose malabsorption
    Secondary
        Infantile infectious diarrhea
        Small-bowel disease
    Polycyclic alcohols used as sweeteners
        Mannitol
        Sorbitol
Laxatives
    Lactulose
    Magnesium salts
    Phosphate salts

the impairment of hydrolysis of the respective substrates to their constituent simple sugars. The unabsorbed compounds produce a marked osmotic effect, which induces a net flow of water and electrolytes into the intestinal lumen. Furthermore, when the unabsorbed sugars reach the colon, organic acids are formed by bacterial fermentation. The consequent acid pH impairs the absorption of water and electrolytes by the colon. The net result is a watery diarrhea.

In clinical practice intestinal lactase deficiency is the most commonly encountered type. In the United States the primary form is present predominantly in blacks (70%–75%), Indians (60%), and Mexicans (74%), but is also found in 5% to 20% of whites. Lactase deficiency may also be secondary to (or borderline deficiency states may be unmasked by) blind loops, gastric surgery, and a host of infectious, inflammatory, and infiltrative disorders. Some patients with abdominal cramps, distention, excessive flatus, and intermittent diarrhea who were thought to have a functional bowel disorder may actually have intestinal lactase deficiency.

Table 2 Causes of Secretory Diarrhea

Cause	Clinical Disorder
Bacterial enterotoxins	
Enterotoxogenic *Escherichia coli*	"Turista"
Vibrio cholerae	Asiatic cholera
Shigella dysenteriae	Bacillary dysentery
Staphylococcus aureus	Food poisoning
Clostridium perfringens	Food poisoning
Drugs	
Caffeine	
Diuretics	
Laxatives [dioctyl sodium sulfosuccinate (DOSS), phenolphthalein]	
Theophylline	
Hormones	
Gastrin	Zollinger-Ellison syndrome
Prostaglandins	Medullary carcinoma of the thyroid
Serotonin	Carcinoid syndrome
Vasoactive intestinal peptide (VIP)	Pancreatic cholera
Miscellaneous endogenous substances	
Dihydroxy bile acids	Crohn's disease
Hydroxylated fatty acids	Malabsorption

Monosaccharide Malabsorption

The inability to absorb glucose and galactose is a rare congenital disorder, usually appearing a few days after birth. The infants develop watery diarrhea and soon become dehydrated. The diarrhea is promptly corrected by a diet in which fructose is substituted for all other sources of carbohydrate. Glucose and galactose absorption may also be impaired in severe infectious diarrhea in infants and, rarely and to a mild degree, in small-bowel disease.

The polycyclic alcohols, mannitol and sorbitol, which are commonly used as sweeteners, are poorly absorbed and, if consumed in quantity, regularly induce diarrhea. Saline laxatives contain polyvalent ions, such as magnesium, sulfate, or phosphate, which are incompletely absorbed and exert an osmotic effect, resulting in an increase in fecal water.

Table 3 **Causes of Diarrhea Due
to Damaged Mucosa**

Infections
    Bacterial (salmonellosis, shigellosis)
    Fungal (candidiasis, histoplasmosis)
    Parasitic (amoebiasis, giardiasis)
    Viral (reoviruses, adenoviruses)
Inflammatory disorders
    Antibiotic-induced diarrheas
    Celiac sprue
    Crohn's disease
    Pseudomembranous enterocolitis
    Ulcerative colitis
    Whipple's disease
Congenital disorders
    Congenital chloridorrhea
    Fatal congenital diarrheas

Secretory Diarrhea

The abnormal secretion can originate from the stomach, small
intestine, or colon. Active ion secretion in the small intestine may
be mediated by high intracellular concentrations of cyclic AMP.
Prostaglandins, vasoactive intestinal peptide (VIP), dihydroxy bile
acids, and the toxins of the *Vibrio cholerae* and some *Escherichia
Coli* species have been shown to activate or stimulate the production
of adenylate cyclase, inducing an increase in mucosal cyclic AMP.

Table 4 **Causes of Diarrhea Due to
Deranged Motility**

Irritable colon syndrome (spastic colitis)
Parasympathomimetic (cholinergic) drugs
Postvagotomy diarrhea
Hyperthyroidism
Diabetic enteropathy
Carcinoid syndrome
Blind loop syndromes

This cyclic AMP-mediated secretion may be operative in other types of secretory diarrhea.

An excess of dihydroxy bile acids may reach the colon and induce secretion in clinical disorders associated with bile acid malabsorption. This may occur in Crohn's disease involving the terminal ileum and after resection of the distal small intestine. Hydroxylation of unabsorbed fatty acids by bacteria occurs in a variety of disorders characterized by steatorrhea, particularly in celiac sprue, and stagnant or blind loops of the small intestine. These fatty acids are potent, irritating cathartics and mimic the action of castor oil, which contains ricinoleic acid, a hydroxy fatty acid.

Diarrhea Due to Damaged Mucosa

In those diarrheas due to bacterial, parasitic, or viral infections the onset is acute, but tends to be more insidious in those due to other causes. The feces contain blood and pus in shigellosis and ulcerative colitis, but not always in salmonellosis. Blood alone is usually seen in amoebiasis. When pus or blood, or both, are detected in the stool, cultures for bacteria and at least three specimens for ova and parasites should be obtained. Direct smears from the rectal mucosa and rectal biopsy during sigmoidoscopy facilitate the diagnosis of amoebiasis.

A pale, mushy, foul-smelling stool that contains excess amounts of fat and undigested food is characteristic of malabsorptive disorders, such as sprue and Whipple's disease. A quantitative fecal fat determination, small-bowel x-ray, and jejunal biopsy will usually identify each of these two diseases. If fungal infections are suspected, direct smears from mucosal lesions and cultures are essential.

Diarrhea Due to Deranged Motility

Aberrations of colonic myoelectric activity have been postulated as operative in the irritable bowel syndrome. A rapid transit time can sometimes be observed at fluoroscopy in hyperthyroidism and the irritable colon syndrome. Distention and spasm due to ulceration and inflammation may also impair normal intestinal motility and significantly contribute to the diarrhea in enteric infections and inflammatory bowel disorders. In diabetic enteropathy the diarrhea may be related to an abnormal peristaltic pattern.

WHAT THERAPY CAN BE PROVIDED IN
THE ABSENCE OF A SPECIFIC DIAGNOSIS?

In cases where a self-limited illness is thought to be present (the disease previously referred to as viral gastroenteritis), it is appropriate to prescribe an antidiarrheal agent. A number of these exist; they operate on one of three mechanisms. These mechanisms and medications are listed in Table 5. With the exception of the bulking agents, these drugs should not be employed in chronic diarrheal states.

Usually patients with diarrhea need not be hospitalized. During the acute illness, inpatient care may be required for patients with toxic disease who have high fevers, dehydration, or electrolyte imbalances. Occasionally hospitalization may also be required for associated pain or bleeding.

Some therapeutic guidelines can be generated based on the underlying pathophysiologic mechanisms. For instance, in osmotic diarrhea states, cessation of the offending agent will relieve the diarrhea. Most commonly these agents are laxatives, lactose, or artificial sweeteners.

Adequate fluid replacement is the mainstay of therapy for all secretory diarrheas. (In Asiatic cholera, as an extreme example, as much as 1 liter of isotonic fluid can be lost per hour during the first

Table 5   **Antidiarrheal Agents**

Agent	Dose
Anticholinergics	
Tincture of belladonna	0.5–1.0 ml q 4–12 hours
Paregoric	4 ml q 4–12 hours
Tincture of opium	0.5–1.0 ml q 4–12 hours
Diphenoxylate with atropine (Lomotil)	1–2 tablets q 4–12 hours
Codeine	30–60 mg q 4–12 hours
Smooth-muscle inhibition	
Loperamide	2–4 mg q 4–12 hours
Bulk agents	
Kaopectate	15–30 ml q 2–8 hours
Psyllium mucilloid	1–2 tsp q 8–12 hours

24 hours, and prompt and vigorous replacement is essential to maintain life.) The diarrheas associated with enterotoxigenic *E. coli* and staphylococcal and clostridial food poisoning are usually of short duration, that is, eight to 12 hours. No antimicrobial therapy is indicated. Secretory diarrhea associated with hormones elaborated by tumors is initially managed supportively until the diagnosis is made by appropriate hormone assays and radiographic localization of the tumors. Thereafter specific surgical or chemotherapeutic modalities are selected. Bile acid diarrheas due to distal ileal disease or resection may respond to a bile acid–sequestering resin, such as cholestyramine.

The treatment of infections that damage the intestinal mucosa is controversial. *Salmonella enteritis* requires antimicrobials only if accompanied by enteric fever, septicemia, or abscesses. Chloramphenicol or ampicillin are usually effective. *Shigella dysenteriae* infections should be treated with antibiotics only if accompanied by significant fever, toxicity, and bloody diarrhea. In such instances appropriate sensitivity testing should be performed, since the organism has been found to be resistant to many of the commonly recommended antibiotics. Metronidazole is the drug of choice for amoebiasis and either quinacrine or metronidazole is effective for giardiasis. Drugs that inhibit intestinal motility, such as antispasmodics and opiates, prolong the duration of the diarrhea and should be avoided. The treatment of the other disorders listed in Table 3 will be discussed in subsequent sections and chapters.

Treatment of motility disorders is directed at the basic disease process. All drugs that could conceivably affect intestinal motility should be discontinued.

ADDENDUM: SPECIAL TYPES OF DIARRHEA

Several forms of diarrhea share a number of special clinical features, which deserve emphasis. Although the mechanisms involved may be interesting and important from a physiologic standpoint, they are of less concern to the clinician, who is faced with the need for a rapid diagnosis and prompt institution of therapy.

Bloody Diarrhea

Bloody diarrhea with an acute or explosive onset is most likely due to bacterial or amoebic infection. Identification of the offending organism by direct smears of the stool or rectal mucus during sigmoidoscopy and appropriate cultures is essential. If the onset of bloody diarrhea is more gradual or insidious, ulcerative colitis, Crohn's disease, ischemic colitis, or malignant neoplasms are the most likely causes. Rarely, polyarteritis and other forms of vasculitis as well as amyloidosis of the colon may present in this fashion. The workup should begin with a plain film of the abdomen, which may reveal multiple ulcerations, suggesting ulcerative colitis; segmental involvement, characteristic of Crohn's colitis; or submucosal edema or fingerprinting, features of ischemic colitis. In all of these disorders, except in obvious ischemic colitis, a sigmoidoscopy is subsequently performed and several biopsies from involved areas are obtained. If the mucosa is normal on sigmoidoscopy, a barium enema should be performed. Diverticular disease of the colon may present as hematochezia and occasionally as bloody diarrhea. The onset of bleeding may be acute or insidious.

Antibiotic-Induced Diarrheas

Almost every antibiotic presently in use may induce diarrhea (Table 6). There is great variability in the severity of diarrhea, which may range from a mild increase in stool frequency without any discernible mucosal changes to profuse, almost constant outpourings of water with mucosal ulcerations and pseudomembranes. At the present time most of the cases of pseudomembranous enterocolitis are related to the administration of antibiotics, particularly clindamycin hydrochloride (Cleocin) and lincomycin hydrochloride (Lincocin).

Antibiotics may cause diarrhea by altering the normal intestinal microflora, selectively inhibiting one or more species and allowing others to proliferate. There may be a superinfection by enteropathogens. In some cases of pseudomembranous enterocolitis, clostridial species, especially *Clostridium difficile,* have been cultured from the stool. Antibiotics may also have a direct effect on the intestinal mucosa and interfere with cellular metabolism.

Table 6 Antibiotics Associated with Diarrhea

Ampicillin
Cephalexin (Keflex)
Cephalosporin (Cephadyl, Ancef, Cephazolin)
Chloramphenicol (Chloromycetin)
Clindamycin (Cleocin)
Cotrimazole
Erythromycin
Lincomycin (Lincocin)
Neomycin
Penicillin
Tetracyclines

The first step in the management of antibiotic-induced diarrheas is the cessation of antibiotic therapy. Stool cultures are obtained and patients are sigmoidoscoped. Of particular importance is the presence of pseudomembranes, which appear as multiple whitish-yellow adherent plaques on the rectal mucosa. Fluids and electrolytes are administered until all signs of dehydration have resolved and the diarrhea has ceased. Antidiarrheal agents should be used cautiously, if at all. They do not shorten, but may actually prolong, the duration of the symptoms. In severely ill patients with pseudomembranous enterocolitis, particularly if clostridia have been cultured from the stool, oral vancomycin, 500 mg four times a day, should be administered.

Surreptitious Diarrhea

The detection of the causative agent in some cases of diarrhea may tax the resources and patience of physicians. When a thorough workup has failed to provide any evidence of organic disease, consideration should be given to the surreptitious use of drugs. Laxatives or other drugs capable of inducing diarrhea may be secretly taken by some patients to gain attention from family and friends, to punish a loved one, or because of other real or imagined needs. Osmotic laxatives (such as magnesium or phosphate salts), secretory laxatives [such as dioctyl sodium sulfosuccinate, or DOSS (Colace), or phenolphthalein] and many others may be used by these patients. If the surreptitious use of a laxative is suspected, alkalinization of a stool specimen and the appearance of a pink color confirms the presence of a phenolphthalein-containing laxative. (A negative test does not exclude the possibility that other laxatives are being used.) Chronic diarrhea is also a paradoxical effect of opiates. In order to verify the suspicion of surreptitious drug use, it may be necessary to search the patients' belongings.

Traveler's Diarrhea

Traveler's diarrhea, or turista, is a common affliction of tourists who visit foreign countries. The frequency of this illness varies with the age of the traveler, the country of origin, and the area visited. It occurs most frequently in persons from northern industrialized nations who visit warmer, less sanitary countries. Tourists have assigned a variety of terms to this syndrome, such as Montezuma's revenge (Mexico), Delhi belly (India), Chiliitis (Chile), Aden gut (Middle East), and Hong Kong dog (China).

The syndrome has been studied most intensively in Mexico, and, in the majority of these cases, it is caused by enterotoxigenic *E. coli*. The infection is spread by contaminated food or water and may be prevented by avoidance of ice, salads, and unpeeled fruit. Drinking only boiled or carbonated water, the low pH of which limits bacterial contamination, may also be beneficial.

Almost all afflicted patients have watery, nonbloody diarrhea with mild to moderate abdominal cramps. Anorexia, nausea, malaise, and feverishness may occur, but temperatures higher than 38 C are distinctly unusual. Symptoms may last two to seven days, but occasionally persist for as long as two weeks, particularly if motility-inhibiting drugs are employed.

Two drugs have been shown effective in preventing traveler's diarrhea. Bismuth subsalicylate (Pepto-Bismol) has been reported to be useful in prophylaxis as well as in relieving the symptoms of enterotoxigenic *E. coli* infections. It may act by neutralizing or inactivating the enterotoxin. Doxycycline (Vibramycin), a long-acting tetracycline, has been shown in two controlled studies to prevent traveler's diarrhea if taken daily in a single dose. However, this antibiotic can itself cause diarrhea and photosensitivity reactions. It should not be used in pregnant women or in children because it can stain developing teeth.

Traveler's diarrhea may also be caused by shigellae, *Giardia lamblia* or, less commonly, by salmonellae, viruses, or amoeba. As a general rule it is recommended that all patients with traveler's diarrhea whose symptoms persist for more than one week or who have blood in their stool seek medical attention for diagnostic studies and treatment.

SELECTED READING

Bartlett JG, Chang TW, Gurwith M, et al: Antibiotic-associated pseudo-membranous colitis due to toxin-producing clostridia. *N Engl J Med* 298:531–534, 1978.

DuPont HL, Sullivan P, Pickering LK, et al: Symptomatic treatment of diarrhea with bismuth subsalicylate among students attending a Mexican university. *Gastroenterology* 73:715–718, 1977.

Markham HD, Rosenberg P, Dettbarn WD: Eye drops and diarrhea. *N Engl J Med* 271:197–198, 1964.

Rambaud JC, Matuchansky C: Diarrhea and digestive endocrine tumors. *Clin Gastroenterol* 3:657–670, 1974.

Read NW, Krejs GJ, Read MG, et al: Chronic diarrhea of unknown origin. *Gastroenterology* 78:264–271, 1980.

Sack RB, Froehlich JL, Zulich AW, et al: Prophylactic doxycycline for traveler's diarrhea. Results of a prospective double-blind study of Peace Corps volunteers in Morocco. *Gastroenterology* 76:1368–1373, 1979.

Sleisinger MH, Fordtran JS: *Gastrointestinal Disease.* Philadelphia, WB Saunders Co, 1978, pp 313–330.

CLINICAL PROBLEMS

I. A 26-year-old man has abdominal pain, fever, and diarrhea of three-weeks' duration. He had similar symptoms one year earlier, and he was diagnosed as having Crohn's disease with involvement of the terminal ileum and ascending colon. At that time he was treated with prednisone and had a symptomatic remission. The steroids were subsequently tapered off and discontinued. Currently, repeat barium x-rays reveal involvement of the same areas of the intestinal tract, and it is believed that the present illness represents an exacerbation of Crohn's disease.

1. What mechanisms are producing the diarrhea?
2. What would be the characteristics of the stool?
3. How could these diarrheal processes be managed?

II. The patient continues to have recurrences of the Crohn's disease and two years later undergoes a surgical resection of the involved intestine (the ascending colon and 50 cm of ileum). Shortly after the start of oral feedings in the hospital, he begins to produce four to five watery diarrheal stools a day unassociated with fever or pain. When he stops eating the diarrhea is substantially reduced to the point that he passes only a small amount of "loose material." This process continues unchanged for the next three months, during which time his weight remains constant.

1. What is now causing the diarrhea?
2. What would be the characteristics of the stool?
3. How could the diarrhea be managed?

III. The diarrhea resolves on treatment and the patient does well for several years, after which he again experiences recurrent exacerbations of Crohn's disease. Because of recurrent bowel obstruction, he undergoes further resection of another 50 cm of ileum. In the months after operation, diarrhea again becomes a significant problem, only now it is associated with progressive weight loss. Cholestyramine, which was useful after the last surgical procedure, is now of only minimal benefit. The diarrhea dramatically lessens when the patient stops eating.

1. What is now causing the diarrhea?
2. What would now be the characteristics of the stool?
3. How could this problem be managed?

Discussion

I. 1. The diarrhea is due to the active intestinal inflammatory process, and is the result in large part of the exudation of fluids. The involvement of the terminal ileum may also be causing bile salt malabsorption; the unabsorbed bile salts cause secretion in the colon. The inflammation may be creating motility disturbances. Secondary lactase deficiency may also be present, supplying an osmotic component.

2. The stool may demonstrate the presence of white and red blood cells. The stool will probably not be hyperosmotic to plasma unless lactose malabsorption is considerable.

3. The principle of management is to reduce the inflammatory process. This can be done with steroids or other techniques, which are described in more detail in the chapter on inflammatory bowel disease. Antidiarrheal agents are not indicated.

II. 1. The diarrhea is unassociated with signs of inflammation and, in fact, arose very soon after all of the apparently diseased intestine was resected. There are some secretory components to this diarrhea (watery diarrhea will persist during fasting), although eating exacerbates the condition. The most likely cause is colonic secretion caused by bile salts that are not absorbed in the remaining ileum. Since the liver can make up for the loss of bile salts by increasing production, malabsorption does not occur.

2. The stool will be an isosmotic fluid.

3. Agents that bind bile salts can be employed, and the dose can be titrated to use that quantity that just prevents the diarrhea. Again anticholinergic agents or other nonspecific antidiarrheal agents are not indicated.

III. 1. The diarrhea is now associated with weight loss, and, assuming the patient's oral intake has been the same, the problem is probably due to the malabsorption of fat. Because of the additional ileal resection, more bile salts are lost and the liver can no longer maintain production. The concentration in the intestinal lumen falls below that necessary to form micelles, and fat can no longer be absorbed efficiently. When the fatty acids reach the colon, they are hydroxylated; these compounds produce a secretory diarrhea. (The bile salts are also still causing colonic secretion.)

2. The stool will contain unabsorbed fats or metabolic products thereof. Again it will tend to be isosmotic to other body fluids.

3. Management of this problem is difficult. Cholestyramine can be used to reduce the amount of free bile acid in the colon. In addition a low-fat diet should be employed. Medium-chain triglycerides can be substituted for the long-chain ones, as these do not require micelle formation for absorption.

4

MARVIN DEREZIN

Constipation

In the United States, it seems that constipation is one of the most popular topics of conversation in the doctor's office. Few physicians, no matter what their discipline, are spared at least one daily encounter with a patient who is concerned about the proper evacuation of their bowels. We can get a glimpse of the enormity of the problem by realizing that over $200 million a year is spent on laxatives and that television commercials for these substances outnumber the ones for oral contraceptives. Large sections of pharmacies are devoted to the evacuation of the bowels, with prominent displays of drugs and various types of enema preparations and apparatuses.

WHAT ARE THE IMPORTANT ASPECTS
OF HISTORY?

The foods that we so lovingly consume with such enjoyment begin a long trip when they drop through the gastroesophageal junction into the stomach. Digestion in the stomach and duodenum allows the nutritious parts of our food and liquids to be absorbed in the small intestine. The residue or "muck" passes distally through the small bowel and only water and unabsorbable material reach the terminal ileum and cecum. The "load" entering the cecum in 24 hours is approximately 1000 cc of water and refuse. Further absorption of liquid takes place in the colon; from the 1000 cc of material that was deposited in the cecum, approximately 250 gm of dehydrated stool is expelled.

I feel it is best to approach the definition of constipation by examining the "normal" person's habit. Usually once a day or every two days there will be an urge to move the bowels that will be answered rapidly. The person will relax the external sphincter and in a short time, a thoroughly formed stool will be evacuated with little difficulty. This will be followed by a sense of completion.

I am struck by the large number of people in our society who are fixated on their bowels, thinking that movements should be under the conscious control of the mind, like driving a car. They feel that evacuation should follow whenever the mental need is present and that the stools should be a predetermined shape, size, and consistency.

Patients have described constipation as "not often enough," "not enough amount," "too narrow," "too hard," and "not totally evacuated." Yet the people with these complaints may not be constipated at all. They may be defining their stools in terms of an ideal that they have learned but that does not exist for them. Certain people will consider themselves "bound up" if their bowels move only every two days instead of every day. Some people feel constipated because they do not evacuate a large enough stool when they feel the normal movement should almost fill a toilet bowl.

Constipation, as defined here, may be considered the inability to move the bowels for a long period of time that results in the feeling of bloating or distention, perhaps associated with cramps and followed by a physically difficult expulsion of stool, which may be far below the "normal" 250 gm a day weight. The constipated stool that was difficult to pass may be very small and hard, in pellet form. The symptoms of constipation may include all of these or any one or more of the components listed. Therefore, it is essential that a careful stool history be obtained to determine if a patient fits the criteria of constipation or if he or she is confused about the tremendous normal variability of bowel habits.

A careful history of laxative and enema use is essential. The detailed dietary history usually assists in determining the type of therapy but dietary factors are rarely the lone etiology for constipation. A drug history is most important, and the physician should ask if the patient has been under care for any systemic disorder (Table 1). Information about prior abdominal surgery or hemorrhoidal surgery may also be helpful. A history of rectocele or cystocele may give a clue to a treatable cause of constipation.

Ascertaining the duration of the constipation will direct attention to certain processes. If the symptom has been present for weeks or months, some obstructive or metabolic disease may be present; functional constipation is usually a lifelong symptom.

Similarly, the presence of weight loss may point to an underlying systemic disorder. Rectal bleeding may imply a luminal mass lesion; it also may be due to local associated rectal disease such as hemorrhoids or a fissure. The presence or absence of abdominal pain will suggest different diagnostic possibilities.

The appearance of the stool may be of diagnostic help. For example, patients with local rectosigmoid spasm, as seen in irritable bowel syndrome, will have narrow stools with mucus, whereas patients with ulcerative proctitis and spasm will have narrowed stools with mucus and blood. Patients with rectal carcinoma will describe progressively narrower stools with blood. Alternating diameter of stools occurs with the benign diseases whereas progressive narrowing occurs with carcinoma. Alternation between diarrhea and constipation is a hallmark of functional bowel disease or irritable colon.

Table 1   **Common Drugs Associated with Constipation**

Anticholinergics (including analgesics with anticholinergic properties)
Antacids containing calcium or aluminum
Antihypertensives (especially ganglionic blockers)
Antidepressants
Diuretics (hypokalemia)
Minerals (iron, bismuth)
Sedatives

WHAT ARE THE IMPORTANT PHYSICAL
FINDINGS TO SEEK?

Physical examination will help to define any systemic disorders. The abdominal examination should be directed at detecting any masses, organomegaly, or tenderness. The tone of the abdominal muscles can be appreciated at this time.

Visual inspection of the perineum and anus will reveal evidence of fissures or hemorrhoids. Rectal examination should be performed to look for masses; a stool specimen should be obtained for occult blood. Digital examination will also give a great deal of information about the muscle tone and thickness of the sphincters. It is a clinical observation that some patients with constipation have a tight anal sphincter, and when asked to bear down and relax, they will have a paradoxical closing of the sphincter. Perhaps this is the same pattern that they use to hold in their emotions (that is, instead of "letting go," they "close off").

WHAT LABORATORY TESTS OR
PROCEDURES SHOULD BE ORDERED?

Sigmoidoscopy is essential for the evaluation of local lesions such as fissures, rectosigmoid carcinoma, or ulcerative proctitis. A barium enema study should follow to look for narrowing due to intraluminal lesions, diverticulitis, or some other inflammatory disease. Extraluminal compression, such as by an ovarian tumor or enlarged uterus, will also be seen.

In cases where laxative abuse (of anthraquinone compounds such as senna or cascara) has occurred, sigmoidoscopy may reveal a dark discoloration of the mucosa. This entity, melanosis coli, carries no pathophysiologic significance, but it should be recognized to avoid more extensive workup. Laxative abuse also may result in the loss of haustrations on barium enema. This condition may be superficially confused with ulcerative colitis, but there is no foreshortening of the bowel and the mucosa is not ulcerated. A screening profile, which includes thyroid studies and a serum calcium and potassium, may expose some hidden metabolic causes.

WHAT ARE THE MAJOR DIAGNOSTIC CONSIDERATIONS?

Many factors affect colon transit and evacuation. These include psychosocial influences, systemic illness, mechanical factors, and drugs (Table 2). At times it is extremely difficult not to be complacent and to look at all patients who arrive at the office with constipation as having a functional complaint. In most instances this is the case, but a simple diagnostic approach will quickly rule out these other causes. Systemic or local disorders must be considered in all patients who find it necessary to seek medical assistance for this distressing symptom.

WHAT SYMPTOMATIC THERAPY CAN BE GIVEN IN THE ABSENCE OF A SPECIFIC DIAGNOSIS?

It is very important during the initial evaluation to describe in detail to the patient that bowel habits vary, that the urge to defecate may occur at any time during the day, and that the frequency may be as little as three times a week in some people. An explanation of the various factors at play, such as described in the next few paragraphs, may provide the patient with a better understanding of the problem.

The ideal for defecation is to evacuate the bowels as soon as the urge arises. The person proceeds immediately to a nearby available facility, that is, in a relaxed quiet place with pleasant surroundings. He or she then relaxes the external sphincter and defecation follows relatively effortlessly and completely; normal activities are resumed. This ideal person has been eating a high-bulk diet that includes salad, fruits, and bran. Unfortunately, in our society these conditions are rarely met.

From the time of childhood, we are taught that anything that relates to the movement of the bowels is obnoxious and disgusting. We are told that we should not talk about our bowels, our bowel movements, or any urges as they relate to the perineal area in general. The description or discussion of bowel movements in public, or even among people who are intimately familiar with one another, is an unacceptable social error. As children, many of us had strict toilet

Table 2 Common Diseases Associated with Constipation

Functional bowel disease (functional constipation)
Organic colonic obstruction
    Diverticulitis
    Stricture (ischemic, postinflammatory)
    Malignancy
    Anal stenosis
    Hirschsprung's disease
Endocrinopathy
    Hypothyroidism
    Hypopituitarism
Pregnancy
Drugs (see Table 1)
Electrolyte disturbance
    Hypokalemia
    Hypercalcemia
Neurogenic
    Spinal cord damage
    Chagas' disease
Depression

training so that we could "stop soiling our diapers" as soon as possible.

We go to school where it is embarrassing to raise our hand to ask the teacher to go to the bathroom. The urge to stool is frequently denied in the hope of finding a more convenient time. As adults, we become involved in our daily activities; our hectic life patterns frequently make it necessary for us to ignore the urge to stool, unless we are at a lull in our schedule or are at home where we can defecate in the calmness and privacy of our familiar environment. If we wander around any major city, we can see why so many people withhold the urge to move their bowels. The toilet facilities are usually cold, austere, and unfriendly looking. They are usually loud; toilet stalls are only moderately private with the tops and bottoms open so that there is constant distraction of people walking by. The shuffling feet and loud noises frequently make the sphincter tighten, and these circumstances also make us voluntarily ignore the urge to evacuate.

The average person now sits down to a dinner that includes a cocktail, small salad, steak with baked potatoes, and a very delicious dessert of pie, cake, or ice cream. This, following the low-residue noon sandwich meal, makes the daily intake of nonabsorbable residue negligible.

In addition to the low-residue diets, environmental influences, and laxative habits, which can cause constipation, a significant segment of the population internalizes feelings. This causes tightness in the perineal area and a general insensitivity to the feeling to evacuate.

Some patients are only troubled with occasional constipation, usually at times of stress. Such patients may appropriately take any of the laxatives listed in Table 3. Even in this situation, however, bulk laxatives are the most physiologic and should be recommended. Only the bulk products are appropriate for long-term use.

Practically speaking, most patients with chronic nonorganic constipation who do not use laxatives will do extremely well with bran, if it is given in increasing doses necessary to effect defecation. Begin with a heaping teaspoon of miller's unprocessed bran mixed in food three times a day and increase to amounts necessary for easy defecation. The patient should be warned that for at least the first two

Table 3 **Classes of Laxatives**

Bulk
    Psyllium mucilloids (Metamucil, Konsyl)
    Bran
    Cellulose

Lubricants
    Mineral oil
    Dioctyl sodium sulfosuccinate (Colace)
    Glycerin suppositories

Saline
    Magnesium salts
    Phosphate salts

Stimulants
    Cascara
    Senna
    Phenolphthalein
    Bisacodyl
    Castor oil

weeks the increased amount of nonabsorbable bulk in the colon will frequently result in gaseousness and cramping. These annoying symptoms pass as the stools are evacuated more readily. For those patients who have difficulty tolerating unprocessed bran, there are many all-bran cereals that can be eaten in large quantities and have a good effect.

The patient is encouraged to eat a diet with a variety of vegetables and fruits and to respond as soon as the urge to evacuate appears. Physical activity should also be encouraged. If needed, stool softeners may be added twice a day for their lubricant effect on the stool, even though scientific evidence for their benefit is unavailable.

For some patients with the early onset of constipation, concentration on the anal area reveals to them the feeling of tenseness in the sphincter; relief may follow the conscious imagining of the muscle relaxing. These patients will sometimes break the cycle when they become aware of the spasm in the perineum. If centers are available that perform anorectal manometry, biofeedback conditioning, which may be helpful for patients with local anal motor disturbance, should be considered.

The laxative habit has become almost epidemic in the United States. Many people become addicted to the use of cathartics at an early age and continue to use them through adulthood. Paradoxically, as time passes, the laxatives have less effect and increasing doses and harsher ones must be added to achieve the goal of a daily bowel movement that is frequently composed of small amounts of stool and mucus. The bowels have become flaccid and relatively insensitive as the doses and varieties of laxatives and enemas have increased. Since the laxatives have become less and less effective and the bowel has become more atonic, it is important to relate to patients the increasing problem. They are already extremely bowel fixated and very resistant to stopping laxatives. However, a detailed and compassionate program such as the one to be outlined, if not curative, is frequently helpful and stops worsening of the laxative habit.

The daily laxatives are eliminated entirely. Should three to four days pass without an evacuation despite the use of stool softeners and bulk, and if the patients are uncomfortable, they are told to evacuate their bowels with a Fleet enema or glycerin suppository. For those patients with a spastic external sphincter, I suggest finger dilatation. They are asked to put a finger cot on the little finger and, with a great deal of lubrication, to use it to dilate the tight sphincter.

They should feel the resistance against the finger and try to relax it before each bowel movement. A single dose of an oral laxative, such as 2 oz of milk of magnesia or 5 oz of magnesium citrate, is reserved for those patients who do not respond to an enema. To allow the use of the laxative eliminates the fear of not being able to evacuate.

I feel it is impossible to expect patients who have spent an entire lifetime taking laxatives and enemas in order to have a "normal" daily bowel movement to suddenly change their habits. They are panicked about moving their bowels and they should be dealt with in a very compassionate manner, with the physician available for telephone consultation. With constant reinforcement, most of these patients can be managed adequately without large doses of laxatives or enemas. For those patients who do not respond to the program, reevaluation for organic disease should be carried out and, if negative once again, referral to a psychiatrist should be encouraged, not as an end in itself but as part of the evaluation and treatment.

Perhaps the most important reminder that we can give the patient, over and over again, is the understanding that constipation and the retention of stool in the colon for long periods of time does not produce disease and that laxative abuse and chronic enemas will make the bowel atonic and will worsen the condition as time progresses. The patient must be given constant reassurance that the constipation habit will take a while to change and that, in the meantime, occasional failure is expected.

SELECTED READING

Devroede, G: Constipation: Mechanisms and Management, in Sleisinger MH, Fordtran JS (eds): *Gastrointestinal Disease*. Philadelphia, WB Saunders Co, 1978, pp 368–386.

Thompson, WG: Constipation, in *The Irritable Gut*. Baltimore, University Park Press, 1979, pp 93–105.

CLINICAL PROBLEMS

I. A 62-year-old woman complains of constipation that has been present "all her life." She denies any recent change in her symptoms, weight change, fever, or pain. She has been evaluated on several occasions in the past 20 to 30 years, and three different barium enemas were all normal except for the presence of diverticulosis. Several sigmoidoscopies have been normal. Her physical examination is entirely normal. A stool specimen is negative for occult blood.

1. What is the cause of the constipation?
2. What further evaluation needs to be done?
3. How should the patient be managed?

II. Another 62-year-old woman complains of constipation of three to four weeks' duration associated with vague lower abdominal pains and occasional blood mixed in with the stool. She has lost five to 10 pounds. She denies fever. Her physical examination reveals a 3 × 4 cm palpable mass in the left lower quadrant and occult blood in the stool.

1. What is the cause of the constipation?
2. What further evaluation needs to be done?
3. How should the patient be managed?

III. A 58-year-old man with unresectable carcinoma of the lung develops severe chest pain and begins to use analgesics. Soon after being switched from aspirin to codeine he notes the onset of constipation. His stool is negative for occult blood and his abdominal examination is unremarkable.

1. What is the cause of his constipation?
2. What further evaluation should be done?
3. How should the problem be managed?

Discussion

I. 1. This woman has the typical symptoms of functional constipation. The presence of the various other diseases mentioned in the chapter (and listed in Table 2) are all made unlikely by the chronicity of the one complaint alone.
   2. No further diagnostic tests need to be performed. Sigmoidoscopies and barium enemas have repeatedly been unre-

markable, and there has been no change in the complaint. If blood had been found in the stool, however, a source would need to be found.

3. The patient should be encouraged to increase her fiber intake and her physical activity. The use of other laxatives or enemas, or both, should be discouraged.

II. 1. In this case the constipation is of recent onset, which points away from a functional process. The abdominal pain, blood in the stool, and palpable mass all point to a colonic obstructing lesion. The most likely possibilities would be a complication of diverticulitis or a carcinoma.

2. The patient should have sigmoidoscopy and barium enema to characterize the site of obstruction.

3. It is likely that this process will need to be dealt with surgically. Increasing bulk in the diet will only accentuate any obstructive symptoms.

III. 1. The temporal relation of the onset of the constipation to the introduction of codeine makes this drug the most likely cause. Although it is possible that the change in bowel habits could be due to intestinal complications of intraabdominal tumor spread, this would be far less likely.

2. No further diagnostic tests need to be performed.

3. Management of the constipation is very difficult. Some type of analgesic is necessary. Bulk laxatives probably will not overcome the anticholinergic effect of the codeine. Physical activity and fluid intake should be encouraged as much as possible. Other laxatives (see Table 3), or even enemas, may be necessary. Fecal impactions should be avoided.

RONALD L. KORETZ

Weight Loss

WHAT ARE THE IMPORTANT ASPECTS
OF HISTORY?

The loss of body mass accompanies a number of illnesses (Table 1). Weight loss may be the presenting complaint or its presence may only be elicited after specific questioning. The common denominator in all states in which weight loss occurs is that the demand for calories exceeds their supply.

Interruption in the supply may happen at several sites. Most commonly the patient simply fails to consume adequate amounts of food. Even in illnesses in which the gastrointestinal tract is primarily involved, and even in situations where frank chemical malabsorption can be demonstrated, a careful dietary history will often reveal evidence of food avoidance. This may, in turn, be the result of a specific

Acknowledgments: I wish to thank Sally Clement and Dorothy Emley for their assistance in the preparation of this manuscript.

60

Table 1 Some Common Considerations in the Evaluation of Weight Loss

Systemic problems producing failure to eat
    Anorexia due to many debilitating illnesses
    Depression
    Drugs
    Anorexia nervosa
    Hypercalcemia
Specific gastrointestinal disorders in which eating produces symptoms
    Pain
        Gastric retention
        Partial intestinal obstruction
        Intestinal ischemia
        Upper gastrointestinal cancer
    Diarrhea (certain malabsorption disorders)
    Vomiting (gastric retention)
Problems with which appetite may be unaffected
    Hypermetabolic (hyperthyroidism)
    Caloric wasting (malabsorption, diabetes mellitus)

intestinal symptom brought about by the ingestion of food (e.g., pain or diarrhea), or it may be due to some more poorly understood phenomenon of the underlying illness (e.g., carcinomatous anorexia).

Thus, a very important aspect of history is a detailed accounting of how much food is consumed each day. The physician should also ascertain the patient's usual daily activity in order to determine whether the caloric intake is appropriate for that patient.

A second component of history, especially important if a pattern of food avoidance is established, is directed at specific symptoms produced by eating. If the patient is afraid to eat because a gastrointestinal disturbance will occur, the presence of primary gastrointestinal disease becomes much more likely. The specific symptoms of concern are abdominal pain, satiety, vomiting, or diarrhea.

Once the food is ingested, it must be absorbed. Both postprandial vomiting and malabsorption result in intestinal calorie wasting. However, among the vast numbers of patients with weight loss, these entities are uncommon, as will be discussed later.

A few patients will lose weight in spite of adequate food intake and no specific intestinal symptoms. Metabolic disorders such as diabetes or hyperthyroidism are found in this population, but even some malabsorptive disorders (especially pancreatic insufficiency) may present without diarrhea.

Patients often cannot quantitate weight losses as they often do not weigh themselves. Questions directed at changes in clothing size or, if old records are available, comparisons of recent weight with previously observed weights, may be helpful in this regard.

In patients with water-retaining states, weight gain should occur. Thus, in the patient with edema, mere maintenance of the total weight should alert the physician to the presence of loss of body fat or protein.

Questions concerning the character of the stool are usually asked, but the answers are often not helpful. Stools that float have a lower density than toilet water, usually as a result of the presence of various gases (not fat). Observations of stool odor are very unreliable. Similarly changes in stool color depend on a number of nondisease factors (diet in particular). However, two questions that may be of help relate to certain malabsorptive states. The presence of oil or grease (in the stool or as a residual in the water–toilet bowl interface) indicates triglyceride maldigestion and suggests pancreatic insufficiency. (If pancreatic lipase splits the triglyceride, the residual monoglyceride and fatty acids are water soluble, so no oil layer occurs.) A large volume of stool that necessitates a second flush to clear the toilet bowl may indicate substantial malabsorption and an increase in the nonwater fecal volume.

Vitamin deficiency states are junior partners of malnutrition. These usually only occur late, if at all. In patients with severe weight loss, however, questions concerning potential vitamin deficiency, especially fat-soluble vitamins, should be posed [e.g., problems with adaptation to dark (vitamin A), tetany (vitamin D), or bruising (vitamin K)]. We are all familiar with the problems of folate or thiamine deficiency in the alcoholic population.

Depression is a common cause of anorexia, although it is sometimes unappreciated in the routine evaluation of the patient. Questions about lifestyle (such as the home situation, sexual activity, sleep habits, etc.) can be revealing in some patients who have no obvious cause for weight loss. Depression is also a part of every chronic "organic" illness, where it is a result and not a cause of the underlying systemic disorder. However, even this secondary depression may contribute to the weight loss problem.

WHAT ARE THE IMPORTANT PHYSICAL FINDINGS TO SEEK?

The principal means of establishing the presence of weight loss is to weigh the patient. If there is any question as to whether a weight-losing process is occurring, serial assessments gathered prospectively may resolve the issue. Sometimes the presence of weight loss can be determined from softer findings, such as loose-fitting clothing, extra holes notched in a belt, or redundant skin folds.

Muscle wasting often occurs in serious catabolic diseases. This wasting is often especially prominent around the face and extremities. Comparison of the current appearance of the patient with old photographs may help if the issue is in doubt.

Nutritional assessment has become very popular as a spinoff of nutritional support. A number of body measurements have been promoted. Sensitive calipers are currently available to determine skin-fold thickness, from which muscle mass can be calculated indirectly. The problem with the anthropometric data is that normal values, especially for older patients, are not well established.

Physical findings that may be associated with particular vitamin deficiencies are listed in Table 2. Many of these findings may be due to other causes or to multiple nutritional deficiencies.

Finally, the findings of any of the diseases that result in the weight loss may be seen. Time and space do not permit an enumeration of all of these processes. However, if a primary gastrointestinal lesion is suspected, close attention must be paid to the abdominal examination. The presence or absence of abdominal bruits, masses, organomegaly, abnormal bowel sounds, or abdominal distention should be noted. Severe malabsorptive states due to intestinal disease may result in dilated fluid-filled loops of bowel that descend into the lower abdomen. The presence of tympany over the upper abdomen and dullness over the lower abdomen may suggest this process.

WHAT LABORATORY TESTS OR PROCEDURES SHOULD BE ORDERED?

As was mentioned previously, a number of attempts have been made to quantify malnutrition (so-called "nutritional assessment"). A variety of laboratory tests have been advocated, including serum

Physical Finding	Possible Vitamin Deficiency
Dermatitis	Riboflavin, pyridoxine, biotin, niacin, ascorbic acid
Cheilosis	Riboflavin, pyridoxine
Glossitis	Riboflavin, niacin, B_{12}
Swollen gums	Ascorbic acid
Xerophthalmia	A
Petechiae	Ascorbic acid, K
Ecchymoses	K
Perifollicular hemorrhages	Ascorbic acid
Peripheral neuropathy	Thiamine, pyridoxine, B_{12}
Ophthalmoplegia	Thiamine
Confusion/dementia	Thiamine, niacin
Muscle weakness	Thiamine, ascorbic acid, E(?)
Ataxia	Thiamine, B_{12}
Poor adaptation to dark	A
Convulsions	Pyridoxine
Anemia	Folic acid, B_{12}
Loss of teeth	Ascorbic acid
Fractures	D
Tetany	D
Congestive heart failure	Thiamine

albumin, serum transferrin, skin testing for common antigens, creatinine-height index, nitrogen balance, and total lymphocyte count. Although some of these studies are relatively simple, others are complex or expensive, or both. For example, an adequately performed nitrogen balance study can usually only be obtained on a metabolic ward. The importance of quantitating the nutritional status of a patient has not been established with regard to any effect on patient outcome. This is because the whole thesis of nutritional support is speculative, at this time, as will be discussed later. Hence, nutritional assessment should not be performed routinely.

Weight loss is only a symptom, and usually a nonspecific one. Thus, most of the diagnostic workup is directed at determining the suspected cause. On the other hand, a complete blood cell count should be obtained routinely for both its diagnostic and therapeutic potential. The presence of anemia, although a late finding, would point to some component of malnutrition or to the presence of a significant coexistent disease. Establishing the cause of the anemia may shed a great deal of light on the etiology of the weight loss. In a similar vein a low serum albumin indicates serious underlying pathology.

Space does not permit an elucidation of all of the tests that could be ordered in any particular case. Rather the emphasis should be placed on establishing a diagnosis or differential diagnosis from the history and physical examination, and then ordering those tests that are appropriate.

Some attention must be paid to one particular test, however, as it is commonly ordered but may often be misinterpreted. This test is the timed fecal fat collection. The fecal fat collection is performed by placing the patient on a standardized fat intake (usually 100 gm) and then having him or her save all of the next three days' stool in a jar. The total fat is measured and, by dividing by three, an average 24-hour fat excretion can be calculated. If the amount of fat the patient consumed is also known (and for this reason the study may have to be performed in an inpatient situation with the hospital dietitian counting the amount of fat the patient ate each day), a ratio between the daily excretion and intake can be calculated. The coefficient of fat absorption, $\dfrac{\text{intake-excretion}}{\text{intake}} \times 100$, should be more than 93%. (Thus, on a 100-gm fat intake, the patient should excrete less than 7 gm of fat a day.)

Several potentials for problems occur. In the hospital, the use of cathartic lipids, such as castor oil, may falsely elevate the daily fecal fat excretion. If the patient is hyperphagic, and fat intake is not quantitated, a fecal fat of 10 gm per day may be perfectly normal if 150 or 200 gm of fat is consumed. (This may be the case in some patients with hyperthyroidism.) On the other hand, a 24-hour fecal fat of 5 gm would indicate marked malabsorption if only 20 gm of fat is consumed. Thus, rather than thinking about stool fat in terms of grams per day, it is much more useful to consider it as a percentage of intake.

Furthermore, if the coefficient of fat absorption is 85% to 90%, even though malabsorption is occurring, the patient should be able to overcome this deficit by eating more. This is often the case in pancreatic insufficiency, where the excess food intake does not produce many symptoms. On the other hand, many patients with only mildly abnormal fat absorption lose weight. Careful dietary history will usually reveal that such people either cannot or will not eat, the point that was made earlier. In the usual circumstance, it is rare to see patients who are losing weight solely because they are failing to absorb after ingesting an adequate quantity of nutritive material.

WHAT ARE THE MAJOR DIAGNOSTIC CONSIDERATIONS?

This material was considered in the first section and will not be repeated here.

WHAT SYMPTOMATIC THERAPY CAN BE GIVEN IN THE ABSENCE OF A SPECIFIC DIAGNOSIS?

Weight loss and malnutrition accompany a number of chronic illnesses. In the eyes of many patients, their families, and even their physicians, this weight loss becomes the symbol of the disease. How many cancer patients have been encouraged to eat, with the idea that an improvement in the nutritional status will cause some improvement in the underlying malignant process? Physicians appear to have accepted this concept and have sought, for decades, ways to provide protein and caloric supplementation to catabolic patients.

Those who live in areas of the world where starvation and malnutrition are a way of life are more susceptible to the ravages of illness, especially infectious disease. Numerous immunologic studies have demonstrated that starving patients or experimental animals have defects in in vitro and in vivo immune mechanisms. Refeeding may improve these mechanisms, and presumably patient (or animal) outcome to the stress of illness would also be improved. Similarly starved experimental animals can be shown to heal subsequent surgical wounds less well than their fed counterparts. This finding has been extrapolated to the clinical situation, where it has been assumed that providing nutritional support will result in a better outcome.

Catabolic diseases arise in well-nourished people, whose malnutrition occurs for reasons other than primary starvation. As intuitively appealing as nutritional support is, it has not been proved that its provision is beneficial in this "secondary starvation." Since nutritional support programs are becoming more widespread, however, it is worthwhile to focus some attention on them.

The provision of nutrients can be accomplished in several ways. Most commonly food is chewed, swallowed, and absorbed. In situations in which this cannot be accomplished, at the other extreme, nutrients can be infused intravenously. If the infusion contains all of the calories, amino acids, vitamins, minerals, and fluid that the organism requires, the technique can be called "total parenteral nutrition" (TPN). If only some of the substances are infused, or if amino acids are used without large amounts of calories (to improve nitrogen balance), the term "peripheral parenteral nutrition" (a peripheral rather than central vein being used) or "partial parenteral nutrition" is appropriate. In between these extremes of feeding are techniques whereby the food is partially dissolved (polymeric chemically defined, or liquid, diets) or even composed of predigested simple chemical compounds (oligomeric chemically defined, or elemental, diets) and either sipped or infused through a tube into the stomach or small intestine.

Since nutritional support is usually used in patients who cannot, or will not, eat normal foods, either parenteral nutrition or one of the various special enteral diets are employed. Among these alternatives, TPN is the one that has generated the most literature, and it will be considered first. The various indications for TPN are enumerated in Table 3. In spite of the wide acceptance of this expensive procedure, only a handful of prospective controlled trials have been conducted in an attempt to demonstrate efficacy. Of more import, these trials have failed to demonstrate a dramatic effect of TPN on clinical outcome.

Of the five studies that have examined perioperative support, none has shown any improvement in survival or morbidity. In one study the patients who received TPN actually seem to have done more poorly with regard to postoperative complications, duration of hospitalization, and overall hospital cost (*Arch Surg* 111:45–50, 1976). In two studies there was no apparent difference between the two groups (*J Surg Res* 23:31–34, 1977 and *Br J Surg* 64:125–128, 1977). The fourth study showed some improvement only in the incidence of wound infection, and the authors felt that this limited

Table 3 **Indications for Total Parenteral Nutrition**

Perioperative support in malnourished surgical patients[a]

Gastrointestinal fistulas

Inflammatory bowel disease[a]

Oncology patients

Acute renal failure[a]

Low birth weight infants[a]

Inadequate bowel ("short-gut") syndrome

Cirrhosis

Burns

Pancreatitis

[a] Controlled prospective clinical trials available for interpretation (see text).

benefit was offset by the risk and expense (*Postgrad Med J* 55:541–545, 1979). In only one study did the data appear to support any use of TPN, and that was in its effect on perineal wound healing after total colectomy (*Lancet* 1:788–791, 1978).

Low birth weight infants gain weight faster when they are given parenteral nutrition. However, this weight gain may be, in large part, edema, and the cost saving in reduced hospitalization time is compensated for by the expense of the treatment. No difference in survival was seen in five prospective studies. TPN is no longer routinely employed in this situation.

One prospective controlled trial (*Gastroenterology* 79:1199–1204, 1980) showed no benefit from TPN in acute colitis. However, one of two controlled trials did demonstrate improvement in survival in acute renal failure when a special TPN formulation, composed of essential amino acids and dextrose, was compared to equicaloric dextrose.

Support for the use of TPN, therefore, comes almost entirely from uncontrolled experiences. One must be very careful in interpreting such data in view of such factors as observer bias or expectation. Since the cost of such support is high (at least $100 a day) and complications occur, perhaps this technique should be used less often until more controlled trials clearly define its place in our therapeutic armamentarium (Table 4).

One special area in which TPN is probably effective is in those patients who have a gastrointestinal tract that is inadequate to maintain life and health. Since, by definition, such individuals would literally starve to death without TPN, controlled trials are not ethically justifiable. Techniques currently exist to provide TPN in a home situation, much in the same manner that home hemodialysis can be employed by patients with end-stage renal disease.

It has been found that the peripheral infusion of amino acids in the early postoperative period will result in less negative nitrogen balance than is seen when glucose alone is employed. It is not uncommon to see hospitalized patients who are not eating being given amino acid infusions. Although this may produce a reduced nitrogen loss over the period of time it is given, again the clinical implications are unknown. It is likely that most patients can tolerate the nitrogen loss without any short- or long-term adverse effects. The one controlled trial studying this demonstrated no difference in patients infused with amino acids as compared to those given standard intravenous fluids. (*Lancet* 1:788–791, 1978). Positive nitrogen balance cannot be achieved with this technique.

More recently, inspired in part by the problems of complications of the central vein catheter, many centers have promoted enteral hyperalimentation. The gastrointestinal tract is intubated, usually using a small-bore tube. The tube may be placed via the oronasal route or it may be implanted surgically into the stomach

Table 4 **Complications of Total Parenteral Nutrition**[a]

Catheter complications

Sepsis

Deficiency syndromes (phosphate, essential fatty acid, copper, zinc, chromium)

Hyperglycemia/hypoglycemia

Hyperammonemia

Electrolyte deficiencies or excesses

Osteomalacia

Jaundice

Fluid overload syndromes

Vitamin deficiencies

[a] In well-run programs, the overall complication rate should be about 5%.

or small intestine. Liquid feedings, usually as "elemental" diets, are infused in a continuous drip. In this case the feeding must be absorbed by the intestinal mucosa. Because the protein is presented as amino acids or oligopeptides, the carbohydrate as simple sugars, and the lipid as dissolved triglycerides, it is assumed that there will be less gastrointestinal stimulation of secretions and easier absorption over shorter lengths of bowel. Unfortunately, these premises are likely not true. The stimuli for pancreaticobiliary or gastrointestinal secretion are all still present and operational. Observed differences between elemental diets and whole foodstuffs are more apparent than real; these differences are due to comparing unlike materials or failing to take into account the slower gastric emptying of high osmotic loads (elemental diets). (Slower emptying produces lower peaks but longer duration of stimulatory drive.)

Elemental diets have been proposed for many of the same reasons as TPN is indicated (Table 5). Again the literature is remarkably absent of prospective controlled clinical trials. Two of three controlled trials in patients with cancer showed no statistically significant differences, and a third trial of patients who received ab-

Table 5 **Indications for the Use of Elemental Diets**

Primary therapy or nutritional support in:
    Perioperative support
    Gastrointestinal fistulas
    Inflammatory bowel disease
    Cancer therapy[a]
    Inadequate bowel syndrome
    Cirrhosis
    Burns
    Pancreatitis
    Chronic intestinal obstruction
    Celiac sprues
    Infantile diarrhea
    Phenylketonuria
Low residue properties in:
    Colon preparation[a]
    Anorectal surgery[a]

[a] Controlled prospective clinical trials available for interpretation (see text).

dominal radiation showed only a reduction in diarrhea in the group that received the elemental diet. Four controlled trials that compared the elemental diet and standard mechanical colonic preparation showed no advantage in using this material for its low-residue properties. One trial in patients undergoing anorectal surgery showed no difference in pain relief.

A number of problems can arise with the use of these diets. Most of these are related to gastric retention, fluid balance, or diarrhea, consequences of the high osmolarity of the fluids. The other difficulties encountered are the relative unpalatability, if they are consumed orally, or discomfort related to the naso/orogastric tube. Very rarely, these mixtures are inadvertently administered intravenously, possibly with disastrous consequences. The 1978 wholesale cost of these diets was approximately $4 per 1,000 calories.

In conclusion, the entire concept of nutritional support is open to serious question, in spite of its widespread use. These techniques are expensive and potentially hazardous. Until efficacy can be established, it would appear inappropriate to apply them routinely.

SELECTED READING

Blackburn GL, Bistrian BR, Maini BS, et al: Nutritional and metabolic assessment of the hospitalized patient. *JPEN* 1:11–22, 1977.

Jeejeebhoy KN, Langer B, Tsallas G, et al: Total parenteral nutrition at home: studies in patients surviving 4 months to 5 years. *Gastroenterology* 71:943–953, 1976.

Koretz RL, Meyer J: Elemental diets—facts and fantasies. *Gastroenterology* 78:393–410, 1980.

Weser E, Kim Y: Nutrition and the gastrointestinal tract, in Sleisinger MH, Fordtran JS: *Gastrointestinal Disease.* Philadelphia, WB Saunders Co, 1978, pp 20–52.

CLINICAL PROBLEMS

I. A 55-year-old controlled alcoholic is seen because of a weight loss of 20 pounds over the past year. He had recurrent bouts of acute pancreatitis for five years until he ceased drinking last year. Since then he has noted that, in spite of a good appetite, his weight has gradually been dropping. In fact, he had to buy a whole new wardrobe because his clothes had become too large. He denies any other gastrointestinal or systemic symptoms. His wife acknowledges that in the past few months she has had to scrape grease from the toilet bowl when she cleaned the bathroom.

The physical examination reveals evidence of weight loss but is otherwise normal. Laboratory tests reveal calcifications of the pancreas (abdominal x-ray), a coefficient of fat absorption of 53%, and a fasting blood sugar of 198 mg%. Abdominal ultrasound and computerized axial tomographic (CAT) scan fail to demonstrate a pancreatic mass or enlargement.

1. Why is the patient losing weight?
2. What further workup should the patient undergo?
3. What can be done with regard to the weight loss?

II. Another 55-year-old controlled alcoholic presents with abdominal pain and weight loss. This man also had recurrent pancreatitis in the past and he stopped drinking four years earlier. For the past six months he has had progressively more severe epigastric and back pain of a constant nature, which is only minimally relieved by sitting forward. During this time he has lost 20 pounds, in large part because of a loss of appetite.

Physical examination reveals evidence of weight loss and a firm, enlarged liver. Further workup demonstrates a solid pancreatic mass (CAT scan and abdominal ultrasound) as well as multiple filling defects on liver-spleen scan. The coefficient of fat absorption is 81%. The fasting blood sugar is 123 mg%. Pancreatic calcifications are present on abdominal flat plate.

1. Why is the patient losing weight?
2. What further workup should the patient undergo?
3. What can be done with regard to the weight loss?

III. A third 55-year-old alcoholic presents with a history of recurrent pancreatitis that he has had "for years." For the past four years, he has experienced daily pain that is indistinguishable from the pain he had with his previous bouts of pancreatitis.

He has been taking progressively greater and greater doses of analgesics, and he is currently using at least three to four grains of codeine per day. During this period of time, he has gradually lost 20 pounds. When asked about his food intake, his response is vague, but it seems that he is eating less now than he did 10 years ago.

Physical examination reveals a disheveled, depressed man with evident weight loss, but with no other abnormalities. An abdominal flat plate demonstrates pancreatic calcifications. The coefficient of fat absorption is 94%. Both CAT scan and abdominal ultrasound are normal. The fasting blood sugar is 97 mg%.

1. Why is the patient losing weight?
2. What further workup should the patient undergo?
3. What can be done with regard to the weight loss?

Discussion

The three problems are presented to highlight superficially similar clinical situations with different underlying mechanisms of weight loss.

I. 1. The patient has a typical presentation for pancreatic insufficiency, in this case both endocrine and exocrine. The retention of appetite is consistent with a lack of symptoms produced by food. The weight loss is predominantly due to a failure of assimilation of foodstuffs in the intestinal lumen related to a deficiency of digestive enzymes. An additional mechanism may be an associated glycosuria.

2. The patient will need to have his diabetes mellitus treated. Although the pancreatic insufficiency could be evaluated more specifically, one could also perform a therapeutic trial with pancreatic enzyme supplementation (see Chapter 19).

3. The weight loss should respond to the treatment just described.

II. 1. Whereas in the previous case the prominent clinical problem was weight loss, in this patient the major symptom is pain. Weight loss appears to be due, for the most part, to decreased intake. Even though the patient has laboratory evidence of mild endocrine and exocrine pancreatic insufficiency, these probably only play a minor role in causing the weight loss.

2. Since the major problem is the abdominal pain, the attention of the workup should be in this direction. The clinical description points toward pancreatic carcinoma (see the chapter on gastrointestinal cancer).

3. The long-term prognosis is related to the extent of the carcinoma, not to the weight loss. Although many physicians would attempt various types of caloric supplementations (orally or parenterally), there is no evidence that the ultimate outcome will be altered significantly.

III. 1. As in case II, the cause of the weight loss is poor oral intake. Unlike both previous situations, however, there is no evidence of pancreatic insufficiency, and malabsorption cannot be implicated. The anorexia in this case may be related to the pain or to associated depression; one frequently overlooked cause is narcotic usage, which is likely a prominent factor in this patient.

2. The patient needs to be evaluated for the abdominal pain. Although is is possible that the pain is due to ongoing pancreatic inflammation, other more likely causes are functional bowel disease or narcotic addiction, or both. (The four-year history makes the presence of carcinoma very unlikely.)

3. The gastrointestinal tract appears to be functioning normally. The thrust of the treatment should be at detoxification and psychological support. If the various factors maintaining the abdominal pain can be reversed, weight gain will ensue.

6

NEIL KAPLOWITZ

Jaundice

WHAT ARE THE IMPORTANT ASPECTS OF HISTORY?

When approaching a jaundiced patient, a history should be obtained to look for a number of key features (Table 1). A careful drug history and quantitation of alcohol consumption should be obtained so as to stop immediately any potentially harmful agent. Drugs and alcohol can produce any clinical pattern of hepatobiliary disease.

The duration of symptoms is a very important feature. For example, chronic hepatitis may be associated with repeated bouts of jaundice over many years, whereas acute hepatitis may be associated with just a few days or weeks of symptoms.

The history of a characteristic prodromal gastrointestinal upset followed by jaundice or preceded by urticaria and polyarthritis may suggest viral hepatitis. The history of exposure to another individual

Acknowledgment: I wish to thank Nick Onstott for his superb administrative assistance.

75

Age

Sex

Family history

Duration (pattern)

Weight loss

Pain—characterize

Fever, rigors

Drugs and alcohol

Exposures, e.g., sexual, transfusions, occupation

Pruritus

---

with viral hepatitis, homosexuality, drug abuse, travel to underdeveloped areas, blood transfusion, or tattoos within the past six months is useful.

Weight loss over several months may point to a neoplasm. Prolonged, unexplained pruritus is sometimes helpful in pointing to chronicity. An etiology of gallstones may be suggested by fever, rigors, or right upper quadrant abdominal pain (perhaps recurrent in nature).

Remember to consider the age and sex of the individual and a family history of jaundice. The elderly patient who presents with jaundice usually has neoplasm, calculi, or a drug reaction, whereas the younger patient is less likely to have these entities and is more apt to have viral hepatitis. Certain diseases are more likely to occur in females (and are rare in males), such as lupoid chronic active hepatitis and primary biliary cirrhosis. A family history may point to fibrocystic disease of the biliary tree (choledochal cyst and Caroli's disease), Wilson's disease, hemochromatosis, α_1-antitrypsin deficiency, or familial benign recurrent intrahepatic cholestasis.

WHAT ARE THE IMPORTANT PHYSICAL FINDINGS TO SEEK?

In the jaundiced patient, there are constellations of signs of chronic liver disease that must be sought (Table 2). The presence of ascites, palmar erythema, gynecomastia, testicular atrophy,

Stigmata of chronic liver disease
  Ascites
  Palmar erythema, spider angiomata, testicular atrophy
Courvoisier's sign (common bile duct obstruction, probably from neoplasm)
Right upper quadrant tenderness
  Hepatic tenderness (diffuse)
    Acute viral hepatitis
    Alcoholic hepatitis (massive, hard liver)
    Primary or metastatic cancer (nodular, hard liver)
  Hepatic tenderness (localized)
    Abscess (pyogenic or amoebic; usually anicteric)
    Neoplasm (benign or malignant; primary or secondary)
  Gallbladder tenderness (localized)
    Acute cholecystitis

and loss of muscle mass suggests a chronic intrahepatic process rather than surgical jaundice. The other useful sign to search for is an enlarged, palpable nontender gallbladder, the so-called Courvoisier's sign, which is virtually pathognomonic of common bile duct obstruction in the setting of jaundice. Usually when the gallbladder is enlarged, one can see it bulge subcutaneously in the right upper guadrant below the liver edge. One should therefore make the inspection in good light with the patient taking deep respirations and follow this with palpation. Courvoisier's gallbladder sign usually indicates a malignant obstruction of the common bile duct. Stone obstructions are associated with chronic cholecystitis and a less distensible gallbladder. However, this rule is not foolproof and, therefore, does not write off the case as incurable if this sign is present.

Another sign often found in the setting of jaundice is tenderness in the right upper quadrant. The key issue is to determine if the tenderness is the result of swelling of the capsule of the liver, as in acute viral or alcoholic hepatitis, or whether it is due to acute cholecystitis. The latter will result in a very localized tenderness whereas the former will be associated with a palpable liver that is tender along its entire margin. Moreover, the "alcoholic" liver is often massively enlarged and hard, making a distinction between benign disease and malignant infiltration difficult. Another possibility to consider in the patient with right upper quadrant tenderness, usually localized and usually without the presence of jaundice, is an intrahepatic abscess, pyogenic or amoebic. The diagnosis is often missed or mistaken for hepatitis or cholecystitis. The liver function tests are usually minimally abnormal and the liver scan–ultrasound combination is diagnostic. One must consider this possibility in the settings described.

The presence of jaundice itself is the most valuable clue that a hepatobiliary problem may exist. The problem of jaundice involves three key junctures in evaluation (Table 3). Is this a noncholestatic jaundice, that is, one based on an unconjugated hyperbilirubinemia? If conjugated hyperbilirubinemia exists, does the jaundice reflect cholestatic or hepatocellular disease? If cholestatic, is this intrahepatic or extrahepatic? In other words, the entire logical sequence is directed at deciding if this is "medical" or "surgical" disease. The progress through these three questions in sequence requires the performance of clinical biochemical tests and certain noninvasive and invasive diagnostic measures.

WHAT LABORATORY TESTS OR PROCEDURES SHOULD BE ORDERED?

In the routine workup of jaundice, it is important to exclude anemia and hemolysis by checking hematocrit or hemogloblin, or both, and reticulocyte count. The urine should be checked for the presence of bilirubin. If no bilirubin is present in the urine in the jaundiced patient, the serum bilirubin should be fractionated to see if there is just unconjugated bilirubin (i.e., indirect representing > 80% of the total). If bilirubinuria is present, there must be excess conjugated or direct bilirubin in the serum, and further fractionation is of no value in the differential diagnosis. Whether 50% or 70%

Table 3 Important Steps in Evaluation of Jaundice

1. Exclude unconjugated hyperbilirubinemia e.g., hemolysis or Gilbert's syndrome
2. Distinguish hepatocellular from cholestatic jaundice
3. Distinguish intrahepatic from extrahepatic cholestasis

                                                                    SYMPTOMS

of the increased plasma bilirubin is direct or indirect has little meaning.

The presence of unconjugated hyperbilirubinemia as an isolated abnormality is almost always accounted for by one of three conditions: (1) pigment overload as in hemolysis (serum bilirubin always < 4 mg/dl); (2) Gilbert's syndrome, a common benign, autosomal dominant, inherited disorder of bilirubin transport into the liver; or (3) congestive heart failure. The documentation of unconjugated hyperbilirubinemia requires exclusion of hemolysis and heart failure (on clinical examination), which leaves the diagnosis of Gilbert's syndrome. No further workup is needed and a liver biopsy is not indicated.

If, as usually is the case, conjugated hyperbilirubinemia is present (e.g., as evidenced by bilirubinuria), attention should next be directed to the serum liver enzyme tests (Table 4). The diagnostic consideration now is whether the jaundice is due to cholestatic or hepatocellular disease. If the serum transaminases are markedly increased (five to 10 times or greater) and the serum alkaline phosphatase is not, hepatitis is suggested. If the opposite pattern is found (alkaline phosphatase elevated more than four to five times), a primary cholestatic disease is the first consideration. Since the alkaline phosphatase originates in organs other than the liver, it is sometimes helpful to order a confirmatory enzyme test, which is more liver specific. The leucine aminopeptidase and 5'-nucleotidase tests are both

Table 4 **Clinical Biochemistry in Hepatobiliary Disease**

Test	Cholestatic	Hepatocellular
SGOT and SGPT	N[a] TO +	+++
Alkaline phosphatase	+++	N TO +
Cholesterol	+ TO +++[b]	N
Albumin	N	N TO +++
Prothrombin time	N	N TO +++
Bilirubin	N TO +++	N TO +++

[a] N, normal.
[b] + TO +++, arbitrary degrees of abnormality.

useful and fairly equivalent in this regard. The other test that is widely employed, γ-glutamyltranspeptidase, is not very useful because it lacks specificity for liver disease and does not correlate well with alkaline phosphatase to point in the direction of cholestasis.

Other test results that are helpful in pointing to hepatocellular disease (acute or chronic) are low serum albumin, elevated gamma globulin, and an abnormal prothrombin time that does not correct with parenteral vitamin K administration. If these test results are normal, one can only conclude that *severe* hepatocellular disease is absent.

There are a variety of tests that are much more specific and strongly suggest the etiology of a liver disease: for example hepatitis serology (covered in the chapter on hepatitis), low ceruloplasmin in Wilson's disease, increased iron saturation in hemochromatosis, α-fetoprotein in hepatoma, and antimitochondrial antibody in primary biliary cirrhosis. In addition, bacteremia documented with blood cultures in a jaundiced patient should lead to the consideration of biliary sepsis until proved otherwise. The difficulty with this observation, however, is that sepsis, probably through the action of endotoxin, can cause intrahepatic cholestasis when the infection does not originate in the biliary tree.

Once the liver enzyme tests and other special tests such as HBsAg have been obtained, many cases will be seen that are obviously hepatocellular such as acute hepatitis, chronic active hepatitis, or certain forms of cirrhosis. In these cases, one may elect to just watch the patient or to pursue the diagnosis with a liver biopsy, particularly if chronic liver disease is suspected.

If the biochemical pattern is cholestatic or ambiguous, or if the preceding history and physical examination are indeterminant or favor obstructive jaundice, the diagnostic approach proceeds to noninvasive tests, which help to decide the approach to invasive tests. It is important to recognize that it is often impossible to decide on the basis of clinical or biochemical findings if a patient with a cholestatic jaundice has intrahepatic or extrahepatic cholestasis. However, when we have reached this point in the evaluation, we have already excluded the typical acute hepatitis, chronic active hepatitis, alcoholic hepatitis, or cirrhosis and drug-induced liver disease. Our aim now is to select the patients who have a surgically remediable extrahepatic obstructing lesion, such as a stone, stricture, or cancer, and to avoid unnecessary surgical exploration in a patient

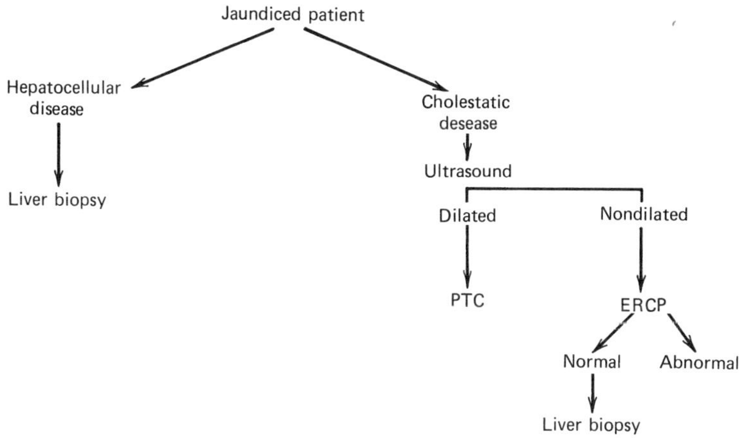

Figure 1 The diagnostic approach to the jaundiced patient. The initial discrimination is made on clinical and biochemical grounds into hepatocellular or cholestatic disease. Indeterminant situations should be added to the cholestatic group. Subsequent studies in the cholestatic group are directed at defining the anatomy of the biliary tree. PTC, percutaneous transhepatic cholangiography; ERCP, endoscopic retrograde cholangiopancreatography.

with cholestasis resulting from an intrahepatic cause (see Fig. 1 for algorithm).

Which Noninvasive Tests Are Useful?

It should be remembered that the oral cholecystogram and intravenous cholangiogram will not visualize in the face of jaundice and should not be attempted. Three noninvasive tests have become available within the past few years: ultrasonography, computerized axial tomography (CAT) scan, and cholescintigraphy.

At the present time ultrasound examination of the abdomen appears to be quite useful and an essential early step in diagnostic evaluations of jaundice. The most important feature sought in this setting is dilatation of either the intrahepatic ducts or the common bile ducts (Fig. 2). When this finding is present, extrahepatic biliary obstruction is almost certainly the cause of jaundice. The basis for this approach is that the biliary tree dilates proximal to a mechanical

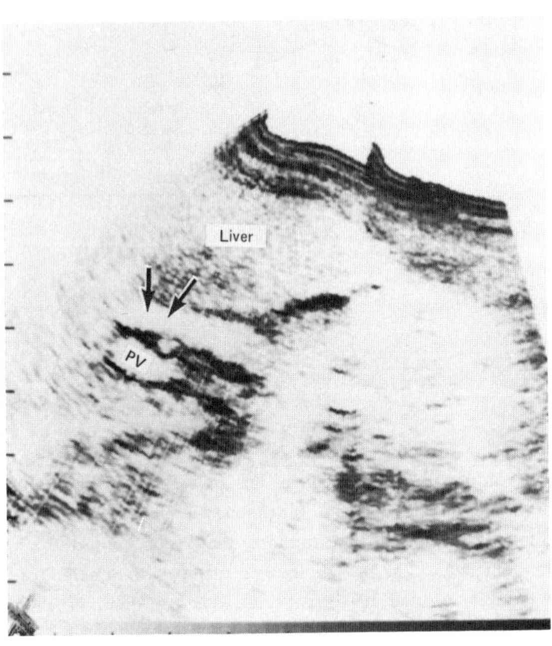

Figure 2 Ultrasound examination of the abdomen demonstrating a dilated common bile duct (arrows) in a longitudinal cut. PV represents portal vein.

obstruction in response to increased pressure. However, the biliary tree often does not dilate in acute calculus obstruction (perhaps because of the acuteness of the situation) and sometimes is strictured throughout, as in primary sclerosing cholangitis. In addition, mild or moderate dilatation of the biliary tree is frequently missed on ultrasound examination. Therefore, the presence of dilatation is highly suggestive of large-duct obstruction whereas the absence of this ultrasound finding means very little. Furthermore, the ultrasound only occasionally gives an important clue as to the specific etiology of the jaundice, such as calculi in the gallbladder or a mass in the pancreas. Therefore, the diagnosis in the jaundiced patient is usually not established by ultrasound. Rather, it plays a key role in deciding which invasive diagnostic test will most likely successfully yield an interpretable cholangiogram.

The other noninvasive tests are of unproved value. The CAT

scan offers no real advantage over ultrasound in evaluating jaundice. Within the abdomen its main use in the future will probably be staging the spread of cancer. Moreover, its cost and availability seriously limit its role. Therefore, under ordinary circumstances, I do not recommend the use of the CAT scan in the evaluation of jaundice.

Cholescintigraphy involves the intravenous administration of a technetium-labeled gamma-emitting radioisotope that is taken up by the liver and excreted into the bile. HIDA and PIPIDA are agents that are currently being evaluated. This approach will demonstrate the biliary tree even in the face of moderate jaundice, but resolution and the ability to interpret dilatation or localize the level of obstruction are doubtful. However, this test does have one important application (unrelated to jaundice): the evaluation of upper abdominal pain related to acute cholecystitis (see chapter on gallstone disease).

What Is the Role of Invasive Tests?

So far, we have evaluated the jaundiced patient with history, physical examination, clinical chemistry, and ultrasound. We then usually proceed to definitive cholangiography. When the ultrasound has demonstrated dilated ducts, this procedure confirms obstruction and localizes it in the biliary tree (distal, middle, or proximal). The cholangiogram determines whether or not mechanical obstruction is present when the ultrasound does not reveal biliary dilatation.

There are two major approaches to the definitive visualization of the biliary tree cholangiographically. One is accomplished by introducing contrast through a thin needle inserted percutaneously into the liver (percutaneous transhepatic cholangiography, or PTC) and the other by introducing contrast through a catheter that has been directed endoscopically into the ampulla of Vater (endoscopic retrograde cholangiopancreatography, or ERCP). The choice of approach is often determined by the expertise available.

Assuming both are performed routinely, most physicians use the result of the ultrasonography in determining which approach to use. If biliary dilatation exists, PTC will be successful in obtaining a cholangiogram in virtually 100% of the cases; if the ducts are not dilated, PTC will successfully visualize the ducts 50% to 60%

of the time. Coagulation disturbances and ascites will limit the needle approach. In contrast, the success of ERCP does not depend on the pathology present but rather on the skill of the endoscopist. Most experienced individuals succeed in 70% to 80% of attempts.

Therefore, ultrasound information determines the subsequent procedure attempted. If the first procedure selected fails, the other can then be attempted. The bonus information from ERCP is as follows: (1) direct visualization of the ampulla in the case of ampullary carcinoma and (2) determination of the pancreatic duct system (pancreatogram) to evaluate the possibility of carcinoma of the pancreas or chronic pancreatitis. In addition, ERCP can be performed more safely in situations in which PTC is contraindicated.

Complications with PTC and ERCP are infrequent ($< 10\%$) and rarely life threatening, particularly if the patients are given prophylactic broad-spectrum antibiotics before and after the procedure to avoid sepsis. PTC can result in bleeding or bile peritonitis. Therefore, it is our practice to alert the surgeons when a PTC is

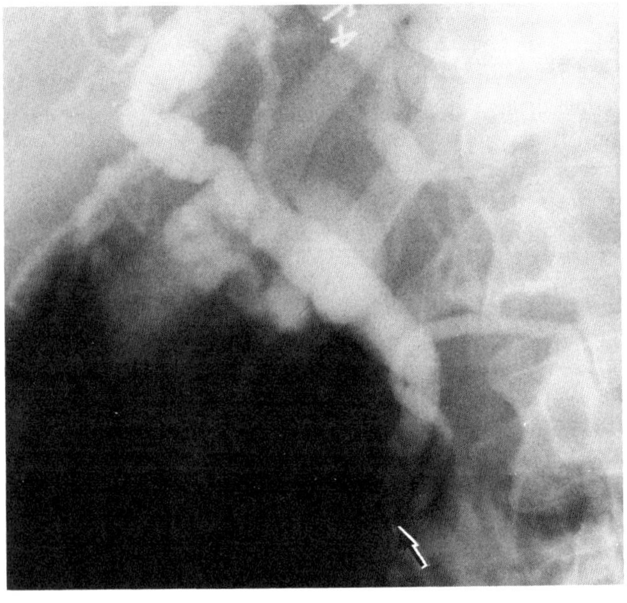

Figure 3 Endoscopic retrograde cholangiopancreatography showing cluster of radiolucent calculi (arrow) in the distal common bile duct.

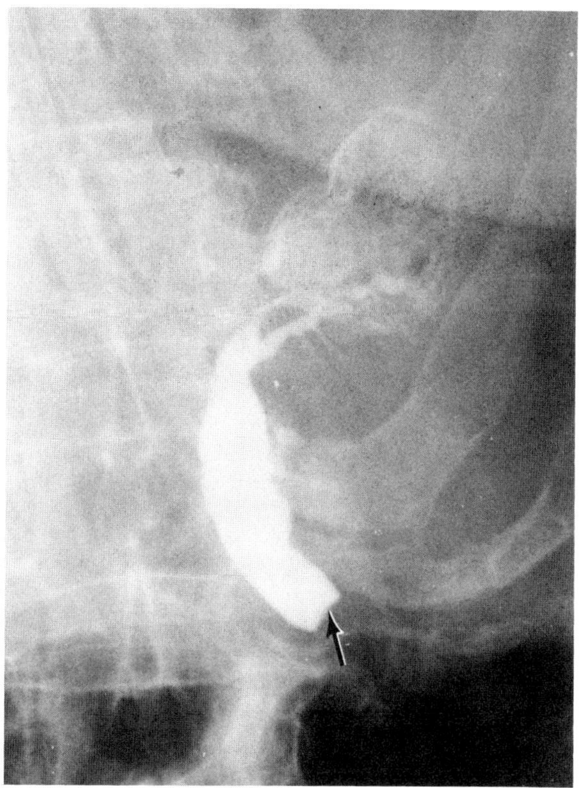

Figure 4 Percutaneous transhepatic cholangiography showing dilated common bile duct obstructed distally by a lesion with a meniscus indicative of a large calculus (arrow).

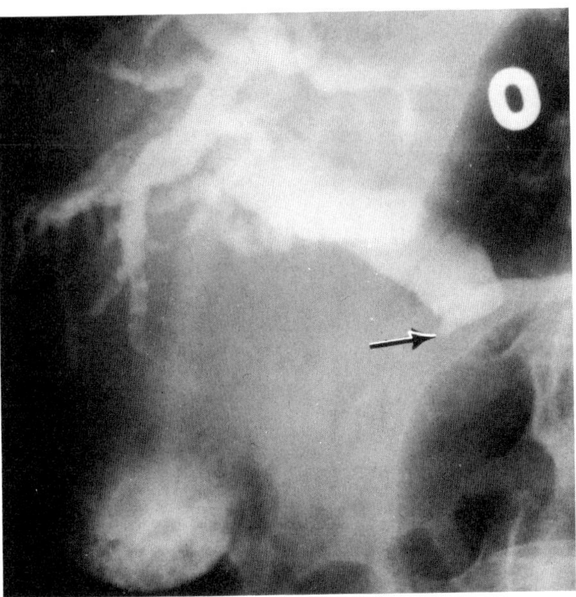

Figure 5 Percutaneous transhepatic cholangiography showing complete obstruction of the mid–common bile duct with a tapering (arrow) indicative of carcinoma of the head of the pancreas. Note the massive proximal dilatation.

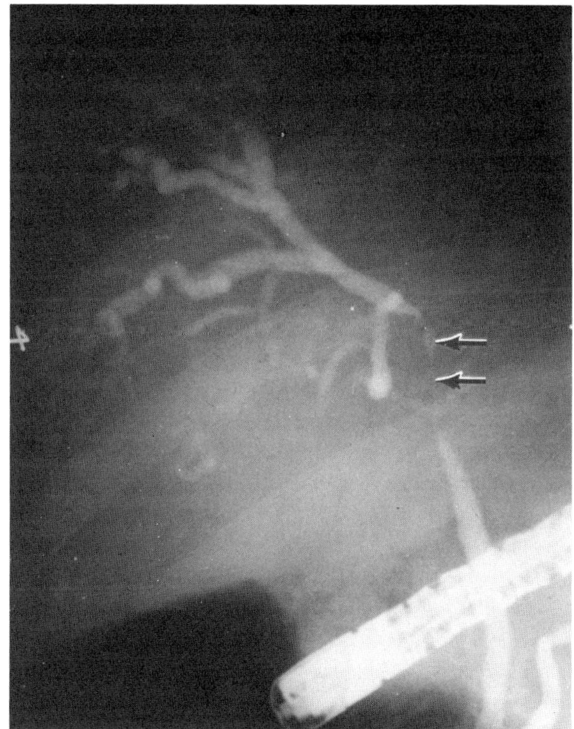

Figure 6 Endoscopic retrograde cholangiopancreatography showing strictured lesion (arrows) in the common hepatic duct and region of the bifurcation without significant dilatation. This lesion was caused by bile duct carcinoma.

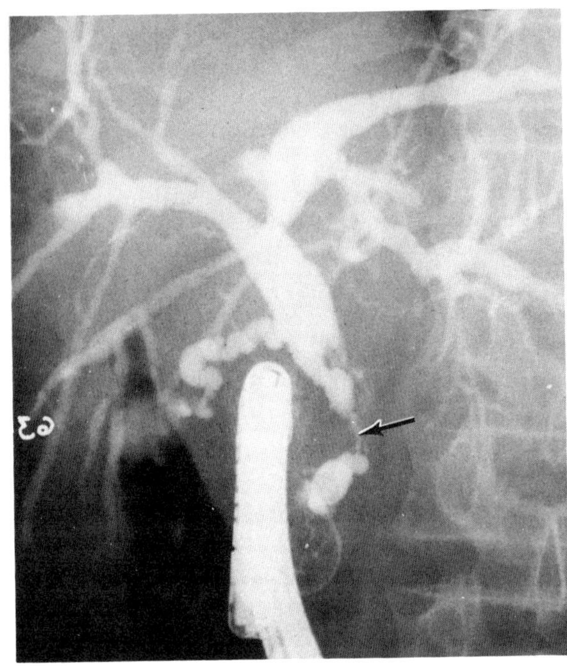

Figure 7 Endoscopic retrograde cholangiopancreatography showing stenotic irregular lesion of a segment of mid–common bile duct (arrow) associated with proximal dilatation due to bile duct carcinoma.

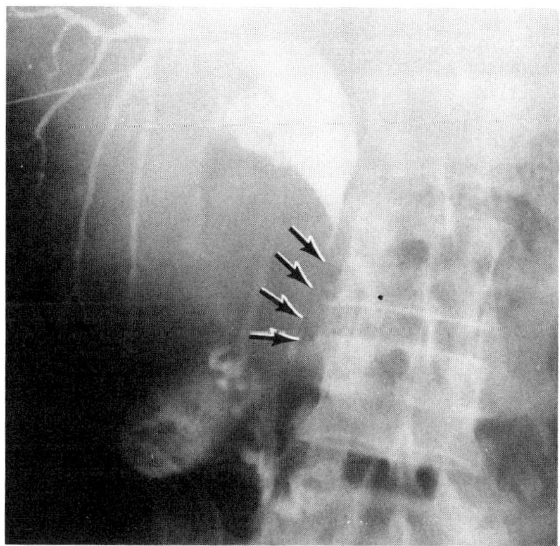

Figure 8 Percutaneous transhepatic cholangiography showing dilated duct system tapering to a very long stenotic common duct (3-cm stricture—arrows) due to extrinsic compression by the pancreas in chronic alcoholic pancreatitis. Note the diffuse intrapancreatic calcification.

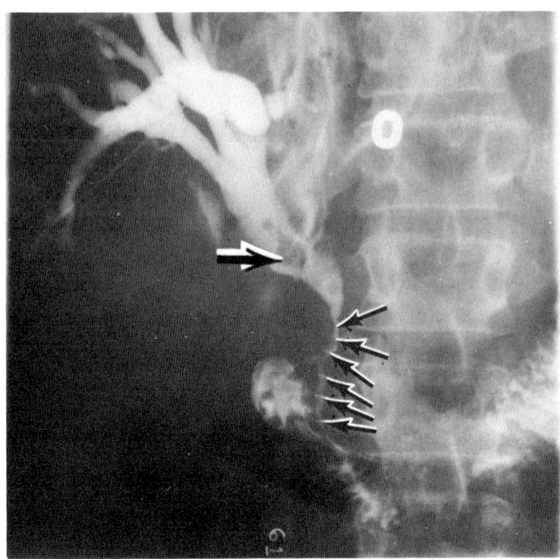

Figure 9 Pecutaneous transhepatic cholangiography showing a long intrapancreatic stenosis of the common bile duct (small arrows) due to alcoholic pancreatitis (note calcifications). Note calculi in the more proximal dilated ducts (large arrow).

performed, thereby aiming for expeditious operative intervention (within a day or two) if a mechanical obstruction is diagnosed.

These approaches to cholangiography offer a road map for the surgeon and allow the health care team an opportunity to make a reasonable judgment about the specific pathology. This is illustrated in Figures 3 to 9, which demonstrate the typical spectrum of lesions seen on the cholangiogram.

Finally, what does the physician do if the cholangiogram is normal? In this case, a very reasonable presumptive diagnosis of intrahepatic cholestasis can be made. Further workup will depend on the patient's course but often culminates in a liver biopsy. When to biopsy patients is an impossible issue to generalize and opinion varies. As is always true in medicine, the diagnostic approach is directed at finding treatable lesions. Thus, there is no need to biopsy the liver in the setting of acute hepatitis, but in chronic hepatitis treatment depends on demonstrating the appropriate histopathology. In the cholestatic situation, persistence of jaundice warrants an examination of the histopathology despite the frequent lack of specificity of the findings, since primary biliary cirrhosis, granulomatous disease, including sarcoid, and neoplastic infiltration may be found.

Summary

Jaundice continues to be one of the most commonly encountered hepatobiliary problems, requiring careful decision making regarding a "medical" versus "surgical" cause. The approach to jaundice is greatly aided by the history and physical examination. Further insight is gained from routine clinical biochemistry. The history, physical examination, and routine clinical biochemistry will correctly establish a diagnosis in medical versus surgical jaundice in 80% to 90% of instances. However, if jaundice persists or is not of clear-cut etiology, definitive evaluation of the biliary tree anatomy is warranted using the newer modalities, ERCP or PTC. The role of ultrasonography and body scanning (CAT) in the workup of jaundice remains ill defined. The more refined noninvasive and invasive diagnostic modalities help in the 10% to 20% of instances in which the clinician cannot determine the cause of jaundice and can also expedite the workup as compared to the old approach of prolonged observation.

WHAT ARE THE MAJOR DIAGNOSTIC CONSIDERATIONS?

The differential diagnosis of cholestatic and hepatocellular disease is given in Table 5. The very rare possibilities are not included so as to limit the consideration to everyday practice.

WHAT SYMPTOMATIC THERAPY CAN BE GIVEN IN THE ABSENCE OF A SPECIFIC DIAGNOSIS?

The important consideration is to establish the diagnosis. In some patients with chronic intrahepatic cholestasis, the major disturbing symptom is pruritus. The mechanism for pruritus is in dis-

Table 5 Working Differential Diagnosis of Hepatobiliary Disease

Hepatocellular disease
  Acute
    Viral hepatitis
    Drug hepatitis
    Alcoholic hepatitis
  Chronic
    Chronic persistent hepatitis (viral)
    Chronic active hepatitis (viral, drug, Wilson's disease, idiopathic)
    Cirrhosis (active or inactive)
      Chronic active hepatitis
      Alcoholic
      Hemochromatosis
      α_1 antitrypsin deficiency
      Wilson's disease
Cholestatic
  Intrahepatic
    Drugs
    Hodgkin's disease (without liver involvement)
    Sepsis
    Benign postoperative
    Alcohol
    Pericholangitis (inflammatory bowel disease)
    Sarcoidosis
    Primary biliary cirrhosis
    Benign familial recurrent intrahepatic cholestasis
  Extrahepatic
    Choledocholithiasis
    Cancer
      Bile duct
      Ampullary
      Carcinoma of the pancreas
    Stricture
      Post-cholecystectomy
      Ampullary
      Chronic alcoholic pancreatitis
      Sclerosing cholangitis
    Stasis
      Choledochal cyst
      Caroli's disease

pute but probably reflects bile acid retention in the skin. This can be treated with an oral sequestering agent such as cholestyramine, which causes the excretion of bile acids in feces and eventually depletes the body of bile acids (or perhaps other substances) responsible for the itching.

SELECTED READING

Berk PD, Javitt NB: Hyperbilirubinemia and cholestasis. *Am J Med* 64: 311 326, 1978.

Kaplowitz N: Cholestatic liver disease. *Hosp Pract* 13(8):83–92, August, 1978.

CLINICAL PROBLEMS

In the following problems, three sets of diagnostic tests will be considered. They will be classified as follows:

    Blood tests: Reticulocyte count
                   Fractionation of bilirubin
                   SGOT, SGPT
                   Alkaline phosphatase
                   Leucine aminopeptidase
                   Albumin and total protein
                   Prothrombin time
                   α-fetoprotein
                   Antimitochondrial antibody
                   Ceruloplasmin
                   Serum iron and iron-binding capacity
Noninvasive tests: Ultrasonography
                   CAT scan
                   Cholescintigraphy
                   Intravenous cholangiography
                   Oral cholecystography
    Invasive tests: Percutaneous transhepatic cholangiography
                   Endoscopic retrograde cholangiopancreatography
                   Liver biopsy
                   Exploratory laparotomy
                   Arteriography

I. A 38-year-old man undergoes a routine physical examination. He has no complaints, and the examination is entirely normal. Routine laboratory work is obtained, and all test results are normal (including the hematocrit, urinalysis, SGOT, and alkaline phosphatase) except for a total bilirubin of 2.5 mg%.

1. What additional blood tests should be obtained at this point?
2. What noninvasive tests would be appropriate?
3. What invasive tests should be performed?

II. A 40-year-old man with chronic alcoholism is admitted to the hospital with a two-week history of jaundice, dark urine, fever, right upper quadrant pain, and ascites. He has been a heavy drinker for at least 15 years. Physical examination demonstrates icterus, spider angiomata, palmar erythema, ascites, hepatosplenomegaly, and peripheral edema. His serum bilirubin is 21 mg%, his white blood cell count is 17,000/mm³ (68% polymorphonuclear leukocytes), and his prothrombin time is 16 seconds (control, 11.5 seconds). A urinalysis demonstrates bilirubin and a normal urinary sediment.

1. What additional blood tests should be obtained?
2. What noninvasive tests would be appropriate?
3. What invasive tests should be performed?

III. A 57-year-old woman presents with a three-day history of epigastric and right upper quadrant abdominal pain, jaundice, and dark urine. She was found to have gallstones two years earlier but refused operation. On physical examination she is icteric and has a tender, mildly enlarged liver. There are no physical findings of cirrhosis. Preliminary laboratory values reveal a normal hematocrit, leukocytosis (13,000), a serum bilirubin of 6.3 mg/dl, an alkaline phosphatase of 225 units (normal, less than 105), and an SGOT of 62 units (normal, less than 40).

1. What additional blood tests should be obtained?
2. What noninvasive tests would be appropriate?
3. What invasive tests should be performed?

Discussion

I. 1. The first step is to determine whether the bilirubin elevation
   is due to hepatic disease. In this case, it is likely that the
   hyperbilirubinemia is due to some prehepatic cause. Thus,
   the bilirubin should be fractionated. It is likely that a raised
   level of unconjugated bilirubin will be found. The normal
   hematocrit makes hemolysis unlikely but a reticulocyte count
   should be obtained to rule out a compensated hemolytic
   anemia.
2. No noninvasive test need be obtained if the bilirubin is almost all unconjugated (indirect).
3. No invasive tests need be performed if the bilirubin is unconjugated. However, if conjugated hyperbilirubinemia is
   present there is a possibility of liver disease and a liver
   biopsy should be considered.

II. 1. The patient has obvious liver disease, very likely due to alcohol, as manifested by the physical findings of cirrhosis.
   The history of dark urine suggests direct hyperbilirubinemia,
   which is confirmed on the urinalysis, and, therefore, a bilirubin fractionation need not be done. An SGOT, SGPT, and
   alkaline phosphatase should be obtained. (An SGOT that is
   three to four times the upper limit of normal and an alkaline
   phosphatase and SGPT that are normal or only minimally
   elevated would be characteristic of alcoholic liver disease.)
   A low serum albumin and elevated globulin would also point
   to chronic severe hepatic damage.
2. The presence of fever, jaundice, and right upper quadrant
   pain also suggests the possibility of extrahepatic bile duct
   obstruction. This should be evaluated with ultrasonography,
   though it should be recognized that a normal study does not
   conclusively exclude obstruction.
3. Assuming the ultrasound examination does not show dilated
   ducts, it would be appropriate not to perform any of the
   listed invasive tests because of the serious hepatic failure. A
   liver biopsy could be obtained when the ascites resolves and
   the coagulation studies return to normal.

III. 1. The patient presents with a typical clinical and biochemical
   picture of obstructive jaundice. Although a leucine aminopeptidase test could be ordered to confirm the hepatic source

of the elevated alkaline phosphatase, this is not necessary in this circumstance.

2. Again, an ultrasound examination should be performed to confirm the presence of a dilated biliary tree. The study may even demonstrate a stone in the common bile duct. An intravenous cholangiogram should not be ordered because it will not visualize with this degree of jaundice.

3. If dilated ducts are demonstrated, it would be appropriate to proceed directly to exploratory laparotomy. Some physicians might prefer to obtain a road map of the biliary tree. If this is desired, a preoperative percutaneous transhepatic cholangiogram could be obtained. (Note that the choice of test is based on the results of ultrasonography.) If the ultrasound does not demonstrate a dilated biliary tree, ERCP should be performed to exclude extrahepatic obstruction.

RONALD L. KORETZ

Gastrointestinal Bleeding

The management of gastrointestinal bleeding encompasses two aspects: control of the hemorrhage and its physiologic effects and ascertainment of its source. The following discussion will focus on these two components separately. Most of this chapter will concentrate on acute overt bleeding processes. At the end, some attention will be paid to other special problems.

WHAT ARE THE IMPORTANT ASPECTS OF HISTORY?

In the patient with acute bleeding, the single most important step is the restoration of an adequate circulating blood volume. Thus, the first few questions of history should be directed at quantitating the volume deficit. The presence of thirst or symptoms relat-

Acknowledgments: The author appreciates the time and trouble taken by Sally Clement and Dorothy Emley in preparing the manuscript.

ing to postural hypotension indicate a significant deficit (over one liter).

The volume of blood lost can usually be grossly estimated by asking the patient how much blood came out as stool or emesis. The rapid exsanguination of a large quantity is more likely to result in hypotension than is a slower but more chronic loss of the same number of red blood cells. Patients with large amounts of blood in their gastrointestinal tract will have not only black stools but also diarrhea. Conversely, patients who have had black but formed stools for several days may have anemia, but their blood volume is more likely to be intact.

The color of the stool only reflects the length of time the blood has remained to be digested in the intestinal lumen. In general, blood traversing the entire small and large bowel is in the intestine longer than is blood emanating from the cecum or sigmoid colon. Usually, bleeding from sites orad to the ligament of Treitz produces black stool and that from the distal small intestine or right side of the colon produces purple or maroon stool; blood from the rectosigmoid area leaves the anus in its native bright-red color. In this regard it must be remembered that stool color is also related to other variables. Hence, black stools may also be seen, in the absence of blood, if iron, charcoal, spinach, or bismuth has been ingested.

Blood that has been in the stomach for an hour or more begins to be digested and any clots that were present begin to dissolve. These processes produce the characteristic dark flecks of blood referred to as "coffee grounds" (in vomitus).

As already noted, determining the source of the bleeding is less important than restoring hemodynamic stability. Once these latter processes are under way, several points of history may lead to an etiologic diagnosis.

Inquiry into previous bleeding episodes and their nature, or into the presence of other illnesses that predispose to bleeding, is an important avenue to pursue. Predisposing illnesses include not only gastrointestinal ones (e.g., cirrhosis, peptic ulcer disease, diverticulosis, inflammatory bowel disease) but also such entities as coagulopathies.

The presence or absence of pain may suggest specific entities (e.g., peptic ulcer disease, reflux esophagitis). Bleeding from varices or diverticula is usually painless.

As will be discussed later, various chemicals may be associated with bleeding. These include medications, such as aspirin, and alcoholic beverages.

A history of an initial nonbloody vomitus, followed subsequently by hematemesis, is classic for a common form of upper gastrointestinal hemorrhage due to a rent in the mucosa at the gastroesophageal junction (the Mallory-Weiss tear). The common sources of upper and lower gastrointestinal bleeding are itemized in Table 1.

WHAT ARE THE IMPORTANT PHYSICAL FINDINGS TO SEEK?

As was true when considering history, the first effort of the physical examination in the acutely bleeding patient should be an assessment of his or her volume status. This should be undertaken even before the history is completed.

Blood pressure and pulse should be ascertained with the pa-

Table 1 Common Sources of Gastrointestinal Bleeding

Upper gastrointestinal bleeding
    Duodenal ulcer
    Gastric ulcer
    Gastritis
    Esophagitis $\pm$ esophageal ulcer
    Duodenitis
    Varices
    Gastric carcinoma
    Mallory-Weiss tear

Lower gastrointestinal bleeding
    Carcinoma of the colon
    Varices
    Diverticulosis/diverticulitis
    Angiodysplasia
    Ischemic enteritis
    Inflammatory bowel disease
    Hemorrhoids
    Colonic polyps

tient in a recumbent position. If these are normal, the patient should be asked to sit, then dangle the feet, and finally stand, with the blood pressure and pulse determined in each position. If the blood pressure drops by more than 10 mm Hg, or if the pulse increases by more than 10 to 20 beats a minute, postural hypotension is present, and this is prima facie evidence of significant volume loss.

Other measurements also reflect volume status and may be employed at times. Urine output directly correlates with the circulating blood volume. Central venous pressure determination will correlate as well, but is usually superfluous.

Blood is a cathartic. Patients with gastrointestinal bleeding will have active bowel sounds. The absence of bowel sounds in the face of bleeding would point to some intraabdominal catastrophe.

Usually patients who complain of bleeding are bleeding. Occasionally it becomes necessary to document the presence of blood in the intestinal lumen. This can be performed most simply by testing a stool specimen for blood. Rarely it may be necessary to pass a nasogastric tube and to test the gastric contents. (More commonly a tube is passed to document that the bleeding is, in fact, coming from the upper gastrointestinal tract.)

The physical examination should also encompass a search for the source of bleeding. Signs of chronic liver disease will be discussed in the subsequent chapter on cirrhosis. Epigastric tenderness may indicate the presence of peptic ulcer disease. An enlarged liver may be appreciated in patients with intestinal cancer and hepatic metastases. Skin ecchymoses are common in patients with coagulopathies.

WHAT LABORATORY TESTS OR PROCEDURES SHOULD BE ORDERED?

The hematocrit or hemoglobin level does not reflect volume status but only what portion of the volume present is occupied by red blood cells. As an example, an individual with an aortoenteric fistula may have a relatively normal hematocrit in spite of being in shock. At the other extreme, patients with iron deficiency anemia and hematocrit values in the teens are usually volume expanded. Furthermore, if serial hematocrits are obtained in patients with recent hemorrhage, the value commonly falls (even if the bleeding has stopped) as the volume is reconstituted with fluids such as saline. Nonetheless it is a standard procedure to obtain a hemoglobin or hematocrit when first seeing the patient.

Other laboratory values may reflect hypovolemia more accurately. These include the serum creatinine or blood urea nitrogen (BUN) and the urine specific gravity. A direct determination of blood volume in the actively bleeding patient is time consuming, unreliable, and not helpful.

Clotting parameters should be obtained in patients with suspected liver disease or with other causes of potential coagulopathies. In patients with liver disease, the bleeding is not, in and of itself, due to the coagulation defect, but it is likely that the severity is, in part, attributable to this coexistent problem.

Before embarking on the issue of endoscopy in upper gastrointestinal bleeding, an interesting point concerning diagnosis should be made. Establishing a diagnosis is not, in and of itself, therapeutic. In fact, the overall mortality from gastrointestinal bleeding (approximately 10%) has not changed in spite of our more sophisticated diagnostic tools. Even prospective controlled trials have failed to demonstrate any difference in outcomes between groups of patients who have had vigorous diagnostic attempts made, usually including endoscopy, and those who have not. Perhaps this should not be a surprise. Most episodes of bleeding stop spontaneously or shortly after hospital admission and do not recur. Mortality is usually related to factors unassociated with the specific bleeding lesion such as age or coexistent disease of other organ systems.

With this caveat, what efforts should be expended toward establishing a specific diagnosis? The principle to be followed is to make those diagnoses that will affect short-term or long-term management.

As has been shown, establishing a diagnosis does not affect the short-term management or outcome of those patients who stop bleeding. For those who do not, and for whom surgical therapy is proposed, it is important to determine the site of bleeding so that an appropriate operation can be performed. Such patients should undergo emergency endoscopy (or whatever other tests are available to make the diagnosis quickly).

In a subpopulation of those who stop bleeding, a specific diagnosis is still important. This includes those thought to have bled from peptic ulcer disease, varices, or esophagitis. Future surgical decisions made on these disorders are based on documentation of bleeding.

Thus, patients thought to have bled from these lesions should receive prompt, though not emergent, evaluation. Since endoscopy is more accurate than are barium studies, it should be the test of first choice.

In patients suspected of having bled from nonrecurring lesions (e.g., erosive gastritis or a Mallory-Weiss tear), the diagnosis is of little import. Even here, one could still be concerned over the presence of peptic ulcer disease. An upper gastrointestinal barium examination, while not as accurate as endoscopy, is usually satisfactory in ruling out the ulcer, and it is considerably less stressful for most patients.

I would propose the following general policy for patients with upper gastrointestinal bleeding. Young patients thought to have a Mallory-Weiss tear or gastritis should be evaluated with a barium study at the next convenient elective time. (The purpose of this study is not to establish the diagnosis but to exclude the presence of another common lesion, ulcer disease.) Those patients believed to have ulcers should be treated for this disease and evaluated radiographically or endoscopically at the next convenient elective time. (If one test is negative, the other should be performed, as the purpose in this case is to establish the diagnosis.) Patients thought to have bled from varices or esophagitis should undergo endoscopy (a more sensitive diagnostic test) at the next convenient time. (If endoscopy is negative, a barium study could then be performed to look for endoscopically missed ulcers.) Patients who continue to bleed after admission and are considered for operation, regardless of the suspected cause of bleeding, should undergo emergency endoscopy. Finally, all patients older than 40 who have upper gastrointestinal bleeding should at least have a barium study to exclude the presence of a malignancy. This protocol is summarized in Table 2.

What about lower gastrointestinal bleeding? Are endoscopic or radiographic tests of value in this situation? In this instance, no controlled trials have looked at the value of establishing the diagnosis, but again it would not be surprising if there was no measurable effect on short-term outcome. On the other hand, it seems intuitively obvious that most of the causes listed in Table 1 should be diagnosed.

The general philosophic approach I employ in these patients is the following. All such patients undergo emergency sigmoidoscopy on admission. Inflammatory bowel disease can be found in this way,

Suspected Source	Diagnostic Evaluation
Young patient with gastritis or Mallory-Weiss tear	UGI[a] electively
Peptic ulcer disease	UGI and/or endoscopy electively
Variceal bleeding	Elective endoscopy (UGI if endoscopy negative)
Esophagitis	Elective endoscopy (UGI if endoscopy negative)
Malignancy	Elective UGI and/or endoscopy
Continued bleeding	Emergent endoscopy

[a] UGI, barium upper gastrointestinal series.

and the source of the bleeding can be determined to be above or below 25 cm from the anus. The standard sigmoidoscope is large enough in diameter to allow the adequate aspiration of blood and debris.

If the bleeding is found to be emanating from beyond the reach of the sigmoidoscope, the patient is observed. Usually the bleeding ceases. If this is the case, the observation is continued without diagnostic intervention for at least 24 hours, after which a barium enema is performed. If this fails to establish a diagnosis, colonoscopy is performed after the patient has undergone suitable preparation.

The use of fiberoptic flexible colonoscopes or sigmoidoscopes in the actively bleeding patient is usually not helpful, as the intestinal contents cannot be cleared rapidly enough. The purpose of the 24-hour delay before embarking on a barium study is to ensure that the hemorrhage has stopped. (Residual barium in the colon will interfere with subsequent diagnostic arteriography.)

If the bleeding does not stop, arteriography is obtained. In order for this to be successful, however, the patient needs to be bleeding at a rate of at least 2 to 3 cc a minute (approximately one unit of blood every three to four hours).

We should pause at this point to mention one particular lesion that has received a great deal of attention in the literature lately, angiodysplasia of the colon. This vascular lesion is probably acquired, occurring predominantly in older patients. It tends to arise near the cecum or proximal right colon and may be a result of repeated bouts of subclinical vascular insufficiency. It is difficult to identify but appears to be composed of dilated small blood vessels, especially capillaries and veins. It is usually diagnosed endoscopically or arteriographically. This may be the lesion that really bleeds in some of the patients who were previously thought to have bled from diverticulosis. (This may explain the observation that, although diverticula arise predominantly on the left side of the colon, bleeding from "diverticulosis" comes from the right side in half of the cases.)

WHAT ARE THE MAJOR DIAGNOSTIC CONSIDERATIONS?

The common causes of bleeding have already been listed in Table 1.

WHAT SYMPTOMATIC THERAPY CAN BE GIVEN IN THE ABSENCE OF A SPECIFIC DIAGNOSIS?

As has been stressed before, the most important consideration is the restoration of a normal circulating blood volume. This is accomplished by the intravenous administration of fluids; under the usual circumstances, saline is adequate. One must be careful, especially in older patients (and possibly also in patients with varices), not to overload the circulation. (Pulmonary edema is one of the more common complications of fluid replacement; burst varices may also be a problem in patients with cirrhosis.) Careful monitoring of orthostatic blood pressure and pulse, urine output, and even central venous pressure, is helpful in this regard.

Attention should be paid to my phrase "circulating blood volume." Note that nothing was said concerning restoration of the hematocrit to normal. As was mentioned earlier, the hematocrit does not measure volume. It is likely that we, as physicians, have tended to overtransfuse our bleeding patients.

The resting adult requires about 250 cc of oxygen (O_2) per minute. This is delivered to the tissues bound to hemoglobin (1.34 cc O_2/gm hemoglobin) and dissolved in the plasma (3 cc O_2/liter). If one assumes that a patient can double his or her stroke volume and pulse rate (thereby quadrupling cardiac output), it can be calculated that the minimum hemoglobin concentration required to deliver that volume of O_2 to the tissues (assuming 100% tissue extraction) is 0.6 gm%, which corresponds to a hematocrit of 2%. I am not advocating that patients be allowed to exsanguinate to that level, but am pointing out that one must be able to distinguish between the signs and symptoms of hypovolemia and those of hypoxia and then react appropriately. These signs and symptoms are listed in Table 3.

Cell death that occurs during bleeding arises from the cardiac output being so reduced that oxygen cannot be carried to the tissues, not from a failure to have enough oxygen in any given milliliter of the blood. Although the situations are not directly comparable, in the chronic state patients can tolerate very low hemoglobin or hematocrit levels. (As an example, consider the occasional patient with chronic anemia who is seen with mild complaints of shortness of breath on exertion and whose hematocrit is less than 10%!)

It is illogical to arbitrarily set a hemoglobin or hematocrit level and transfuse all patients to that level. Even the argument that one wants a high hematocrit in case the patient rebleeds is not appropriate, as the problem in rebleeding is the same as in the initial hemorrhage, hypovolemia.

This would not be as major an issue if blood transfusions were

Table 3　**Signs and Symptoms of Hypovolemia and Hypoxia**

Hypovolemia
Hypotension
Tachycardia
Thirst
Oliguria
Hypoxia (normovolemia assumed to be present)
Confusion
Angina pectoris
ECG changes of ischemia
Lactic acidosis

innocuous. However, in addition to using a scarce commodity, transfusion reactions and posttransfusion hepatitis frequently occur. The problems of volume overexpansion have already been mentioned.

How does one decide to transfuse? My first admonition is not to select an arbitrary hematocrit level. Rather, begin by establishing a normovolemic state as quickly as possible. If, in this state, evidence of oxygen deficiency is present, the patient needs red blood cells no matter what the hematocrit level is. On the other hand, hematocrit levels below 25%, and even below 20%, can be tolerated comfortably by many patients. Within a few days of the bleeding, assuming the patient has adequate iron stores, reticulocytosis will begin and patients will restore their hemoglobin levels to normal on their own over the next few weeks.

There is not much evidence to support the technique of iced-saline lavage. Its main function may be to clean out the stomach for subsequent endoscopy.

Most patients can also be managed without nasogastric suction. Although this can be used to monitor for recurrent bleeding, other clinical parameters (bowel sounds, stool output, vital signs, urine output, and even hematocrit levels) are equally effective and not as uncomfortable. On occasion such tubes can be used to instill antacids, although I personally would prefer to drink them if I were a patient given the choice. The tubes may be indicated in patients with cirrhosis to prevent the blood from entering the bowel and producing encephalopathy. (The tubes probably do not cause the esophageal varices to rebleed.)

In the absence of a specific diagnosis, antacids or cimetidine are frequently used to reduce acidity, even though there is no evidence that they are of value during active bleeding. (If peptic ulcer disease is present, these agents may be justified for their efficacy in ultimately healing the lesion.) On the other hand, these agents probably do not do much harm unless an overabundance of magnesium-containing antacids is employed, in which case diarrhea ensues. (If antacids are used, they should be given hourly, as they empty rapidly from the stomach.)

What about emergency surgical intervention? It has been my policy to seek a surgical consultation for any patient admitted with bleeding, even though the vast majority of these patients never reach the operating room. There are no strict guidelines as to when or if operation should be undertaken, and the decision is individualized for each patient. In general, patients who continue to bleed and who lose four to five units of blood in the first day or two after admission become strong candidates for surgical intervention. Patients with gastritis are evaluated for longer periods rather than being subjected to gastrectomy. In the rapidly bleeding patient, considerations such as availability of a rare blood type might force an earlier operation. (Yes, I do transfuse at times!) The patient's age and any coexistent medical problems also enter into this consideration.

SPECIAL PROBLEMS

Occult Blood Found in Stool on Routine Examination

Testing for occult blood does not measure red blood cells per se, but rather the presence of an enzyme from the cell cytoplasm, peroxidase. (For this reason, the ingestion of iron does not interfere with the test.) Red cells that enter anywhere in the gastrointestinal tract, and which subsequently degenerate, provide peroxidase. Thus, occult blood in the stool may result even from nosebleeding.

Large studies have revealed that a substantial proportion (approximately 50%) of asymptomatic, middle-aged, or older (over 40 years) patients with positive Hemoccult slides will, on extensive workup, reveal organic causes for the occult blood. Although most of these causes are benign, a significant minority (perhaps 10% of those with positive tests) have demonstrated carcinoma of the colon, often in early stages.

Debate exists as to the role of diet in creating false-positive or false-negative reactions. Some investigators have felt that meat can cause a false-positive reaction, and have advocated meat-free diets. Others have claimed that high-fiber diets should be consumed for several days before testing, as the bulk will traumatize any luminal lesion and cause it to bleed. Antioxidants, such as ascorbic acid (vitamin C) in large doses, may interfere with the chemical reaction and produce false-negative results.

In general, it has been my policy to include stool testing for occult blood as part of the complete physical examination. Those who have positive results and no readily apparent cause (such as aspirin use or a recent nosebleed) are asked to go on a meat-free, high-bulk diet for several days and then submit three separate specimens. If blood is present in any of these specimens, a workup is undertaken. If no blood is found, the three-stool routine is repeated in six months. If it is again negative, no further evaluation is pursued.

Since the source of the blood may be anywhere in the gastrointestinal tract, examination of both the upper and lower systems is in order. If barium studies (upper gastrointestinal series and barium enemas) and sigmoidoscopy are negative, more stool specimens are obtained. Those patients whose tests remain positive undergo endoscopic examinations (gastroscopy and colonoscopy). Otherwise the workup ceases at that point.

If the entire workup is negative and the stools are positive, it is important not to neglect future examination. In such cases, repeat evaluation (especially with regard to the colon) should be undertaken six months later and one year after that. The failure of any lesion to make itself apparent in this 18-month period would argue for a benign process, which is not likely to have any significant impact on the patient.

Unexpected Iron Deficiency

Iron deficiency is not a "normal" finding in any male or in a premenstrual or postmenopausal female. The most likely cause for this is blood loss in the gastrointestinal tract. Thus, such patients with occult blood in the stool must be evaluated as already described. Those with iron deficiency without demonstrable occult blood should also be evaluated similarly if the following comments do not apply.

Other causes of iron deficiency exist. Most importantly, a careful dietary history must be obtained. Obviously a lack of iron intake will ultimately lead to deficiency of this mineral. Such a problem is commonly seen in young children kept on a milk diet. Rarely adults may also advertently or inadvertently neglect to include iron in their diet. Iron deficiency may be a complication of excess starch consumption, either because not enough iron is consumed or because it is chelated by the starch itself. (The chelated iron precipitates and cannot be absorbed.) Pica is often not readily admitted by patients, and this history should be sought specifically but in a nonthreatening manner.

Iron malabsorption is a very uncommon cause of iron deficiency. Occasionally this can be seen in mucosal disease of the small intestine, classically of the proximal small bowel, such as celiac sprue. The claim has been made that antacids interfere with iron absorption. Although this may be true in a biochemical sense, it is not usually a clinical problem. Postgastrectomy patients often develop iron deficiency years after their operation. Other causes of hypochromic microcytic anemias are listed in Table 4.

Intermittent Overt Bleeding with a Negative Diagnostic Workup

Intermittent overt bleeding with a negative diagnostic workup is a rare but perplexing and frustrating experience for the clinician. Such patients undergo multiple barium, endoscopic, and angiographic studies. Usually some small vascular lesion is responsible. One can only recommend persistence in the workup. Another diagnostic tool, which may be of use in those with rectal bleeding, is the passage of a long nasogastric tube during the bleeding episode. Every 10 cm, aspiration is performed until blood returns. The tube is clamped and located radiographically; barium can even be instilled to visualize that one particular area specifically.

Obscure Causes of Gastrointestinal Bleeding

Table 5 lists a variety of rare causes for gastrointestinal bleeding. A discussion of the evaluation for these lesions is beyond the

Table 4   **Causes of Hypochromic Microcytic Anemias**

Microcytic, hypochromic:
   Iron deficiency
   Thalassemia
   Anemia of chronic disease
   Sideroblastic anemia
   Benign mesenteric lymphoid tumors
Microcytic
   Copper deficiency

Table 5   Rare Causes of Gastrointestinal Bleeding

Neoplasms
  Benign: leiomyoma, lipoma, hemangioma, hamartoma (including Peutz-Jegher syndrome)
  Malignant: lymphoma, carcinoid, sarcoma, melanoma, leukemia
Vascular
  Aortointestinal fistula
  Rendu-Osler-Weber syndrome
  Ehlers-Danlos syndrome
  Pseudoxanthoma elasticum
  Blue rubber-bleb nevus syndrome
Infection
  Granulomatous: tuberculosis, fungal
  Parasitic
Miscellaneous
  Radiation
  Ulcer of the small intestine or colon
  Eosinophilic gastroenteritis
  Meckel's diverticulum
  Uremia
  Amyloidosis
  Trauma
  Blood dyscrasias
  Hemobilia

scope of this text. However, one should be aware of the mucocutaneous findings associated with some of these disease states. These are enumerated in Table 6.

Drugs and Gastrointestinal Bleeding

A number of medications have been implicated in the etiology of gastrointestinal bleeding. Foremost among these is aspirin; a large number of other nonsteroidal antiinflammatory agents are also thought to predispose to erosive gastritis, perhaps as a result of their action on prostaglandins. Usually aspirin is the only drug associated with clinically relevant hemorrhage.

Many drugs cause nonspecific gastrointestinal symptoms such as nausea or vomiting. It should not be inferred, however, that these drugs therefore cause a discrete hole (ulcer) or erosions in the intestinal mucosa.

 Mucocutaneous Manifestations of Rare Syndromes Associated with Gastrointestinal Bleeding

Syndrome	Manifestations
Peutz-Jegher	Melanin deposition around and in oral cavity (especially buccal mucosa), palms, soles, perianal area
Rendu-Osler-Weber	Telangiectasias of lips, tongue, skin
Ehlers-Danlos	Hypermobile joints; lax skin; wide scars over bony prominences
Pseudoxanthoma elasticum	Yellow macules in skin folds (especially in the neck, axillary, inguinal, and periumbilical areas; similar in appearance to chicken skin); retinal angioid streaks
Blue rubber-bleb nevus	Hemangiomas of skin (especially of the trunk and arms)

Hemobilia

Hemobilia is an obscure cause of gastrointestinal bleeding that is also beyond the scope of these considerations. It should be considered when, in addition to hemorrhage, the patient describes bouts of classic biliary colic. (These episodes of pain may be due to blood clots traversing the common bile duct.)

Prophylaxis for Stress Bleeding

A number of illnesses, characterized by severe physiologic insult, are associated with gastrointestinal bleeding. Such patients usually require confinement in an intensive care unit. Bleeding will be seen hours to days after the initial insult. It is thought that a variety of hemodynamic, neurologic, and/or endocrine factors predispose to this "stress bleeding."

This section will not discuss the pathophysiology or evaluation of patients with stress bleeding. However, it should be pointed out that several studies performed on a variety of critically ill patients have shown that the incidence of bleeding would appear to be less in those who received either prophylactic antacid (usually as an hourly intragastric titration) or cimetidine, as compared to control subjects not so treated. It is important to emphasize that much of the bleeding prevented in these studies was probably of no clinical consequence; nonetheless such prophylaxis is commonly employed in the critically ill patient.

SELECTED READING

Boley SJ, Sammartano R, Adams A, et al: On the nature and etiology of vascular ectasias of the colon. *Gastroenterology* 72:650–660, 1977.

Cotton PB, Russell RCG: Diseases of the alimentary system. Haematemesis and malaena. *Br Med J* 1:37–39, 1977.

Eastwood GL: Does early endoscopy benefit the patient with active upper gastrointestinal bleeding? *Gastroenterology* 72:737–739, 1977.

Hastings PR, Skillman JJ, Bushnell LS, et al: Antacid titration in the prevention of acute gastrointestinal bleeding. *N Engl J Med* 298:1041–1045, 1978.

Law DH, Watts HD: Gastrointestinal bleeding, in Sleisenger MH, Fordtran JS (eds): *Gastrointestinal Disease*. Philadelphia, WB Saunders Co, 1978, pp 217–240.

Tedesco FJ, Waye J, Raskin JB, et al: Colonoscopic evaluation of rectal bleeding. *Ann Intern Med* 89:907–909, 1978.

CLINICAL PROBLEMS

I. A 27-year-old man with a past history of uncomplicated duodenal ulcer disease comes to the emergency room after having passed black stools for two days; he then vomited "coffee-ground" material. He states that for the past two weeks he has been having his usual ulcer pain, for which he has taken antacids. He denies alcohol or aspirin use.

A rapid physical examination reveals resting tachycardia (pulse of 110) with a blood pressure of 115/80. When he stands his blood pressure drops to 95/70 and his pulse increases to 125. Other than mild epigastric tenderness, the examination is negative. His stool is black and positive for blood.

1. What resuscitative measures are in order?
2. What lesions could be responsible for the bleeding?

3. What further information is necessary to care for this patient?

II. A 21-year-old college student comes to the emergency room with his friends. They had been involved in an ice cream eating contest all day and the patient, feeling quite bloated, induced vomiting. About 30 minutes later he became nauseated and, with another emesis, produced a "bowl full" of red blood and clots. He has had no previous gastrointestinal problems.

His examination is unremarkable. His vital signs are normal and no postural changes occur. A stool specimen is negative for occult blood. A nasogastric tube is passed and the gastric contents have a few dark flecks that are positive for blood.

1. What resuscitative measures are in order?
2. What lesions could be responsible for the bleeding?
3. What further information is necessary to care for this patient?

III. A 66-year-old man presents with a three-hour history of the painless passage of maroon diarrheal stools. He has no past history of any intestinal problems, but he has a long history of arteriosclerotic coronary vascular disease with angina and a previous myocardial infarction. He noted an episode of angina as he entered the emergency room; it was relieved with nitroglycerin.

His physical examination reveals a blood pressure of 110/70 and a pulse of 90. When he sits up and dangles his feet his blood pressure drops to 75/50 and his pulse increases to 130. He again complains of angina. His cardiac and abdominal examination is unremarkable. His stool is maroon and positive for blood. A nasogastric aspirate shows no blood present in the stomach.

1. What resuscitative measures are in order?
2. What lesions could be responsible for the bleeding?
3. What further information is necessary to care for this patient?

I. 1. The patient presents with apparent hypovolemia as manifested by his tachycardia and postural hypotension. His most emergent problem is the restoration of his blood volume, for which he should be given intravenous fluids. Because of his age and otherwise good health, saline alone would be appropriate. He should be hospitalized for further observation.

2. The most likely source of the blood loss is a duodenal ulcer. The other entities listed in Table 1 are much less likely.

3. For the immediate time period, no other information is necessary, although a baseline hematocrit should probably be obtained. A presumptive diagnosis of ulcer disease could be made and the patient could be begun on appropriate therapy. If the bleeding ceases, an emergency evaluation is not necessary. However, it is important to document the source of bleeding. Endoscopy or a barium upper gastrointestinal series, or both, should be obtained for this reason.

II. 1. In this instance no evidence of hypovolemia is present. The patient should be admitted to the hospital and an intravenous line should be established in the event of further bleeding. He will require only maintenance fluids unless other evidence of hypovolemia becomes apparent.

2. A Mallory-Weiss tear is the most likely cause of the bleeding. This lesion typically bleeds once and then ceases. There is no reason to suspect ulcer disease or liver disease.

3. Again a baseline hematocrit should probably be obtained, but no other immediate information is necessary. If the bleeding ceases, there is no reason to attempt to prove the diagnosis. An upper gastrointestinal x-ray will adequately exclude the presence of an ulcer.

III. 1. This patient has evidence of hypovolemia and complicating angina. The myocardial ischemia is probably caused by the volume deficit, and that should be corrected. Many physicians might be concerned over the angina and would use blood in addition to saline. (There is no indication, however, for the use of uncrossmatched O-negative blood in this case.)

2. The etiology of this bleeding is unclear and may be due to ischemic bowel disease, diverticulosis, angiodysplasia, or neoplasm. (Inflammatory bowel disease and varices are much less likely; hemorrhoidal bleeding is usually bright red.)

3. The immediate care of the patient necessitates close monitoring of his volume status. This patient should appropriately be placed on continuous cardiac monitoring and be evaluated for myocardial damage. Establishing the site of bleeding, while important, can be delayed if the bleeding stops. Sigmoidoscopy should be performed, however. If bleeding does not stop, and especially if surgical therapy is contemplated, preoperative arteriography may be necessary.

8

MARTIN A. POPS

Dysphagia

Dysphagia, which means difficulty in swallowing, is an important symptom that almost always signifies some disorder or disease process involving the pharynx or esophagus; it requires evaluation and, eventually, treatment. Odynophagia refers to pain associated with swallowing and may or may not accompany difficulty in swallowing. Globus hystericus, which refers to the sensation of a lump in the throat, must also be differentiated from dysphagia. This sensation, which may be due to a contraction of the cricopharyngeal muscle (the upper esophageal sphincter), transiently disappears when the patient swallows. Serious underlying pathologic processes are not associated with globus hystericus.

WHAT ARE THE IMPORTANT ASPECTS
OF HISTORY?

Three distinct patterns of dysphagia can be appreciated historically and are important to differentiate. Progressive dysphagia describes a situation in which the patient has initial difficulty only with solid, especially chunky, food. However, as time goes on, smaller and softer material also produces symptoms. Such dysphagia is associated with a narrow mechanical obstruction, such as carcinoma or a peptic stricture (Figs. 1, 2).

Total dysphagia applies to the simultaneous occurrence of dysphagia to both solids and liquids. This history suggests a neuromuscular defect in the esophagus so that either propulsion is impaired or one of the sphincters will not open. Achalasia and diffuse esophageal spasm are examples of this.

Fixed dysphagia describes difficulty in swallowing boluses only of a certain size or greater. Unlike progressive dysphagia, the size or malleability of the symptom-producing food does not change. As an example, a patient may have problems only if he or she swallows a chunk of meat without chewing it. This history implies an ob-

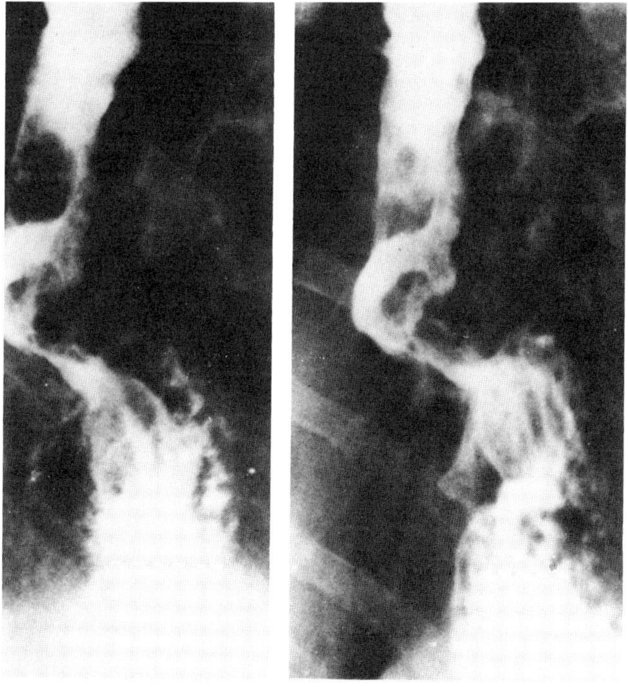

Figure 1 Carcinoma of the esophagus; note narrowing and irregularity of distal esophagus.

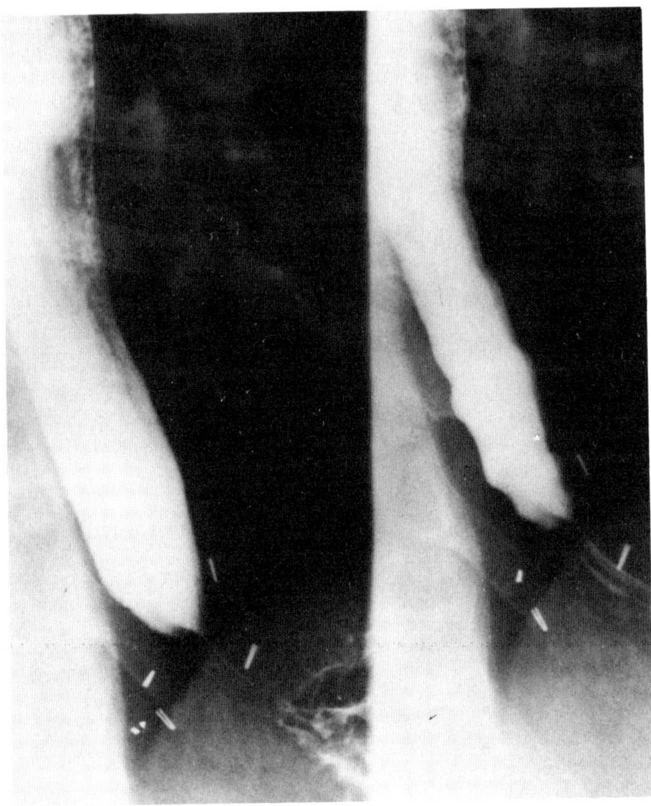

Figure 2 Benign (peptic) stricture of esophagus; note tapered narrowing without mucosal irregularity.

struction of a fixed size that is not becoming smaller, such as an esophageal ring.

Questions should also be directed to the apparent location of the impedance in swallowing. Patients with obstructive lesions of the distal esophagus near the esophagogastric junction will most often point to the xiphoid area to answer the question, "Where does the food seem to stick?" The site may be referred higher, however, especially as the duration of the disorder lengthens. When a patient does point to the xiphoid area, one usually can conclude that a distal esophageal problem is present. Referring the point of sticking to a region higher up in the chest does not reliably indicate the level of the lesion. However, the patient who immediately regurgitates food or liquid into the mouth or more characteristically through the nostrils should be suspected to harbor some disorder in the hypopharynx or most proximal portion of the esophagus.

The sudden onset of dysphagia would occur with obstruction (e.g., a foreign body or very large bolus of food). Severe dysphagia that develops over hours might suggest some traumatic injury to the hypopharynx or esophagus. Dysphagia that is present for many weeks or months is typical of an underlying chronic disease.

Another important question is whether the dysphagia is accompanied by pain (odynophagia) or if it is painless. Inquiry should also be made as to the presence of heartburn (pyrosis), which is often not perceived as actual pain by many patients.

The coexistence of other symptoms may provide clues to the diagnosis. For example, a patient may complain of having trouble swallowing. Closer questioning may reveal that the actual complaint is difficulty or hesitancy in initiating the act of swallowing and at the same time some difficulty in forming words. Such symptoms would be highly suggestive of a neuromuscular disorder involving not the esophagus but the skeletal musculature of the pharynx and tongue. Similarly, complaints of odoriferous breath (halitosis) may suggest chronically retained foodstuffs, possibly in a pouch (Zenker's diverticulum) or even in a grossly dilated esophagus.

In this regard it is very important to inquire about symptoms of aspiration. These may not be appreciated by the patient, especially if the aspiration occurs some time after the food ingestion. Aspiration may present as a nocturnal cough, recurrent pneumonia, unexplained fevers, or chronic obstructive pulmonary disease. The presence of recurrent bouts of aspiration should encourage an expeditious workup.

Peculiar swallowing maneuvers may suggest specific entities. The classic example of this is achalasia, in which the obstruction to the passage of food is a lower esophageal sphincter that fails to relax. This resistance can be overcome by hydrostatic pressure; the patient may report having to consume large quantities of liquids to "flush the food through." (Standing erect, lifting the head and neck, and performing Valsalva's maneuver will also increase the hydrostatic and intrathoracic pressures.)

Collagen vascular disease is a rare cause of dysphagia. However, among these patients, Reynaud's phenomenon is a commonly associated disorder. Hence, the presence of Reynaud's phenomenon and dysphagia should suggest scleroderma or some other vasculitis.

WHAT ARE THE IMPORTANT PHYSICAL FINDINGS TO SEEK?

Careful examination should be directed at the mouth, tongue, pharynx, and hypopharynx to look for any mucosal lesions such as ulceration or erosion, presence of muscle twitching (fasciculation), or atrophy or apparent weakness of throat and neck muscles. Examination of the chest should exclude the obvious presence of pulmonary or mediastinal disease, which could impinge on the esophagus. General physical examination should include the skin and joints to look for collagen disorders, which can involve the esophagus. Finally the abdomen is examined for the presence of subxiphoid or epigastric tenderness, a mass, or an enlarged liver.

A very simple test is helpful in confirming the existence of some impedance to swallowing. The patient is told to hold a mouthful of water while the doctor places the diaphragm of the stethoscope on the left lower anterior rib cage over the stomach. On signal from the doctor, the patient swallows the water; the answers to several questions are then sought. Is the water swallowed or regurgitated through the nostrils? Is there trouble initiating swallowing? What is the time duration from swallowing to entrance (signified by gurgling heard over the stomach) of the water into the stomach? A normal swallowing time for water is 5 to 13 seconds. A markedly prolonged swallowing time (15–25 seconds) often signifies high-grade impedance of esophageal peristalsis.

WHAT LABORATORY TESTS OR PROCEDURES SHOULD BE ORDERED?

The majority of procedures relevant to the consideration of dysphagia are detailed in the chapter on esophagitis. The most important diagnostic test is a contrast (barium or water-soluble dye) radiographic study of the hypopharynx and esophagus. (Water-soluble contrast is used when perforation of the esophagus is suspected; otherwise barium is more useful.) Both anatomic (e.g., cancer or stricture) and motility (e.g., achalasia or scleroderma) disorders may be visualized. Cineradiography is useful in detecting motor disorders including those of oropharyngeal origin. If a routine barium swallow does not reveal a cause for the dysphagia, a bolus of bread or meat or a barium-filled capsule should be given with barium in an attempt to reproduce dysphagia.

Esophagoscopy and biopsy together are most valuable in detecting intraluminal mucosal lesions such as esophagitis or carcinoma. This procedure is not recommended for all patients but should be performed in those whose disease has not been diagnosed by less invasive methods.

Other procedures have limited and very specialized values for certain esophageal disorders and are not generally applicable. For example, esophageal manometry is of value in confirming a diagnosis of achalasia (cardiospasm) or diffuse esophageal spasm (Figs. 3–5). It is often not necessary in a patient who gives a clear history of the problem and in whom esophagography is confirmatory.

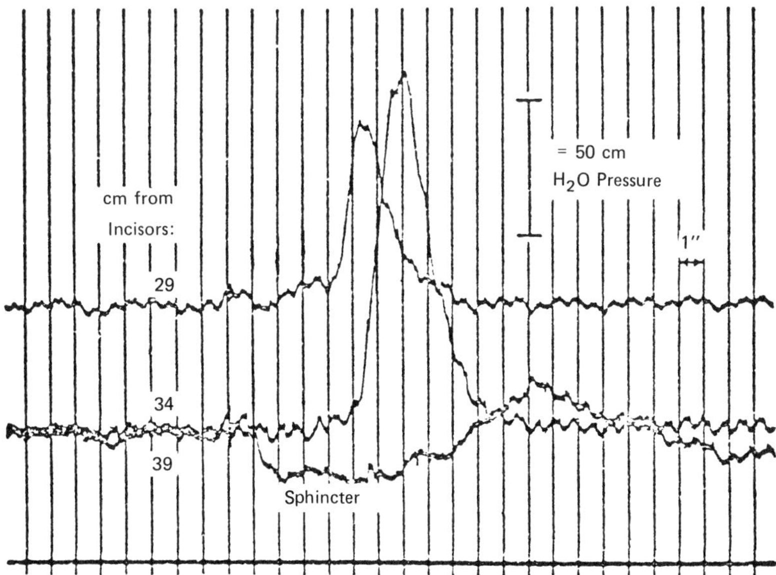

Figure 3 Normal manometric tracings. Note the contraction of the esophagus in response to swallowing passes as a peristaltic wave. This tracing demonstrates the reduction in pressure in the lower esophageal sphincter in advance of the wave.

Table 1 lists the major diagnostic tests used in evaluating dysphagia along with the disorders diagnosed most frequently by these tests. It is stressed that a good history is the most important of all "tests."

WHAT ARE THE MAJOR DIAGNOSTIC CONSIDERATIONS?

Table 2 lists and classifies the known causes of dysphagia. Esophageal rather than oropharyngeal causes are encountered far more frequently by the family practitioner. Some of the more important diseases will be discussed briefly.

Cancer of the Esophagus

Most carcinoma of the esophagus is squamous cell in type. Three-fourths of adenocarcinomas occur in the distal esophagus and probably originate in the proximal fundic portion of the stomach. Regardless of cell type, dysphagia is the most important symptom. It is initially intermittent but then becomes continuous and progressive. At first dysphagia is noted for solid foods such as meat or vegetables with high cellulose content, then for soft foods, and finally even for liquids. Pain occurs late.

Several esophageal diseases are thought to be premalignant.

Table 1 Major Diagnostic Tests in Dysphagia[a]

Test	Most Frequently Diagnosed Disorder
X-ray study	Carcinoma, cardiospasm, esophagitis, stricture, diffuse spasm, esophageal ring
Esophagoscopy and biopsy	Carcinoma, achalasia, esophagitis, stricture
Exfoliative cytology	Carcinoma
Manometry	Achalasia, diffuse spasm, esophagitis
Acid perfusion (Bernstein test)	Esophagitis
Acid reflux (Tuttle test)	Esophagitis

[a] See chapter on esophagitis for descriptions of these tests.

Oropharyngeal diseases
  Mechanical obstruction
    Tumors
    Esophageal web (Plummer-Vinson syndrome)
  Motility abnormalities
    Neuromuscular (cricopharyngeal achalasia, polymyositis, myositis, myasthenia gravis, dystrophia myotonica, amyotrophic lateral sclerosis, Parkinson's disease, cardiovascular accident, bulbar polio)
    Loss of tongue function (myasthenia gravis, dystrophia myotonica)
Esophageal diseases
  Mechanical obstruction
    Intraesophageal lesions
        Carcinoma (squamous cell, adenocarcinoma)
        Stricture (peptic, alkali)
        Lower esophageal ring (Schatzki's)
        Leiomyoma
    Extraesophageal compression
        Mediastinal tumors (carcinoma, lymphoma)
        Vascular abnormalities (aortic aneurysm, aberrant right subclavian artery)
        Cervical osteoarthritis (exophytes)
  Motility abnormalities
    Loss of peristalsis (achalasia, scleroderma, other collagen vascular diseases, diabetic neuropathy)
    Excessive contractions (diffuse esophageal spasm)
  Miscellaneous disorders
    Infections (Monilia, herpes simplex)
    Large esophageal diverticulum

These include achalasia, Barrett's esophagus, Plummer-Vinson syndrome, and lye strictures. The diagnosis should be suspected in patients presenting with dysphagia who are older than 45 years. The barium x-ray shows an irregular shelf-like defect in the barium column when the tumor projects into the lumen. Some patients develop a scirrhous or submucosally infiltrating tumor that may be confused with a benign stricture on x-ray. Esophagoscopy and biopsy and/or cytology are indicated. Frequently, especially in infiltrating lesions, a biopsy will reveal either normal tissue or inflammation. If the suspicion for cancer remains high, operation may be the only way to establish the diagnosis.

Operation is the treatment of choice for carcinoma of the

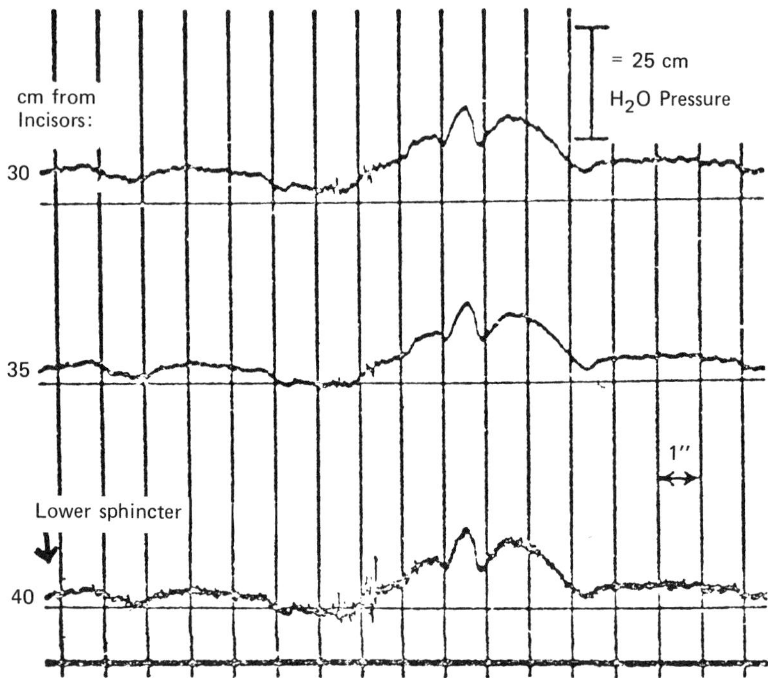

Figure 4 Manometric tracings of achalasia. Note weakened peristaltic action that occurs over the length of the esophagus simultaneously. Also note the failure of the lower sphincter to relax.

lower one-third of the esophagus. High-dose external radiation is the preferred therapy for squamous cell carcinoma above this area.

Benign Strictures of the Esophagus

Most often the result of long-standing reflux esophagitis, these strictures are usually seen in the distal esophagus but may extend upward to involve a long segment if reflux and subsequent inflammation are severe. The diagnosis is usually suspected when a patient gives a chronic history of heartburn. Dysphagia is at first noted for solid foods; liquid dysphagia occurs as the stricture continues to narrow the esophageal lumen.

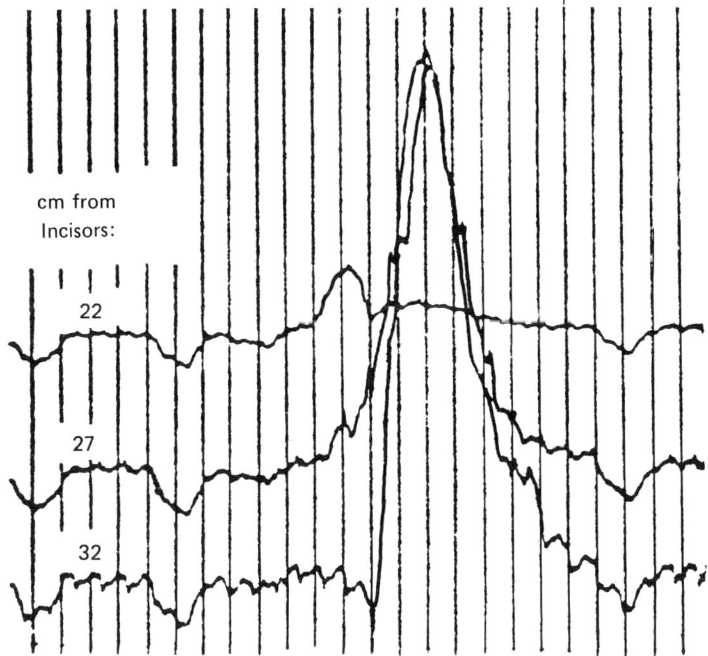

Figure 5 Manometric tracings of diffuse esophageal spasm. Patient demonstrates high-pressure simultaneous contractions.

X-ray and esophagoscopy are indicated in these patients. It is sometimes difficult to differentiate these lesions from carcinoma of the scirrhous type.

Treatment is twofold: at the same time that the stricture is being dilated mechanically, the patient is placed on an adequate antireflux program. (See chapter on esophagitis.) Operation is warranted for those patients whose reflux is severe and resistant to medical management.

Achalasia

Both abnormal motility of the esophagus and disturbed lower esophageal sphincter function lead to dysphagia in achalasia, a puzzling disorder. Achalasia may develop at any age; it is the most common cause of dysphagia in young people (late teens, twenties, and thirties). Initially, dysphagia is intermittent and tends to occur for both solids and liquids. Characteristically, the patient with achalasia complains of pressure and retrosternal fullness after eating. Regurgitation, or even aspiration of esophageal contents, may occur, especially at night. The patient often drinks water to "wash down the meal."

The radiographic appearance of achalasia is very characteristic; dilatation, impaired emptying, a beak-like tapered narrowing of the distal segment, and loss of motility (i.e., absence of peristaltic waves) are seen. Manometry is confirmatory and shows absent or reduced peristalsis in the distal one-half of the esophagus, high resting pressure in the lower esophageal sphincter, and a failure of relaxation of the sphincter in response to swallowing.

Medical therapy on a long-term basis is ineffective in achalasia. Pneumatic dilatation of the lower sphincter with a hydrostatic bag is preferred by most gastroenterologic specialists. The dilatation ruptures the sphincter but does not improve the abnormal motility. In patients who fail to respond to dilatation, operation (the Heller myotomy) is indicated.

Cricopharyngeal achalasia and a complicating pulsion diverticulum (Zenker's diverticulum) should be suspected in an elderly patient who feels food sticking in the suprasternal area and who regurgitates foul-tasting material, especially at night after retiring and lying on the side. The diverticulum, located just above the upper esophageal sphincter, may grow to an enormous size ($\geqq$ 6 cm). Although a cricopharyngeal myotomy may relieve the dysphagia, large Zenker's diverticula are symptomatic and may need to be resected surgically.

Diffuse Esophageal Spasm

In diffuse esophageal spasm, a motility disorder, there is a synchronous contraction of the esophageal musculature rather than an orderly peristaltic wave. Consequently, a bolus (solid or liquid) cannot be conducted down the esophageal lumen. In some patients, this abnormal motility pattern may be triggered by reflux esophagitis; in others, it appears to be a primary motor disorder.

Often chest pain accompanies the spasm. This pain may be very similar to cardiac angina, and nonspecific ECG changes can even occur. The elicitation of a history of dysphagia during an episode of pain is quite helpful.

Esophagography may demonstrate "tertiary" contractions in patients with diffuse esophageal spasm. However, these contractions may also be seen in normal patients (especially the elderly, in whom this is referred to as "presbyesophagus").

Treatment is directed at the reflux esophagitis if those symptoms are also present. Nitroglycerin may relieve both the pain and the dysphagia. If the problem is incapacitating, pneumodilatation or myotomy may need to be performed.

WHAT SYMPTOMATIC THERAPY CAN BE GIVEN IN THE ABSENCE OF A SPECIFIC DIAGNOSIS?

In general, it is a mistake to attempt to treat a patient with dysphagia symptomatically without knowing the diagnosis. Dysphagia almost always means organic disease and should not be interpreted as a neurotic complaint. Patients who complain of a lump in the throat and say they cannot swallow but who are otherwise healthy have globus hystericus (which can usually be managed with explanation and reassurance).

The initial efforts of the physician should be directed toward making a diagnosis and not toward symptomatic therapy (e.g., diet manipulation, antispasmodics, sympathomimetics, etc.). Such treatment may tend to obscure the diagnosis and delay the definitive treatment needed once a specific diagnosis is made. Dysphagia is a most revealing and specific gastroenterologic symptom that localizes the disease process in most cases, suggests the correct diagnosis, and definitely indicates the need for prompt action by the physician.

SELECTED READING

Cohen S, Lipshutz WH: Lower esophageal dysfunction in achalasia. *Gastroenterology* 61:814–820, 1971.

Kramer P: The esophagus, in Keefer C, Wilkins R (eds): *Medicine: Essentials of Clinical Practice.* Boston, Little, Brown and Co, 1970, pp 455–488.

Seaman WB: Pharyngeal and upper esophageal dysphagia. *JAMA* 235: 2643–2646, 1976.

Ventrappen G, Hellemens J: Diffuse muscle spasm of the esophagus and the hypertensive lower esophageal sphincter. *Clin Gastroenterol,* 5: 59–72, 1976.

CLINICAL PROBLEMS

I. A 45-year-old man complains of occasional food sticking in his chest. He has had four or five episodes over the past four years of hurriedly swallowing a piece of meat only to feel it getting caught in the lower esophagus. It will only pass with difficulty and, on two occasions, he has had to induce vomiting to bring the bolus back up. His physical examination is normal.

   1. What type of dysphagia is he describing?
   2. What further diagnostic tests should be done?
   3. How should he be managed?

II. Another 45-year-old man complains of problems with swallowing that have been becoming worse over the past two years. Before that he had a long history of heartburn, but he thinks that that may have become "a little better" since the dysphagia began. Two years ago he noted that, if he did not chew meat well, it would occasionally get stuck. The problem gradually worsened so that by 3 months ago, he was forced to eat only liquids. Currently even thick liquids are not passing readily. He has lost 25 pounds in the past year. His physical examination is unremarkable except for evidence of weight loss.

   1. What type of dysphagia is he describing?
   2. What further diagnostic tests should be done?
   3. How should he be managed?

III. A third 45-year-old man is seen for dysphagia. For the past 20 years he has had episodes in which food seems to stick. From the beginning, it made no difference whether the food was liquid or solid. These episodes are becoming more and more frequent. He is able to sometimes "push" the food through by drinking large quantities of water. Two years ago he was seen by another physician, who told him he had a "stricture." He underwent dilatation without success. He has lost 20 pounds.

He has also noted that he has trouble sleeping at night. Further questioning reveals that he frequently wakes up choking and cannot catch his breath. He has had two episodes of pneumonia in the past year that he attributed to smoking.

Physical examination demonstrates evidence of weight loss but is otherwise unremarkable.

1. What type of dysphagia is he describing?
2. What further diagnostic tests should be done?
3. How should he be managed?

Discussion

I. 1. The patient is describing fixed dysphagia. It occurs only with solid food, and there is no historical evidence indicating progressive terminal narrowing. The most likely cause for this symptom is a fixed narrowing in the distal esophagus such as a Schatzki's ring.

2. Esophagography will likely confirm the diagnosis. However, care must be taken to have the patient swallow a large bolus of barium so that the distal esophagus is forced to distend. Otherwise, it may not spread wide enough to identify the one small area that cannot open appropriately.

3. The treatment would consist of removing the cause of obstruction. In the case of a Schatzki's ring, dilatation with a large mercury dilator (48 or 50 French) or biopsy of the ring through an endoscope is usually sufficient.

II. 1. This is the classic description of progressive dysphagia. One clearly gets the impression of an esophageal lumen that is gradually becoming smaller. The slow rate of occlusion (two years), as well as the history of reflux, would argue for a benign peptic stricture.

2. The confirmatory diagnostic test would be an esophagogram. Once the anatomy was defined, endoscopy and biopsy would be carried out.

3. The initial problem is to dilate the esophagus. This procedure is usually performed by a gastroenterologist or surgeon. Once the lumen has been opened, the patient will need treatment for reflux esophagitis; he will probably be a surgical candidate. (See the chapter on esophagitis for a description of these procedures.)

III. 1. The fact that from the beginning the problem has been present with both liquids and solids implies total dysphagia. This, in turn, implicates a motility disorder. The ability of water to flush the food down points to an obstruction, such as a lower esophageal sphincter that cannot relax, that can be overcome by a hydrostatic column. Of concern in the history is the nocturnal aspiration. This is an important area about which to question dysphagic patients, and its presence should prompt an expeditious evaluation.

2. As before, esophagography should be performed first. An area of narrowing, probably where the barium trickles through the lower esophageal sphincter, may be inappropriately called a stricture. Endoscopy is usually the next step. (Before performing endoscopy, the excess fluid should be aspirated from the esophagus to reduce the chance of aspiration.) A narrow sphincter is seen through which the endoscope will pass if pressure is exerted. The definitive test, however, is esophageal motility. This was shown in Figure 4, and it demonstrates the failure of the lower esophageal sphincter to relax.

3. Once the diagnosis is established, the lower esophageal sphincter is ruptured either with pneumatic dilatation or myotomy. Patients with total dysphagia require close follow-up study, even after a successful treatment. Since the sphincter is no longer intact, they become victims to reflux esophagitis. Furthermore, achalasia is a premalignant lesion.

ARTHUR D. SCHWABE

Gas

WHERE DOES GAS COME FROM?

A variety of symptoms may be attributed to an excessive amount of gas in the gastrointestinal tract and "too much gas" is a common complaint of patients consulting a physician. In recent years we have learned a great deal about the origin and composition of intestinal gas and have developed a sound approach to management. The primary sources of gas in the gastrointestinal tract are air swallowing, intraluminal production, and diffusion into the lumen from the blood stream. The major gases—nitrogen, oxygen, hydrogen, methane, and carbon dioxide—make up more than 99% of intestinal gas and have no odor. The pungent smell associated with the passage of flatus is due to gases such as indoles, skatoles, and hydrogen sulfide, which are present only in trace amounts.

Approximately 600 ml of gas is passed daily through the rectum in normal subjects. Large amounts may be excreted after the ingestion of nonabsorbable oligosaccharides and polysaccharides and in the presence of several malabsorptive disorders. However, most of the patients who have symptoms attributed to gas neither produce more gas nor have an excessive amount of gas present in their GI tracts. Before we examine the clinical features of the intestinal gas syndromes, a brief examination of the major intestinal gases is in order.

Nitrogen

Nitrogen (N_2), the predominant bowel gas, is found throughout the GI tract. Almost all the N_2 in the stomach is taken in during swallowing and is subsequently regurgitated. When a person is in the upright position, very little of this swallowed N_2 passes into the intestine; rather N_2 arrives there primarily by diffusion from the blood stream. There is no evidence that any N_2 is produced by colonic bacteria. Thus, the N_2 in flatus, approximately 400 ml per day, is produced almost entirely from diffusion and occasionally from swallowed air.

Oxygen

Oxygen (O_2) is present only in extremely low concentration in the colon, since it is utilized rapidly by aerobic bacteria. The low O_2 concentration is of no significance in the clinical gas syndromes.

Hydrogen

Hydrogen (H_2) is produced solely by bacteria in the colon. Excess H_2 production takes place only when large amounts of unabsorbed carbohydrates or proteins, or both, reach the colon. In normal subjects excess H_2 is generated after the ingestion of beans and other oligosaccharides and polysaccharides, which cannot be digested and absorbed (Table 1). These sugars pass into the colon, where they are readily fermented by the colonic bacteria liberating H_2. Excessive H_2 production is also an important feature of intestinal lactase deficiency and other malabsorptive disorders, such as sprue and pancreatic insufficiency.

Table 1 **Foods Containing Gas-Producing Oligosaccharides**[a]

Barley
Broad beans
Chinese artichokes
Coconut meat
Cotton seed
Crucifers and crucifer seeds
    Brassica
    Brussels sprouts
    Cabbage
    Kohlrabi
    Mustards
Dwarf beans
Figs
Fruit plant shoots
Honey
Molasses
Mulberries
Nuts
Raw beet sugar
Rye seeds
Soybeans
Sugar beets
Sugar cane
Wheat
Yeast

[a] All of these foods contain raffinose or stachyose, or both.

Methane

Only one-third of the adult population is capable of methane (CH_4) production and, like H_2, CH_4 is derived solely from the metabolism of colonic bacteria. Unlike H_2, however, the production of CH_4 is unrelated to food ingestion and persists during fasting. The tendency to harbor CH_4-producing bacteria runs in families and appears to be determined by early environmental factors. The stools of CH_4 producers consistently float in water.

Carbon Dioxide

Carbon dioxide (CO_2) is found in all parts of the GI tract. In the upper small intestine, CO_2 is produced when hydrochloric acid or organic acids are neutralized by bicarbonate. Each mEq of bicarbonate that interacts with 1 mEq of H+ yields 22.4 ml of CO_2. Almost all of this CO_2 is absorbed rapidly during its passage through the small bowel and does not appear in the flatus. Colonic bacteria are capable of producing CO_2 from sugars and fatty acids. Excessive amounts of CO_2 are produced after the ingestion of beans and other unabsorbed oligosaccharides. The CO_2 in flatus thus originates entirely from colonic bacteria.

WHAT ARE THE IMPORTANT ASPECTS OF HISTORY?

There are three clinical gas syndromes that may be recognized by characteristic historical features and symptoms.

Aerophagia and Excessive Belching

Normal individuals deposit 2 to 3 ml of air in the stomach with each swallow and belch occasionally during or after meals or after the ingestion of carbonated beverages. This eructation, recognized as gastric belching, represents a release of air from the gastric air bubble. It is involuntary and pleasurable, occurs at irregular intervals, and is not preceded by a swallow.

In many people the rate of air swallowing is increased during periods of emotional stress, anxiety, and nervousness. Some of these people will consult their physician because of excessive belching and are convinced that they have a serious underlying disease. Description of the belching process will usually identify some of these patients as esophageal belchers. Esophageal belching occurs when air is swallowed halfway down the esophagus and is then forcefully and voluntarily expelled. Esophageal belches are loud, occur repeatedly at more or less regular intervals, can often be demonstrated on command, require effort, and are always preceded by a swallow.

Gas Pain Syndrome

Patients was gas pain syndrome complain of bloating, distention, cramping abdominal pain, or merely "too much gas." The abdominal pain usually occurs in the lower part of the abdomen but may be localized to either side. Recent studies have demonstrated conclusively that these patients do not have excessive amounts of gas in their intestinal tracts, but that they have a decreased tolerance to bowel distention as well as disordered motility that interferes with the orderly passage of gas through the bowel. The patients usually incriminate a variety of foods as responsible for their symptoms. However, with the exception of a few patients who have intestinal lactase deficiency and therefore should be on lactose-restricted diets, no other foodstuff has been shown consistently to precipitate or aggravate the symptoms.

Excessive Flatus

Normal individuals pass flatus an average of 14 times a day in amounts averaging 600 ml per day (range, 200–2,000 ml/day). A marked increase in the frequency or the total amount of flatus may be observed by the patient or, on occasion, the patient's family. Once air swallowing and excessive ingestion of oligosaccharides and polysaccharides have been excluded by a careful history, consideration should be given to intestinal lactase deficiency. Some patients, when questioned in depth, will recall that during a period of abstinence from milk, the amount of flatus passed per anum was markedly less or that consumption of more than a pint of milk per day regularly induces diarrhea and abdominal cramps. More generalized and serious malabsorptive problems may exist in some patients with increased amounts of flatus, although they will usually have primary complaints other than the flatulence, such as diarrhea or weight loss. (See the chapter on weight loss.)

WHAT ARE THE IMPORTANT PHYSICAL FINDINGS?

Esophageal belchers can be recognized by the loud, repetitive noises emanating from their mouths and the accompanying swallows preceding each belch. The strain of the voluntary effort may be visible on their faces. Patients with gas pain syndrome usually have diffuse abdominal tenderness and hyperactive bowel sounds without visible distention. On the other hand, patients who actually do produce excessive flatus may have moderate distention, diffuse tympany, borborygmus, and, if they have steatorrhea, evidence of weight loss.

WHAT LABORATORY STUDIES SHOULD BE ORDERED?

Patients with aerophagia, excessive belching, or esophageal belching (but no other symptoms) require only reassurance and an explanation of the condition. If other symptoms, such as abdominal discomfort and nausea, coexist, an upper gastrointestinal x-ray should be obtained.

Patients with the gas pain syndrome should have a lactose tolerance test to rule out intestinal lactase deficiency. If production of excessive flatus is suspected, patients should also be tested for steatorrhea. Theoretically gas chromatographic analysis of rectal gas could be performed, in order to verify the source of the gas. (A high concentration of N_2 in rectal gas indicates that air swallowing is the major source. High concentrations of H_2 and CO_2 in rectal gas are characteristic of increased colonic gas production from one or more unabsorbed foodstuffs.) Such analyses are not generally available, however.

WHAT ARE THE MAJOR DIAGNOSTIC CONSIDERATIONS?

Patients who complain of excessive belching, whether of esophageal or gastric origin, usually have emotional disturbances, such as anxiety, depression, or hysteria. Patients with the gas pain syndrome may also have functional diarrhea or constipation, or both. The diagnostic considerations for those complaining of excessive flatus include primary or secondary intestinal lactase deficiency, impaired digestion or absorption of fat, or consumption of the flatulogenic oligosaccharides enumerated in Table 1.

WHAT SYMPTOMATIC THERAPY CAN BE GIVEN?

Esophageal belchers usually only require reassurance and an explanation of the voluntary nature of their symptoms. Mild sedation may be useful adjunctive therapy.

Gastric belchers should be advised to eat their food slowly and to avoid carbonated beverages. In addition, neutralization of gastric hydrochloric acid with antacids between meals may help to reduce the formation of CO_2 and the frequency of belching.

Patients with the gas pain syndrome should be advised to take hydrophilic colloids, such as psyllium seed preparations (Metamucil, Konsyl, Effersyllium, etc.). (Remember that when these colloids are first ingested an increase of flatus may develop. This problem usually resolves itself with time.) Since even normal volumes of gas may induce pain in these patients, they should be counseled to avoid lactose and the gas-producing oligosaccharides (see Table 1). It might be assumed that since these patients have disordered intestinal motility anticholinergics should be the logical initial therapeutic agents. However, no controlled studies supporting the efficacy of these drugs are available. Most patients in my experience have obtained only partial symptomatic relief, usually only for a short time, or have reported no change in pain and bloating after receiving anticholinergic therapy.

Patients with excessive flatus due to intestinal lactase deficiency respond readily to lactose restriction. If the problem is due to malabsorption, specific therapy, such as a gluten-free diet for celiac sprue, eventually eliminates the excessive flatus. If lactase deficiency and malabsorption have been ruled out, empiric restriction of carbohydrates, including lactose, may be beneficial. In the occasional patient with excessive flatus due to air swallowing, simple counseling usually suffices to eliminate the problem.

SELECTED READING

Lasser RB, Bond JH, Levitt MD: The role of intestinal gas in functional abdominal pain. *N Engl J Med* 293:524–526, 1975.

Levitt MD: Volume and composition of human intestinal gas determined by means of an intestinal washout technic. *N Engl J Med* 284:1394–1398, 1971.

Levitt MD, Lasser RB, Schwartz JS, et al: Studies of a flatulent patient. *N Engl J Med* 295:260–262, 1976.

McNally EF, Kelly JE Jr, Ingelfinger FJ: Mechanism of belching: effects of gastric distension with air. *Gastroenterology* 46:254–259, 1964.

Nohain J, Caradec F: *Le Petomane. A Tribute to the Unique Act which Shook and Shattered the Moulin Rouge.* London, Souvenir Press, 1967.

Steggerda FR: Gastrointestinal gas following food consumption. *Ann NY Acad Sci* 150:57–66, 1968.

CLINICAL PROBLEMS

I. An anxious 45-year-old man complains of "excessive belching." He denies any systemic or gastrointestinal symptoms other than this. He is observed to swallow repeatedly and then eructate loudly. He states that this is the same problem that he has all of the time.

   1. If rectal gas analysis were performed, what would be the composition of the patient's gas?

   2. What is causing the symptoms?

   3. What treatment might be effective?

II. A 52-year-old woman complains that she has had "excessive gas" all of her life. When asked to describe her gas symptoms, she relates multiple vague descriptions of abdominal pain and bloating. She denies weight loss or diarrhea. Results of her examination are completely normal except for tenderness throughout the abdomen and hyperactive bowel sounds. She has no visible abdominal distention.

1. If rectal gas analysis were performed, what would be the composition of the patient's gas?
2. What is causing the symptoms?
3. What treatment might be effective?

III. A 46-year-old woman complains that she has had "excessive gas" for at least the past 10 years. When asked to describe her symptoms, she relates that she passes flatus during the entire day, and that it is very embarrassing for her and her coworkers. She denies weight loss or other systemic problems. She enjoys milk and ice cream and consumes them frequently even though they seem to cause diarrhea. Her examination is unremarkable except for some mild abdominal distention and tympany.

1. If rectal gas analysis were performed, what would be the composition of the patient's gas?
2. What is causing the symptoms?
3. What treatment might be effective?

Discussion

I. 1. This patient's problem is related to aerophagia. He might demonstrate high concentrations of nitrogen.
2. The symptoms are caused by the patient's own voluntary aerophagia, which he demonstrates during the examination.
3. The most effective treatment is an explanation of the symptoms and reassurance that no major pathologic process is at work. It would be appropriate to explore some of the underlying reasons for the patient's anxiety, and to relate them to the aerophagia.

II. 1. Since the patient's problem is not caused by a quantitative or qualitative abnormality in gas production, her fecal gas analysis will be normal.

2. This patient's symptoms are actually a variant of functional bowel disease and are due to deranged intestinal motility. (See the chapter on functional bowel disease.)

3. The treatment should consist of supportive care (including psychologic support), the avoidance of flatulogenic substances, and a trial of some type of bulk preparation, such as bran or psyllium mucilloids. Anticholinergics (including analgesics) should be avoided.

III. 1. It is likely that this patient is malabsorbing lactose, and her rectal gas will show increased quantities of hydrogen and carbon dioxide.

2. The symptoms, as noted, are due to the malabsorption of lactose.

3. The patient should be tried on a lactose-free diet. Although she could be cautioned to avoid the various other flatulogenic substances listed in Table 1, lactose deprivation alone is likely to be successful. Since the problem has been present for many years, it is unlikely that any serious intestinal disease is present, and this patient probably has a primary lactase deficiency.

PART II

DISEASE ENTITIES

10

MARTIN A. POPS

Esophagitis

HOW DO I MAKE THE DIAGNOSIS?

Symptoms related to the backward flow of gastric acid into the esophagus (gastroesophageal reflux) are among the most common complaints related to the gastrointestinal tract. The patient with symptomatic reflux esophagitis complains predominantly of "heartburn," discomfort, fullness, or true pain in the substernal area of the chest. This may be accompanied by other symptoms of a varied nature that are usually not constant.

Typical reflux esophagitis pain is a substernal pressure that comes on more frequently when the patient lies down, especially after a large meal, and that is relieved by sitting up. Bending over may also precipitate episodes of pain. Regurgitation of gastric acid into the esophagus gives rise to the burning sensation of "heartburn." Prompt relief of this pain by antacids is typical for reflux esophagitis.

The diagnosis is usually established on the basis of history. Unless some complication of the disease has occurred (see later section), the physical examination is unremarkable. A stool specimen should be tested for occult blood.

An upper gastrointestinal series should be obtained to look specifically for a hiatal hernia and evidence of esophageal reflux. Although the relationship between reflux esophagitis and hiatal hernia is debatable, it is a fact that most patients with esophagitis also have a hiatal hernia. At this point, it would be appropriate to give the patient a trial of medical therapy. If relief is prompt and complete, the diagnosis of reflux esophagitis can be accepted.

In cases of atypical esophagitis, which may not be associated with the classic symptoms, or when simple therapeutic measures fail, other diagnostic tests may be necessary. These tests are enumerated in Table 1.

The most widely used and reliable test for reproducing the symptoms of reflux esophagitis is the Bernstein test. A nasogastric tube is passed into the esophagus with its opening in the upper one-third of the esophagus. The tube is connected by a three-way stop-cock to two infusion bottles, one containing normal saline, the other 0.1N hydrochloric acid (HCl). The esophagus is first perfused with saline at a rate of 100 to 120 drops per minute for 10 minutes with the patient in the upright position. Then, without the patient's knowledge, the acid is perfused at the same rate for up to 30 minutes or until symptoms appear. If the patient develops his or her usual symptoms, the drip is switched back to saline. If the symptoms then disappear, a second attempt is made to reproduce them with more acid. The correlation between heartburn and a positive Bernstein test is almost 100%. However, a positive test does not prove reflux but rather provides evidence that the pain is a result of sensitivity of the esophageal mucosa to acid.

Table 1   **Diagnostic Tests for Reflux Esophagitis**

Bernstein test

Esophageal manometry

Acid reflux test (Tuttle test)

Esophagoscopy and biopsy

Indwelling esophageal pH probe

Radioisotope scanning

Manometry is the technique by which the lower esophageal sphincter was first identified. In suspected esophagitis, a measure of the competence of the lower sphincter can be made. Also, abnormal peristaltic waves, which may result from reflux, can be found. If the pressure within the sphincter is low at rest, reflux, though not proved, is suggested, since most patients with peptic esophagitis have lower than normal sphincter pressures (below 15 mm Hg). Manometric study is unnecessary in patients with typical reflux symptoms but can be very useful in patients with atypical symptoms or unexplained chest pain.

The acid reflux test (Tuttle) offers the most direct measure of spontaneous reflux. A pH electrode on a manometric plastic catheter apparatus is passed into the stomach and 180 to 200 cc of 0.1N HCl is infused through the manometric catheter. With the patient supine the pH electrode is withdrawn until it is 4 cm above the upper margin of the lower esophageal sphincter. Normally, the pH should rise to above 6.0. If reflux is present, the pH probe will register sustained periods during which the pH falls to 4.0 or below. This test is both highly sensitive and highly selective and is thus a reliable method for confirming spontaneous acid reflux.

An atypical history, failure to respond to treatment, or the development of a complication would justify endoscopy and biopsy of the lower esophagus. It should be emphasized, however, that the endoscopist may see a perfectly normal esophageal mucosa in a patient with reflux esophagitis, and, therefore, endoscopy should not be considered the final or definitive diagnostic test. Biopsy increases the diagnostic yield but here again it cannot be considered the definitive test. The changes (classically consisting of inflammatory reaction and extension of the dermal pegs to or almost to the free surface of the epithelium) may be spotty and missed in the biopsy. They may also not be present in up to one-third of patients with esophagitis.

It is evident from the foregoing that there are a great many ways to evaluate a patient with suspected reflux esophagitis. The history alone will establish the correct diagnosis approximately 80% of the time. Since several tests are available, some difficult and expensive, and since each does not give the complete answer, some direction is needed. To put this into perspective, the following recommendation is made. If a clear history of reflux is obtained, order a barium swallow to confirm reflux since patients who show free reflux on barium swallow while supine will show positive results on all the other tests. The next step is a therapeutic trial. If the history is atypical or confusing, a Bernstein test will, if positive, confirm that the symptoms are esophageal in origin. If the patient responds poorly or not at all to medical management, an acid reflux test and measurement of the lower esophageal sphincter pressure are indicated. Esophagoscopy and biopsy may also be useful at this point.

WHAT ADDITIONAL WORKUP DOES THE PATIENT REQUIRE?

The diagnosis of esophagitis cannot be separated from that of chest pain of cardiac origin, specifically from coronary angina, with which esophagitis may be confused. It is sometimes impossible to separate esophageal from cardiac pain by symptoms alone. The pain fibers follow a common pathway. One cannot be sure that the patient with esophagitis does not have coronary artery disease. One is frequently confronted by a patient who complains of chest pain or discomfort. He or she is middle-aged and overweight, may be a "type A" personality, may be a heavy smoker, and may even have a family history of coronary artery disease.

Generally, three types of patients are encountered when one considers the question of chest pain due to coronary artery disease versus that due to reflux esophagitis. The first patient has either reflux esophagitis or angina pectoris. The second one has both reflux esophagitis and angina. The third patient has chest pain that is neither angina pectoris nor reflux esophagitis, but is convinced that something is wrong with the heart. In the first instance, the evaluation will proceed along the lines discussed in the previous section if esophagitis is suspected.

A complete discussion of coronary angina is beyond the scope of this chapter. However, typical angina is usually a substernal, constricting chest pain that is classically brought on by exertion or tension and sometimes by eating. Radiation of the pain down the left arm, more commonly noted in angina, can occur in esophagitis. A very helpful maneuver may be the obtaining of an electrocardiogram during an episode of pain. If the history is questionable and the ECG does not change during episodes of pain, one can be more comfortable that the patient does not have angina. On the other hand, if ST and T wave sagging are seen on the ECG during pain, and recede when the pain goes away, angina is very likely.

In the patient with both reflux and angina pectoris, the history is extremely important. Sometimes patients can tell the difference between the two types of pain or realize that different maneuvers help the pain. If the pain is relieved by rest at times while at other times it is relieved by sitting up or taking antacids, the physician must question the patient about the minute details of the pain in either situation. Such careful history taking often clarifies the situation. Since it is common for patients to have both problems, evaluation should be undertaken to rule in or out both conditions. An ECG during pain or an exercise test may confirm a diagnosis of angina while an acid perfusion test (Bernstein) is a very useful provocative test for reflux esophagitis.

The third situation deals with the patient with substernal discomfort who has neither condition. Such patients may be very anxious and fearful that they have something wrong with their hearts. In addition to the appropriate diagnostic and therapeutic tests previously described, look for other things such as chest wall tenderness or pleuritis or some intraabdominal condition such as peptic ulcer or gallbladder disease.

HOW SHOULD I TREAT THE PATIENT?

Management for the vast majority of patients will be successful. It can be divided into three components: postural, dietary, and medical.

Initially, the patient has to be educated about the disease so that he or she will cooperate in its management. Failure to comply due to poor understanding by the patient is the most frequent reason for therapeutic failure. This will be discussed further in a later section.

Postural therapy is easily explained. Reflux is more likely to occur when the patient is flat and the counter effect of gravity is lost. To get gravity working the patient should be instructed to elevate the head of the bed on four- to eight-inch blocks. He or she should be warned to omit frequent bending forward such as occurs during certain exercises and pastimes such as gardening, as this maneuver results in the loss of gravity forces as well as an increase in intraabdominal pressure.

If the patient balks at using blocks under the bed, elevation can be accomplished by a triangular bolster made of thick foam rubber on a firm mattress or a plywood wedge under the mattress. Sleeping on several pillows does not make up for these other techniques; it may increase intraabdominal pressure and worsen reflux symptoms. In addition, it is important to advise the patient to avoid recumbency for at least three hours after a meal because this is the time when there is a greater tendency for reflux to occur as a result of gastric distention and increased intragastric pressure. (A logical extension of this advice is the avoidance of bedtime snacks.)

Dietary therapy is also fairly simple. In general, extremes of hot and cold should be avoided. Fat can cause the release of both secretin and cholecystokinin, which may further reduce lower esophageal sphincter pressure. Alcohol and coffee (even decaffeinated brands) are harmful and should be avoided. Acid pH beverages, such as citrus juices, may directly injure the acid-damaged epithelium. Foods that contain garlic, onion, or mint should be discouraged, as these substances all contain chemicals (carminatives) that reduce lower esophageal sphincter pressure. Finally, any food or beverage that the patient repeatedly cannot tolerate should be avoided. The simplicity is: eat what you can and don't eat the things that characteristically cause heartburn. A summary of the dietary restrictions is seen in Table 2.

Most experts urge weight reduction for obese patients with reflux esophagitis simply because almost everyone's experience is that symptoms lessen dramatically. Finally, smoking should be stopped if at all possible. Cigarette smoking has been shown to reduce lower esophageal sphincter pressure.

The third component of conservative management is medical and usually consists of either antacids or pharmacologic agents, which act to block gastric acid secretion, reduce reflux by stimulating lower esophageal sphincter contractility, or hasten gastric emptying. Since antacids are the most commonly used agents, a few words about their selection are in order.

The aluminum hydroxide/magnesium hydroxide preparations are the most palatable and best tolerated. Dosage can be manipulated using one or more antacids so as to avoid either constipation or diarrhea as distressing side effects (reducing the aluminum intake in

Table 2 Dietary Restrictions in Reflux Esophagitis

Restricted Dietary Component	Pathophysiologic Effect of Component
Extreme temperatures of food or beverage	Alteration of esophageal motility; direct mucosal injury
Fat	Reduction of LESP[a] via release of hormones
Alcohol	
Coffee	
Acid pH beverages	Direct mucosal injury
Garlic, onion, mint	Reduction of LESP via carminative content
Other foods/beverages to which the patient is intolerant	Individual, nonspecific mechanism

[a] LESP, lower esophageal sphincter pressure.

the former and the magnesium in the latter). We discourage the use of calcium carbonate antacids. These compounds are effective in the relief of symptoms, but they may increase the secretion of acid by the effect of the calcium ion on the gastric parietal cell.

An important consideration in the choice of an antacid is its sodium content. This can be a problem in patients who require salt restriction. Fortunately, there is a good choice of effective antacids that have a low sodium content (Table 3).

Opinion is divided on liquid versus tablet antacids. Here again the major consideration is patient acceptance. I prefer liquid antacids, but if the patient is unwilling or unable to take them, tablets usually suffice. The usual dose is one ounce of liquid or one to two tablets chewed one-half hour after meals and at bedtime. For more intensive therapy, if that regimen is not initially effective, an additional dose is given three hours after each meal.

For patients who do not tolerate antacids or do not adhere to a good antacid program or for those who obtain incomplete relief of their symptoms, the next move is to prescribe a single dose of cimetidine, 300 to 600 mg, as prebedtime medication. This has now been approved for chronic treatment of reflux esophagitis and when used in conjunction with antacids or alone, it is often dramatically effective in relieving symptoms. Higher doses of cimetidine are not currently advocated for long-term use of acid-peptic disorders.

Two other agents being used experimentally may soon be ap-

Table 3   **Sodium Content of Various Antacid Preparations**

Drug	Unit	Mg Sodium
Moderate to High Sodium Content		
Alka Seltzer	Tablet	532
Aludrox suspension	30 ml	28
Amphojel suspension	30 ml	50
Basaljel suspension	30 ml	36
Di-Gel	30 ml	48
Gaviscon	Tablet	20
Rolaids	Tablet	53
Titralac	30 ml	76
Very Low Sodium Content (Less than 10 mg/unit)		
Aludrox	Tablet	
Gelusil II	30 ml	
Maalox Plus	30 ml	
Mylanta II	30 ml	
Riopan	30 ml	
Riopan	Tablet	

proved for treatment of reflux. Bethanechol (Urecholine) is effective and it may work by increasing lower esophageal sphincter pressure. Metaclopramide increases lower esophageal sphincter pressure and also facilitates gastric emptying. This latter drug may eventually assume a major role in the treatment of reflux.

Anticholinergic drugs have long been employed in treatment for two theoretical reasons: they may decrease acid secretion and they may counteract spasm of the esophagus that occurs secondary to the reflux. However, it has been shown that anticholinergics reduce the lower sphincter pressure and actively permit more reflux. These medications also retard gastric emptying. For these reasons they should be considered to be contraindicated in the modern treatment of esophagitis due to reflux. Considerations of the surgical therapy are discussed in the section dealing with the management of complications.

WHAT SHOULD I EXPECT FROM
SUCCESSFUL TREATMENT?

As mentioned previously, a favorable response can be expected in more than 80% of patients in whom a combination of postural, dietary, and medical therapy is used. It should be remembered, however, that medical therapy does little or nothing to correct the underlying, abnormal physiologic mechanisms that contribute to reflux; it is thus logical to assume that a patient who lapses back into old ways will suffer relapses of the disease. Education of the patient therefore assumes a major role in prognosis of reflux esophagitis. The goal of therapy should be complete relief of pain. The goal of long-term follow-up study should be to prevent relapses or to promptly reverse them by intensifying therapy.

WHAT MIGHT CAUSE A FAILURE
OF TREATMENT?

In general, patients in whom treatment fails fall into two general categories. The first and most important is the patient who will not or cannot comply with the prescribed regimen. These patients should be counseled as to the importance of following some program so as not only to reduce or eliminate symptoms but also to avoid complications of the condition such as hemorrhage or stricture formation. Sometimes it is necessary to compromise the medical or dietary program to conform to a more realistic assessment of the patient's compliance capability. For example, it is very common for patients to fail to adhere to an antacid regimen because of problems with palatability. Such a patient may respond equally well to a nighttime dose of cimetidine.

The second group of patients who fail to respond are those with reflux that is very severe. These patients may fail to respond to medical therapy completely despite adherence to a strict medical program. This group includes the small percentage of patients with Barrett's esophagus, which will be discussed later. Such patients are appropriately considered candidates for gastroenterologic consultation and surgical therapy.

Occasionally patients are confronted with severe reflux esophagitis caused by underlying systemic diseases. The classic example of this is scleroderma. Patients with this disorder are treated in the previously noted manner but they usually require gastroenterologic consultation.

HOW SHOULD THE PATIENT BE FOLLOWED?

In general, the frequency of office visits is dictated by the severity of symptoms and the presence of complications, if any. Initially, visits at two to four weeks are appropriate in order to assess the patient's response to therapy. Follow-up laboratory examinations are usually not necessary but would be dictated by response or complications. Significant pain or dysphagia that presents beyond the first two weeks of therapy suggests severe disease or noncompliance. Under these circumstances a repeat x-ray or endoscopy may be indicated.

After four to six weeks of therapy, the patient who has had a good symptomatic remission can be told to reduce the frequency of antacid dosage to morning and bedtime. If this is tolerated, the antacids can often be discontinued entirely as other measures such as dietary and postural methods may suffice. These, however, should be carried out indefinitely to prevent further episodes. Asymptomatic patients should then be seen at six- to 12-month intervals in order to reinforce the concept of preventing further reflux.

WHAT COMPLICATIONS OF THE DISEASE CAN OCCUR?

The major complications of peptic esophagitis can be grouped into two categories: short term and long term (Table 4). Esophageal ulcers behave similarly to other peptic ulcers of the gastrointestinal tract. The presence of an ulcer indicates severe reflux disease and it should be investigated to exclude the presence of a malignancy. (The ulcers, however, are not premalignant in and of themselves.) Esophageal ulcers may bleed or perforate although the latter is a rare event. Usually patients with these ulcers ultimately require surgical therapy.

Bleeding may arise from erosions or ulcerations. The bleeding may be macroscopic or microscopic. The incidence of hemorrhage is

Table 4 **Complications
of Reflux
Esophagitis**

Short term
  Esophageal ulcer
  Hemorrhage
  Aspiration
Long term
  Stricture
  Barrett's esophagus

unknown, and the frequency or severity of episodes is variable and difficult to predict.

Reflux by itself or combined with stricture of the esophagus may lead to pulmonary aspiration. This should be strongly considered with any episode of unexplained pneumonia in a patient with a hiatal hernia or reflux. Proven pulmonary aspiration should be an indication for antireflux operation.

Barrett's esophagus is a condition associated with reflux in which severe esophagitis leads to columnar metaplasia in the formerly squamous cell portion of the esophagus, esophageal ulcers, and stricture formation. In addition, there are many reports of adenocarcinoma of the esophagus arising from Barrett's epithelium. It is important to remember that the metaplastic change arises as a consequence of the severe inflammation and not as a congenital disorder of the esophageal mucosa.

The major long-term complication of reflux esophagitis is the development of a peptic stricture. Stricture formation is usually heralded by the insidious onset of dysphagia. At first the dysphagia is produced only by solid, chunky foods that are swallowed as large boluses. The dysphagia becomes progressive in untreated patients and eventually the lumen of the esophagus becomes so narrow as to impede the passage of liquids as well as solid foods.

HOW SHOULD THESE COMPLICATIONS BE MANAGED?

Management of the short-term complications of esophagitis should initially consist of intensification of the medical measures previously discussed. Medical management usually leads to healing and repair of the damaged esophageal mucosa. Therefore, esophageal ulcers or bleeding are rarely indications for more stringent immediate measures unless the conservative medical approach using positioning, antacids and/or acid-blocking agents, and dietary measures is unsuccessful. As noted, many of these patients will ultimately require operation, however. Patients with esophageal strictures should undergo endoscopy and biopsy to exclude a malignant process. The initial therapeutic approach to a benign peptic stricture is usually gentle dilatation of the narrowed area using a mercury-weighted rubber dilator (of the Hurst or Maloney type), a woven silk or reed dilator, or, in more severe stricture, a metal olive passed over a thin wire (Peustow).

Such procedures are usually performed by a gastroenterologist or surgeon. Using mild local anesthesia the physician passes a dilator down the esophagus until resistance is met. Using gentle pressure he or she passes the dilator through the stricture. Dilators are sized on the French (Fr) scale. Very narrow strictures may permit the passage of only a small-bore dilator, such as Fr 19 or 20. The usual procedure is to pass dilators of progressively larger size until the esophageal lumen can be traversed by a dilator of at least size Fr 40. This will usually result in relief of dysphagia and permit a patient to eat normally. Several days or even weeks may be required to dilate a patient to a reasonably sized esophageal lumen since most patients do not comfortably tolerate the passage of more than two or three dilators at each session.

Dilatations are carried out two to three times a week initially and then as necessary to maintain an adequate sized lumen. The frequency of dilatations required is highly variable and depends on the severity of reflux and the adequacy of continued medical treatment. Thus, some patients require frequent dilatations, perhaps as often as once or twice a week; the majority of patients require much less frequent dilatations and may do well with one every two or three months. An occasional patient may not require dilatations at all subsequent to initial bougienage.

No discussion of the management of reflux esophagitis or its complications would be complete without some mention of the role of operation. The newer surgical fundoplication operations have been a major advance in the management of these patients. The question most frequently asked about therapy of esophagitis is "What are the indications for operation?" This is a difficult question to answer; most simply stated surgical candidates would include those patients with recurring complications, either short or long term, despite adequate medical management or those who fail to respond symptomatically to a conscientious, well-planned medical regimen. While the majority of patients with esophagitis will never require surgery, there remains a definite subgroup of patients who fail to respond to medical measures and who, either because of persistence of symptoms or because of recurring complications, are candidates for operation.

For many years, the main surgical treatment was aimed at anatomic correction of hiatal hernias, based on the assumption that hiatal hernias and reflux were synonymous. The results of such repairs, although anatomically successful, were largely disappointing from the standpoint of symptomatic improvement. The modern operations share one feature: they combat reflux by creating a type of anatomic barrier to strengthen the lower esophageal sphincter by a valve-like mechanism. Three types of operations are currently being performed. The Belsey operation, performed via a thoracotomy incision, involves reduction of the hiatal hernia and wrapping of the fundus of the stomach around the distal esophagus to achieve a valve-like effect. The Nissen operation is done through the abdomen and also involves the creation of a valve at the gastroesophageal junction by a wraparound procedure. The Hill operation involves closure of the hiatus followed by fixation of the gastroesophageal junction posteriorly to the median arcuate ligament to assure restoration of an intraabdominal segment of esophagus. In general, these operations have proved successful in approximately 75% of patients.

Some surgeons advocate an ulcer-type operation (vagotomy and gastric drainage procedure) combined with an antireflux procedure. However, there is no evidence that this enhances improvement after surgical therapy unless the patient suffers from coexistent gastric or duodenal peptic ulcer disease.

SELECTED READING

Bernstein LM, Fruin RC, Pacini R: Differentiation of esophageal pain from angina pectoris: role of the esophageal acid perfusion test. *Medicine* 41:143–162, 1962.

Cohen S: Esophageal reflux: new concepts in medical management. *Hosp Prac* 11(5):131–137, May 1976.

Cohen S, Harris LD: Does hiatus hernia affect competence of the gastro-esophageal sphincter? *N Engl J Med* 284:1053–1058, 1971.

Pope CE II: Reflux esophagitis, in Sleisenger MH, Fordtran JS (eds): *Gastrointestinal Disease. Pathophysiology, Diagnosis, Management.* Philadelphia, WB Saunders Co, 1973, pp 83–112.

CLINICAL PROBLEMS

I. A 42-year-old obese man complains of a substernal burning sensation that has been occurring on and off for several years. He notes the discomfort especially at night shortly after he goes to bed and especially if he has eaten a heavy meal late in the evening. He denies weight loss, dysphagia, or bleeding. He has noted that baking soda or antacids relieve the pain within a few minutes. Orange juice ingestion often reproduces the pain "as it goes down." His physical examination is entirely normal. The stool is negative for occult blood.

1. What is wrong with the patient?
2. What further tests should he undergo?
3. How should he be managed?

II. Over the next few months, the same patient pursues the proposed therapeutic course and symptoms resolve without the need for operation. Five years later, shortly after stopping his anti-reflux treatment program, he notes the onset of substernal chest pain, which he describes as "squeezing" in nature and always coming on in association with his usual heartburn symptoms. (He also has his typical heartburn symptoms at other times without the new pain.) This new pain often radiates to the jaw and is relieved by antacids or by nitroglycerin (which was given to him by a friend). On occasion he has noted that, when he swallows cold water during an episode of this new pain the liquid seems to stick in his midchest. Again his physical examination is normal and the stool is negative for occult blood.

1. What new problem is now occurring?
2. What tests should be done?
3. How should he be managed?

III. The patient takes your advice and has a remission of his symptoms. Over the next few years, however, he falls back on his old habits and notes the recurrence of the problem. Because of "pressures," he cannot return to a therapeutic regimen and over the next year his symptoms increase. He now returns to you because his retrosternal burning has become more prolonged, less responsive to antacids, and more frequent. His physical examination is still normal, but his stool is now positive for occult blood. A barium swallow demonstrates an esophageal ulcer and minimal narrowing of the esophageal lumen.

1. What problem may have developed?
2. What tests should now be done?
3. How should this patient be managed?

Discussion

I. 1. This is a typical case of reflux esophagitis.
   2. A barium upper gastrointestinal series should be obtained to confirm the presence of reflux. No other tests need be performed at this juncture. (Note that the patient relates, in the history of orange juice intolerance, a positive "pseudo-Bernstein" test.) A trial of therapy can be initiated.
   3. The patient should be instructed to raise the head of the bed and to avoid bending over or wearing tight abdominal binders. He should go on a weight reduction diet, also altering his dietary intake as described previously in this chapter. He should begin antacids one-half hour after meals and at bedtime.
II. 1. The patient is now describing a pain that has some characteristics of coronary angina. However, it is related to the esophagitis symptoms and he has noted dysphagia. Although coronary artery disease should be considered, he probably is experiencing diffuse esophageal spasm that is triggered by the reflux.

2. An electrocardiagram should be obtained during an episode of pain or, less preferably, an exercise test should be obtained. (It should be noted, however, that diffuse esophageal spasm can produce nonspecific ST-T wave changes on the ECG.) Of more utility, however, will be the confirmation that the pain is due to diffuse esophageal spasm. This can be accomplished with esophageal manometry. (If necessary, one can even attempt to provoke an episode of spasm by perfusing the esophagus with acid or by having the patient drink hot or cold liquids.)

3. If the patient is indeed having spasm secondary to reflux, the therapy should be the same as outlined in chapters 8 and 10. (In addition, nitroglycerin can be used to relieve the spasm pain when it occurs; if this is done, it must be explained carefully to the patient that he does not have coronary artery disease.)

III. 1. The patient now probably has a complication of reflux esophagitis, an esophageal ulcer, and possibly an early stricture. Both Barrett's esophagus and esophageal carcinoma should also be considered.

2. Endoscopy and biopsy should be undertaken to rule out the latter two diagnoses considered.

3. The patient should be put back on the previous treatment regimen with additional doses of antacids three hours after meals. (Cimetidine may also be given.) If a symptomatic stricture is present, dilatation may also be needed. If response to conservative therapy is poor, operation will be indicated.

WILFRED M. WEINSTEIN

Peptic Ulcer Disease

HOW DO I MAKE THE DIAGNOSIS?

The history is still the most important way to narrow the differential diagnosis to peptic ulcer disease and to help determine how vigorous the initial investigative approach should be. Life would be simple if every patient complained of a high epigastric burning pain that began one to two hours after meals and was relieved by food or antacids within 30 minutes. However, many patients do not have these typical symptoms. Nevertheless other important clues are often available to indicate duodenal or gastric ulcer as a diagnostic possibility. Sometimes the patient's pain extends horizontally to the right along the costal margin or vertically along the right rectus sheath. The patient may describe the discomfort as burning, gnawing, boring, hunger, pain, or just plain discomfort. Those with duodenal ulcer often report that their pain is relieved by food or antacids within 30 minutes. However, others experience provocation or worsening of pain by eating. This is especially true in patients with juxtapyloric ulcers. Juxtapyloric refers to ulcers that are located adjacent to the pylorus or within the pyloric canal itself. Many patients report clear-cut precipitation or exacerbation of symptoms by aspirin, caffeine, alcohol, or increased smoking.

A patient's ulcer may be unassociated with pain and the patient may present with a complication such as anemia, gastric outlet obstruction, or massive upper gastrointestinal bleeding. Some asymptomatic ulcers are detected in the course of an investigation for occult gastrointestinal bleeding. Some ulcers are detected incidentally when patients have barium x-rays or endoscopy performed for other reasons.

The physical examination is often normal. The most important abnormal finding is localized tenderness to palpation in the upper or midepigastrium. This physical sign is even more relevant when the tenderness is elicited with only mild or moderate pressure on palpation. Novices often elicit epigastric tenderness in all individuals because they press too hard and massage the aorta. When a peptic ulcer is suspected, a stool specimen should be tested for occult blood.

In my utopia all patients with a first or second attack of what I believe to be uncomplicated peptic ulcer would proceed directly to a trial of therapy. After two weeks of therapy, I would check to ensure that symptoms had improved dramatically and would reinforce the need to continue therapy for a total of six weeks. At that point, if the patient had remained symptom free, therapy would be discontinued and the patient would be instructed concerning long-term management, as outlined later in this chapter. Investigation would be required if a patient failed to become completely symptom free or if a major relapse in symptoms occurred soon after cessation of therapy. This empiric, reasonable approach has been abandoned by most physicians. Unfortunately those who may still practice this method are made to feel guilty by their colleagues or by professional teachers.

Clearly, an empiric therapeutic trial does not establish a "specific" diagnosis, but is a more specific diagnosis really necessary? I think not in a patient with a first or second attack of what appears to be uncomplicated peptic ulcer. We cannot predict the natural history of peptic ulcer in a given patient and we have no simple way to modify the natural history. It is appropriate to wait until the natural history declares itself in the minority of patients who will have a more complicated course.

WHAT ADDITIONAL WORKUP DOES
THE PATIENT REQUIRE?

A baseline hemoglobin is useful. Patients who fail the initial therapeutic trial or have a major relapse of symptoms soon after discontinuation of therapy require further investigation. Two tests are available, flexible fiberoptic endoscopy and barium x-ray. At present, the most widespread practice is to obtain a barium x-ray of the esophagus, stomach, and duodenum as the initial diagnostic test. Then, endoscopy is done if the x-ray is negative, equivocal, or suggests cancer.

Endoscopy is infinitely more precise than x-ray, which has a combined 20% incidence of false-positive and false-negative diagnoses. The major limitation of endoscopy in the United States is that the market value of the test is high and only a limited number of competent endoscopists are available. This has prohibited its general use in the evaluation of patients with suspect duodenal or gastric ulcers. However, it is only a matter of time before endoscopy will replace barium x-ray as the first test in the evaluation of peptic ulcer.

Other investigations in the patient with a proven duodenal or gastric ulcer depend on whether the patient's symptoms suggest a concomitant disease. Peptic ulcer is common and we sometimes detect a gastric or duodenal ulcer in the course of evaluating patients with upper abdominal symptoms. Sometimes we remain unconvinced that the gastric or duodenal ulcer is the real cause of the symptoms. In such circumstances ulcer therapy can be started to see if the symptoms change significantly. Alternatively, investigations can be initiated to rule out the other suspect disorders, concomitant with the ulcer therapy trial.

A frequent consideration in patients with high epigastric or lower retrosternal pain is symptomatic gastroesophageal reflux. This may coexist with ulcer disease or may represent the primary diagnosis in patients with these symptoms. Since treatment is essentially the same for symptomatic gastroesophageal reflux as for peptic ulcer, one can proceed with therapy even when it is impossible to determine whether peptic ulcer or symptomatic reflux is the primary cause of symptoms. In some instances symptoms may mimic symptomatic cholelithiasis or recurrent pancreatitis. Pancreatitis is not usually an important diagnostic consideration unless the patient is an alcoholic or has had recurrent bouts of pancreatitis in the past.

Functional dyspepsia, a "nonentity," merits comment in this discussion of differential diagnosis. Functional dyspepsia generally refers to a pain syndrome similar in character or location, or both, to that of more classic peptic ulcer. Patients have no demonstrable ulcer but some respond to conventional ulcer therapy (*N Engl J Med* 291:567–569, 1974). Other patients do not respond to such therapy. Many consider that these patients have psychological problems. Some do, but so do some patients with any disorder. We should not adopt the universal "cop-out" by labeling these patients as having psychosomatic or functional disease simply because we cannot find a "lesion" in the light of today's knowledge. This is not meant to minimize the importance of the psychosocial evaluation of patients. On the other hand we should not build up a case for functional disease in retrospect simply because the "tests" are normal.

When should we screen for the Zollinger-Ellison syndrome? These rare gastrin-secreting tumors should be suspected when patients have intractable ulcer disease refractory to conventional therapy, frequent ulcer recurrences in various locations (i.e., esophagus, stomach, and duodenum) at different times, ulcers in atypical locations, such as the postbulbar duodenum, or diarrhea accompanying ulcer symptoms. Suspicion should be heightened when there is a strong family history of ulcer disease or when some family members have had pancreatic or parathyroid endocrinopathy. The best tests to screen for the Zollinger-Ellison syndrome are a fasting serum gastrin and a one-hour basal gastric acid secretion. A basal acid output greater than 15 mmole per hour and an elevated fasting serum gastrin strongly suggest the Zollinger-Ellison syndrome.

HOW SHOULD I TREAT THE PATIENT?

In order to put this and subsequent questions into perspective, we need to review the question of natural history. A Pandora's box of important questions has been reopened because of the introduction of cimetidine. The introduction of this drug accelerated the use of prospective controlled trials in peptic ulcer disease. In addition, the use of fiberoptic endoscopy in these trials has provided more precise information concerning healing rates and natural history.

We now have confirmation that antacids heal duodenal ulcers as quickly as cimetidine; there is a high placebo healing rate; discordance between the presence of an ulcer crater and symptoms is common, that is, a crater may be present without symptoms and, conversely, symptoms may occur without the crater; and posttreatment recurrence of duodenal ulcer craters is common but is often not associated with major relapses of symptoms. We should not feel discouraged by these observations. Our mandate is to control symptoms adequately and not to worry too much whether the duodenal ulcer is completely "healed." The majority of patients with duodenal and gastric ulcers will never require operation and will be symptom free for long intervals. Our dilemma is that we cannot order a "serum natural history" in order to single out those who will develop complications, have frequent relapses, and ultimately require surgery.

When we assess peptic ulcer therapy, we need to bear in mind the high placebo healing rate. This does not mean that placebos necessarily heal the lesions but reflects the fact that the natural history of the peptic ulcer is to wax and wane spontaneously, perhaps even when a placebo is withheld. The spontaneous remissions in peptic ulcers have led to a host of claims that different kinds of intervention are successful, such as elaborate unpalatable diets, sedation (which can endanger patients when driving), amateur recommendations to change lifestyle, and others. Fortunately, a more sensible and less meddlesome therapeutic approach is in vogue.

Our current approach may be modified in the future, especially if we can obtain predictors of the natural history in a given patient. Perhaps then we could tailor the intensity of our therapy accordingly. Of course this presumes that more intensive or new therapy would modify the natural history of peptic ulcer, and this question remains open. The current approach to therapy is discussed in the following paragraphs.

An ulcer is a hole or "break" in the lining of the duodenum or stomach. The cause is unknown but we do know that neutralizing some of the acid (antacids) or preventing secretion of some of the gastric acid (with cimetidine) promotes healing. Patients must be forewarned that their symptoms will likely vanish or improve significantly within a few days or weeks. The importance of continuing the treatment course for approximately six weeks needs to be reinforced. It is useful to warn patients in advance that they will tire of this therapy. Ask patients to phone after one, two, and four weeks of therapy, ostensibly to report how they are doing. In reality, the phone call can be used to cheer the patients up and to urge continuance of therapy.

Many patients have the ingrained belief that life stress and ulcer disease are intimately related. I generally preempt their questions or misconceptions by discussing this point at the outset. I indicate that stress is no more or less of a risk factor in the development of ulcer disease than it is in many other conditions. There are times when pain may be provoked by increased stress but at other times this relationship will not hold. Patients should clearly understand that they have not "brought this upon themselves." I also add that they will continue to hear a lot about the relationship between stress and ulcer disease but this merely reflects the persistence of outdated concepts whereby we used to blame "nerves" as the cause of many conditions for which there was no known etiology.

Patients should be advised to avoid foods that predictably precipitate or worsen attacks of pain. The only specific modification in diet is avoidance of caffeine-containing products during the initial treatment phase. These products include coffee, tea, and cola beverages. We used to think that decaffeinated beverages were safe but even these are now in doubt.

Aspirin-containing compounds should be avoided and if patients have taken these on a casual basis for headaches then acetaminophen should be taken in moderation as a substitute. Alcohol should be withdrawn during the initial treatment phase. Patients should be encouraged to stop smoking or at least to drastically reduce the number of cigarettes they smoke. Some patients find all of these proposals too Spartan and become disturbed. When a physician senses this, certain negotiations need to be made to balance benefit versus risk.

Antacid Therapy

Antacid therapy is the preferred initial approach in patients with duodenal and gastric ulcers. Table 1 gives the composition and relative potencies of some antacids. Some of these antacids theoretically require larger doses than are practical in order to achieve optimal buffering of acid. For this reason they are not considered first choice. Some patients will have a distinct prejudice based on prior experience with less potent antacids. When they express a distinct preference, one has to balance potential compliance with common

Table 1   Composition and Neutralizing Capacity of Some Antacids[a]

Antacid	Content	Therapeutic Dose (ml)[b]
Delcid	Al and Mg hydroxides	18
Mylanta II	Mg and Al hydroxides, simethicone	30
Gelusil II	Mg trisilicate, Al hydroxide gel	32
Titralac	Ca carbonate, glycine	40
Camalox	Ca carbonate, Al and Mg hydroxides	42
Maalox	Mg and Al hydroxide gel	56
Di-Gel	Al and Mg hydroxides, simethicone	61
Riopan	Mg and Al hydroxides	69
Trisogel	Mg trisilicate, Al hydroxide gel	76
Amphojel	Al hydroxide gel	117

[a] Data taken from Dutro MP, Amerson AB: *N Engl J Med* 302:967, 1980 and McCarthy DM: Peptic ulcer: antacids or cimetidine? *Hosp Pract* 14:52–64, 1979. A more complete list of antacid formulations is available from these two reference sources.
[b] Milliliters to neutralize 152 mEq of hydrochloric acid.

sense, that is, let them take their antacid of preference if they insist.

Based on previous studies concerning antacid efficacy and taking into account palatability and cost, I generally recommend Mylanta II, one ounce (two tablespoons) one hour and three hours after meals and at bedtime. The one- and three-hour after-meal timing of antacids is important because it yields a more prolonged buffering effect. I also recommend that patients stock up on lesser amounts of constipating antacids such as Amphojel. They can take them part of the time to prevent the diarrhea that may develop when they take Mylanta II. The magnesium in antacids promotes diarrhea and the aluminum promotes constipation. Liquid antacids are more effective than tablets. Patients who cannot keep bottles of liquid with them during working hours may take two tablets instead of one ounce of the liquid antacid.

Calcium-containing antacids are in disrepute because they may cause a greater acid rebound than do noncalcium-containing antacids. Nevertheless, they are often useful when taken occasionally in a treatment course in order to offset the diarrhea produced by antacids with a high magnesium content.

Cimetidine

Many physicians now use cimetidine instead of antacids as the first approach. One reason they do so is their own problems with compliance. Physicians find the prescription of antacids boring, and they are not able to muster enough enthusiasm to educate patients properly concerning the proper use of antacids or to take the time required to monitor compliance. Antacids have an additional strike against them from the physician's and the patient's perspective because the mystique of healing is compromised with a therapy that is advertised routinely on television and can be purchased without the blessing of a prescription. Also, it is simpler to take a pill four times a day rather than antacids seven times a day. Many patients have already heard through acquaintances or the media that a "wonder drug" pill is available to treat ulcer disease and this makes them even more reluctant to take antacids. Therefore, cimetidine probably raises the therapeutic response overall because physicians and patients are inherently more enthusiastic about it and because less patient education is required than with antacid therapy.

My preference for antacids over cimetidine as the first choice in therapy is based simply on the fact that cimetidine has only been used widely for a few years, compared with a much longer experience with antacids. The full spectrum of cimetidine side effects and untoward reactions is not yet defined. The dose of cimetidine is 300 mg before meals and at bedtime for an average of six weeks. The dose needs to be reduced in the presence of renal failure: when serum creatinine is 2 to 4 mg%, give 300 mg three times a day; when serum creatinine is greater than 4 mg%, give 300 mg every 12 hours.

Anticholinergics

Anticholinergics should be avoided in patients with gastric ulcer because gastric stasis may delay gastric ulcer healing. In duodenal ulcer they may be useful as adjunctive therapy when patients continue to be wakened at night with pain after institution of therapy with antacids or cimetidine. The anticholinergics can be given at night in double the usual dose since the patient can sleep through the side effects and avoid the inevitable dry mouth, dry eyes, and so forth. Anticholinergics should be avoided in all patients with a history of glaucoma or symptomatic prostatism.

WHAT SHOULD I EXPECT FROM SUCCESSFUL TREATMENT?

At least 75% of duodenal and gastric ulcers will heal during a six-week course of therapy. Symptoms usually disappear much earlier. Approximately 15% of patients with duodenal ulcer will ultimately require an operation either because of intractability (frequent symptomatic recurrences) or because of complications. Overall, complications occur in approximately 25% of patients with duodenal ulcer at some point in their lives. The need for operation in gastric ulcer, especially in the body of the stomach, is probably greater than it is for duodenal ulcer.

From a pathophysiologic and complication point of view, prepyloric ulcers of the stomach behave more like duodenal ulcers than do ulcers located more proximally in the stomach. Aspirin-associated ulcers often improve dramatically if the aspirin can be withdrawn.

WHAT MIGHT CAUSE A FAILURE OF TREATMENT?

Failed treatment is usually represented by frequent symptom relapses after appropriate courses of therapy. When these relapses interfere with a patient's life, the term intractability is applied. We do not understand the reason why some patients pursue this course and we cannot predict at the outset who will have frequent symptom relapses.

Sometimes the reasons for failure become apparent: failure to take therapy as prescribed, continued smoking, alcoholism, or aspirin ingestion. Corticosteroids may delay healing. The role of nonsteroidal antiinflammatory agents is less clear in this regard.

A much less frequent form of failed treatment is failure to control symptoms and heal an ulcer during a given course of therapy. Sometimes the combination of antacid and cimetidine therapy will "break the cycle." If not, one should consider three possibilities:

the ulcer is too deep (i.e., penetrating), the patient's pain may be due to something other than the ulcer, or an underlying Zollinger-Ellison syndrome is present. A tiny group of patients has none of these problems and we do not know why their ulcers fail to heal after many months of therapy.

WHAT ARE THE SIDE EFFECTS OF TREATMENT?

Antacids

Altered bowel habit is the major complication of antacids and has been discussed previously. In addition, certain drugs given concomitantly may not be absorbed optimally. Most antacids contain substantial amounts of sodium and must be used with caution in patients with heart disease, hypertension, renal disease, and ascites. All antacids and probably cimetidine enhance the absorption of dicoumarol and L-dopa and reduce the absorption of other drugs such as phenothiazines, isoniazid, nitrofurantoin, penicillin G, and sulfonamides. To help avoid drug interactions, have the patients take other medications at least one hour removed from their last or next dose of antacid. This reduces the possibility of drug interactions especially with the seven-times-per-day antacid regimen.

Cimetidine

The reported complications to date are uncommon or rare. They include elevation of liver enzymes, minor elevations in serum creatinine, gynecomastia, mental changes (especially in the elderly), and drug fever. The effects of sedatives, such as diazepam, and anticoagulants may be enhanced. Rare complications are reversible hepatitis, impotence, and serious confusion. As with any new drug, the best approach is to consult the most recent reviews of cimetidine from time to time and more importantly to have patients promptly report new symptoms while they are receiving cimetidine.

Physician-Induced Side Effects

Physician-induced side effects are common and fall into two categories. One is the patient who is inadequately taught what a peptic ulcer is and the rationale for therapy. This patient either fails to comply with therapy, or becomes dependent and panics with any minor flare in symptoms. The second category of physician-induced side effects occurs when sedatives are prescribed for patients or when arbitrary recommendations are given to change lifestyle, spouses, and so forth, simply because the patient has a peptic ulcer. In other words, some patients are inadequately educated concerning their disease and others are needlessly frightened or mistreated. Side effects of treatment occur when patients are not taught how to juggle the diarrhea-inducing with the constipation-inducing antacids or when antacids are used in a potentially dangerous setting, such as in the presence of renal failure or heart disease. In patients receiving cimetidine, problems may occur if they are not told that they are on a new drug and therefore must promptly report new symptoms.

HOW SHOULD THE PATIENT BE FOLLOWED?

In patients with duodenal ulcer, if symptoms have remitted within the usual two or three weeks, therapy can be arbitrarily stopped at six weeks and no further tests are required. There is no evidence yet that a more vigorous approach with endoscopy at six weeks and continued therapy in the asymptomatic patient with a persistent tiny defect in the mucosa modifies the long-term natural history. Barium x-rays are useless in the follow-up study of duodenal ulcers because they inevitably result in misdiagnoses. Once a duodenal bulb becomes deformed, it is virtually impossible to differentiate a persistent duodenal crater from a healed duodenal ulcer with an x-ray.

In patients with gastric ulcer, a "healing test" is required. This means that at six weeks an endoscopy (or barium x-ray if endoscopy is not available) should be performed to ensure complete healing. If endoscopy is performed biopsies should be taken from any persistent gastric ulcer to rule out the possibility that it has been malignant all along. Another six weeks of treatment are required if healing of a gastric ulcer is incomplete. We do not know whether this kind of vigorous approach changes the natural history, compared with a more cavalier approach in which patients simply have gastric malignancy ruled out and have treatment terminated at six to eight weeks assuming there has been an initial prompt remission of symptoms and a "significant" reduction in ulcer size at six or eight weeks. Gastric ulcers that appear benign at the outset with either a barium x-ray or endoscopic examination are not likely to represent malignant ulcers.

Once the initial treatment course is complete, I give the following recommendations to patients. I tell them to avoid aspirin-containing products unless they subsequently develop conditions (such as certain forms of arthritis) that make aspirin a first-line drug. If that happens they are reminded to tell their physician that they have had an ulcer in the past. If they have been in the habit of taking aspirin-containing compounds for nonspecific flu-like symptoms or occasional headaches, they should take acetaminophen in modest doses instead. I tell them to drink alcohol only in moderation and warn them again that cigarette smoking is a major risk factor in ulcer disease and that they should make every attempt to stop.

The essence of follow-up study is to educate patients. The natural history must be explained. They can expect minor symptom flare-ups from time to time that frequently occur in the absence of a specific recurrence of the ulcer itself. The explanation that I use is that, once healed, ulcers leave behind sensitive areas in the stomach or duodenum, analogous to a sensitive scar on the skin. Patients are told to take antacids (one ounce of liquid or two tablets) as needed for occasional symptoms. On the other hand, if symptoms recur in clusters, and especially if patients are wakened at night, they are told to resume the seven-times-per-day antacid regimen on their own and to continue it for at least 48 hours after the last symptom cluster. If they find that clusters recur frequently, they should return for reevaluation. The physician must then decide whether another formal course of therapy is required and whether investigations need to be made. Finally, patients should be advised to inform the physician if they have black stools or develop pain that radiates to the back (ulcer penetration) or pain that is not relieved with antacids.

WHAT ARE THE COMPLICATIONS AND HOW ARE THEY MANAGED?

Intractability

As discussed earlier, intractability does not refer to the rare situation in which symptoms cannot be controlled with a given course of therapy. Rather, it refers to frequent relapses that require such frequent formal courses of therapy that they seriously interfere with patients' lives or with their perception of their ability to cope with the discomfort or the therapy. The final judgment concerning intractability is subjective and requires the best elements of a sound physician-patient relationship, preferably one in which a single physician has followed the patient over a number of years.

An individual who is a mercenary soldier and does not wish to change his occupation might judge (rightly so) that two or three flare-ups over a two- or three-year period constitute intractability. His occupation takes him to remote areas where it is dangerous to be disabled by discomfort and where it is impossible to obtain medical care. On the other hand, an internist with a morbid fear of surgery might be quite content to put up with many relapses and frequent courses of therapy in order to avoid operation.

In assessing the question of intractability, it is extremely important to determine in advance what the patient's reaction to surgery will be. Some patients are relieved to be given the surgical option because they have friends or relatives who had eminently successful results from ulcer surgery. Others may have a great fear of surgery because a friend or relative has died directly or indirectly from operation for peptic ulcer.

Severe recurrent disease (intractability) constitutes the most common indication for operation. Preoperative assessment should include endoscopy.

Chronic maintenance therapy with cimetidine is now used in those who would normally require operation for intractability but are very old or are poor surgical risks because of other medical problems. Maintenance cimetidine is also indicated in some patients with rheumatic disorders who are receiving drugs that may be promoting peptic ulceration and in whom these drugs cannot be withdrawn. The efficacy of long-term maintenance cimetidine therapy in these circumstances is unknown.

Bleeding

Approximately 20% of all patients with duodenal or gastric ulcer will bleed at some time in their lives. Bleeding is a much more common complication than obstruction or perforation. It may occur without any antecedent pain or may be the first presentation of a gastric or duodenal ulcer. The bleeding may be massive with hematemesis and watery melena or it may be more insidious and present as iron deficiency anemia or melena, or both.

For massive bleeding the initial approach is to resuscitate the patient, give blood, and start ulcer therapy. Endoscopy should be performed to define the bleeding site.

When bleeding has stopped I use cimetidine as the first-line therapy in all patients, extend the course to eight weeks, and use endoscopic follow-up to ensure complete healing. The hope with this more vigorous follow-up approach is that it may somehow modify or improve the long-term natural history and prevent further bleeding episodes. However, there are no data to support this approach.

How many times should a patient bleed before surgery is recommended? The standard number is two. However, in younger patients it is reasonable to assess how serious the bleeding incidents have been and how widely spaced in time. On the other hand sometimes a severe first bleed makes operation imperative. The mortality and morbidity from gastrointestinal bleeding increase dramatically in older individuals. For that reason one might opt for surgery during or after the first major bleeding incident in an older individual because continued or subsequent bleeding poses major threats to the heart, kidney, and brain.

It has become fashionable to use intravenous cimetidine as initial treatment for gastrointestinal bleeding. However, there is no evidence that it modifies the course. Fortunately, most patients who present with bleeding from a gastric or duodenal ulcer stop within 24 hours of admission to the hospital.

Obstruction

Obstruction occurs because of slow progressive scarring in the region of the pyloric canal. Sometimes it is precipitated by a recurrent ulcer so one has the combination of previous scarring and an active ulcer with inflammatory swelling. Patients may present with complete obstruction in which there is marked gastric retention and frequent vomiting. Sometimes the symptoms are more subtle and progress slowly with early satiety or heartburn. The latter symptom is presumably due to the increased amount of gastric contents available for reflux into the esophagus, so-called secondary reflux.

For complete obstruction, fluid and electrolyte replacement and nasogastric suction are the first approaches. Endoscopy must be performed at some point to determine the cause of the obstruction and to ascertain that the obstruction is in fact due to benign outlet ulcer disease rather than gastric malignancy. In many instances operation will be required. Sometimes the obstruction resolves promptly and standard medical therapy is successful, at least for that episode. Such patients must be followed more frequently to determine whether they are redeveloping signs of gastric outlet obstruction. If surgery is required, adequate preoperative decompression is important so that the normal size and tone of the stomach can be restored. This minimizes the risk of breakdown at anastomoses and permits better positioning of certain kinds of anastomoses.

Perforation

Perforation may be the first presentation of a duodenal or gastric ulcer or may occur in patients with a previous history of perforation. If a duodenal ulcer on the anterior wall perforates, the patient will present with symptoms of generalized peritonitis. A duodenal ulcer on the posterior wall may present with boring pain radiating to the back, that is, a reflection of penetration into the lesser sac and pancreatic bed. In this setting the patient's symptoms actually suggest pancreatitis. Gastric ulcer perforations usually present with generalized peritonitis.

Sometimes gastric ulcers penetrate into the colon and present as a gastrocolic fistula. Duodenal and gastric ulcers rarely penetrate into the biliary tree.

Operation for Peptic Ulcer

Operation is reserved for the complications of peptic ulcer (Figs. 1, 2). In duodenal ulcer the objective of operation is to reduce acid secretion. In the past the standard approach has been to perform a truncal vagotomy. The vagal trunks are interrupted at the diaphragm. The vagotomy is combined either with a pyloroplasty (widening) to facilitate drainage or with antrectomy. Antrectomy and vagotomy are associated with fewer ulcer recurrences than are vagotomy and pyloroplasty. When antrectomy is performed, the

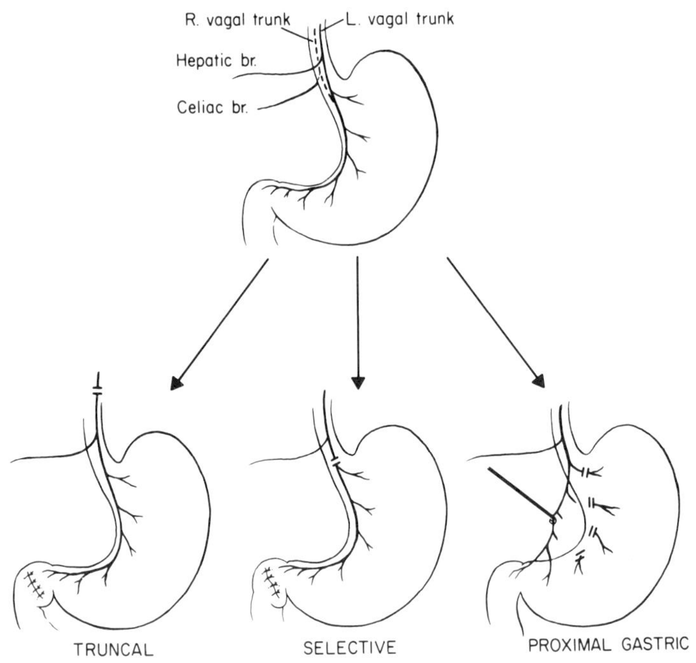

Figure 1 Vagotomy. In truncal vagotomy the vagal trunks are severed just below the diaphragm. Selective vagotomy spares the celiac and hepatic branches; it is rarely performed. In proximal gastric vagotomy only those branches to the acid-secreting part of the stomach are severed. The hepatic, celiac, and gastric antral branches are spared. Points of severance are shown by two short parallel lines.

conventional type of anastomosis used is the joining of the gastric remnant to the first part of the duodenum (Billroth I). If this is impossible because of duodenal scarring, a Billroth II (gastrojejunostomy) anastomosis is fashioned.

A new approach in duodenal ulcer operation is proximal gastric vagotomy. This more technically demanding operation consists of severing only those vagal fibers that supply the acid-secreting part of the stomach, that is, the proximal portion. This operation reduces acid secretion, leaves gastric antral innervation intact, and avoids the need for a drainage procedure. It eliminates the effects of truncal vagotomy on other organs, such as the pancreas, gallbladder,

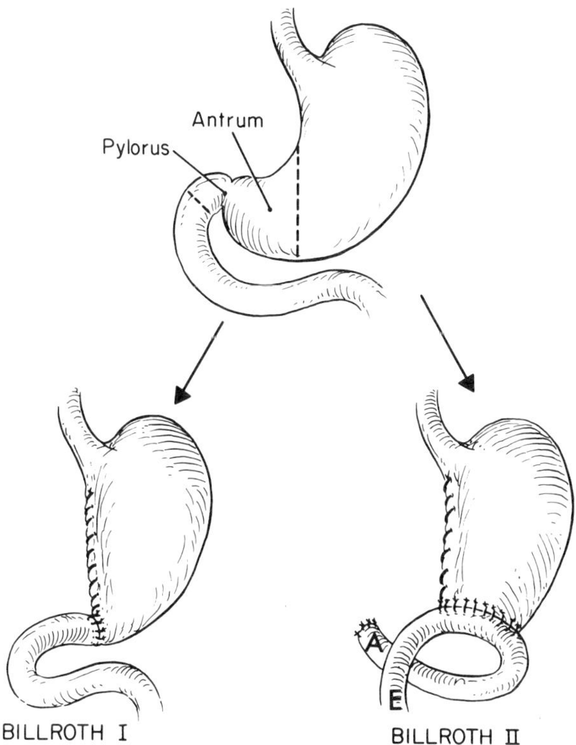

Figure 2 Anastomoses after antrectomy. The Billroth I is a direct end-to-end hookup of the gastric remnant to the duodenum. The Billroth II entails oversewing the proximal duodenum and performing a gastrojejunostomy. The afferent and efferent limbs are labeled A and E, respectively.

and so forth. Long-term follow-up studies will tell us how successful this seemingly more rational approach to duodenal ulcer surgery is. One limiting factor is that the operation is technically more difficult. Hence, many surgeons are justifiably reluctant to employ it because of their lack of training and experience with the procedure. Ulcer recurrence is more common after this operation than after antrectomy and vagotomy.

For gastric ulcer, antrectomy without vagotomy is successful in most instances. When operation is required for recurrent prepyloric (distal gastric) ulcers, the same surgery is employed as for duodenal ulcer, usually vagotomy and antrectomy. This is because prepyloric gastric ulcers behave physiologically more like duodenal ulcers.

When operation is performed under emergency circumstances, the surgical approach may be modified. For example, a perforated ulcer might be dealt with by simply oversewing the perforation.

SELECTED READING

Isenberg J: Long-term medical management of duodenal ulcer. *Hosp Pract* 15(1):63–81, January 1980.
McCarthy DM: Peptic ulcer: antacids or cimetidine? *Hosp Pract* 14(12): 52–64, December 1979.
Silverstein FE: Peptic ulcer: an overview of diagnosis. *Hosp Pract* 14 (11):78–87, November 1979.
Spiro HM: Moynihan's disease? The diagnosis of duodenal ulcer. *N Engl J Med* 291:567–569, 1974.

CLINICAL PROBLEMS

I. A 25-year-old man complains of an epigastric burning pain that occurs one or two hours after eating and is relieved by food or antacids. He has had this discomfort on and off for three weeks. There have been no symptoms of bleeding, vomiting, or diarrhea. His family history is indeterminate, as he was adopted as a baby. His physical examination is normal except for mild epigastric tenderness. His stool is negative for occult blood.

1. What are the diagnostic possibilities?
2. What tests should be ordered?
3. What therapeutic modalities should be employed?

II. The patient becomes symptom free after using the antacids for two weeks. He completes a six-week course, then stops the medication. Six months later he presents with pain that has been present for three days and he states that he has vomited blood that morning. His vital signs are stable, his physical examination is normal, and his stool is black and positive for occult blood.

1. What are the diagnostic possibilities?
2. What tests should be ordered?
3. What therapeutic modalities should be employed?

III. The patient makes an uneventful recovery and completes his eight-week course of therapy. Over the next three years, he has frequent recurrences of the epigastric pain, necessitating seven-times-a-day antacid courses on 10 or 12 different occasions. Two barium upper gastrointestinal x-rays during this period have revealed "active ulcer craters in the duodenum." For the past year he has taken nocturnal cimetidine; this has reduced the frequency of the pain episodes, but they still occur. At the age of 30 he is requesting that "something be done."

1. What are the diagnostic possibilities?
2. What tests should be ordered?
3. What therapeutic modalities should be employed?

Discussion

I. 1. This is a typical case of duodenal ulcer disease. Other diagnostic considerations include erosive gastritis, gastric ulcer, and esophagitis.

2. The patient has no evidence of any complication of ulcer disease. As such it would be appropriate to forego a diagnostic evaluation and begin a "trial of therapy." (See the next question.) If the patient responds and his symptoms disappear, it is unimportant, from a practical point of view, to differentiate the various diagnostic possibilities. The actual diagnosis only becomes important if a more aggressive therapy is entertained, that is, if the symptoms persist or recur on a frequent basis or if a complication ensues. Occasionally a patient may request that a specific diagnosis be established. Under these circumstances an endoscopy or a barium study, or both, could be obtained.

3. The patient can be begun on a course of antacids as previously described in this chapter (seven times per day). The educational process previously described should also be be-

gun. The use of aspirin, caffeine, alcohol, and cigarettes should be discouraged.

II. 1. The most likely source of the upper gastrointestinal bleeding is a peptic ulcer. Some of the other lesions, such as esophagitis and erosive gastritis, may also need to be considered.

2. Since it is important to establish the presence of a bleeding ulcer, because of the future implications of surgical therapy, the patient should undergo endoscopy. If the bleeding stops, however, the endoscopy need not be performed on an emergent basis.

3. The patient should be admitted to the hospital and begun on volume supportive therapy. Ulcer therapy should be begun (nasogastric suction, antacids, or cimetidine). When the bleeding has stopped, the patient should complete an eight-week course of cimetidine. He or she should also have endoscopic confirmation of ulcer healing.

III. 1. The patient has developed intractable ulcer symptoms, in his mind and probably in the physician's. An important consideration in such patients is the possibility of a gastrinoma (Zollinger-Ellison syndrome).

2. Since false-positive barium studies can occur, where the "crater" is actually a deformed region of the bulb, the patient should have endoscopic confirmation of the "intractable ulcer" before surgical therapy. He or she should also be evaluated with a fasting serum gastrin and one-hour basal acid secretory study.

3. If the ulcer is indeed present, the patient appears to have developed aggressive peptic ulcer disease that has failed reasonable medical management. If a gastrinoma is ruled out, he or she should be referred for one of the surgical therapies previously described in this chapter.

12

WILFRED M. WEINSTEIN

Postgastrectomy Syndromes

Most patients do extremely well after operation for peptic ulcer. Many experience some symptoms, but they are usually transient or mild. They include dysphagia (associated with vagotomy), early satiety or postprandial fullness relative to the preoperative state, mild change in bowel habit with more frequent loose stools, inability to tolerate alcohol compared to preoperative intake levels, inability to regain the weight lost in association with surgery, and inability to tolerate certain foods (especially milk) because diarrhea or abdominal pain ensue. These symptoms often improve significantly in the first year after operation or remain mild, and patients do not consult a physician.

At the other end of the spectrum is a small group of patients with intractable symptoms identical to those they had preoperatively. These patients may have had ulcer disease, but after gastric operation it is clear that the ulcer disease was not responsible for their symptoms. This group emphasizes how important it is to select patients for elective surgery carefully to ensure that the operation is not performed for symptoms that are not related to peptic ulcer.

179

Hopefully, the more precise diagnostic capability provided by fiberoptic endoscopy will reduce the numbers of patients with this so-called "albatross syndrome."

After conventional operation for peptic ulcer, 5% to 10% of patients have symptoms of sufficient severity to warrant consultation with a physician. Table 1 outlines the symptoms and syndromes that will be considered. Clear-cut definitions of these symptom complexes are difficult because overlap is frequent. Nevertheless, one group of symptoms generally predominates. The most common categories are those in which symptoms are precipitated by eating.

MULTIPLE POSTPRANDIAL SYMPTOMS

Early Gastrointestinal and Systemic Symptoms

The most common symptom complex is a feeling of early satiety or fullness that occurs during or shortly after a meal. This may be associated with nausea and occasionally with vomiting. Abdominal pain may be an accompaniment, often a crampy or bloated sensa-

Table 1 Side Effects of Operation for Peptic Ulcer

Multiple Postprandial symptoms
    Early
    Late
Predominant pain and/or vomiting
    Defined causes
        Recurrent ulcer
        Mechanical obstruction
        Bezoar
        Afferent loop syndrome
    Ill-defined "causes"
        Nonobstructive delayed emptying
        Reflux gastropathy
Depression and anxiety
Anemia
Diarrhea/malabsorption
Other problems
    Metabolic bone disease
    Gastric cancer

tion. Sometimes the symptoms are followed by lower abdominal cramps, described as "gas pains," and diarrhea. The associated systemic symptoms often include a feeling of weakness, drowsiness, flushing, and sweating. Many patients report that they feel an urge to lie down; while supine, their symptoms are relieved in part. In some patients with these early postprandial symptoms, the gastro-intestinal manifestations predominate, and in others the systemic manifestations predominate.

Multiple factors are operative. These include disturbances in gastric motor function, rapid gastric emptying, and "dumping" of food and fluid into the small bowel. Sometimes patients can identify specific precipitants. These are commonly carbohydrates, especially lactose-containing (dairy products) and sugar-containing foods or fluids.

Investigations are usually not required. The therapeutic approach is to have the patient take frequent small meals, reduce carbohydrate intake, and take liquids between meals rather than with meals. Those with severe systemic symptoms who find it necessary to lie down after meals often avoid eating during working hours. These individuals should ensure adequate nutritional intake during nonworking hours. When early satiety and vomiting are the predominant symptoms, metoclopramide taken orally before major meals may improve symptoms. This drug, which should be available soon in the United States, has a central antinauseant effect and promotes gastric emptying. Its major potential side effects are drowsiness and extrapyramidal symptoms.

Late Postprandial Symptoms

The predominant symptoms are similar to those of hypoglycemia. They generally arise one to three hours after meals and consist of sweating, weakness, and even confusion at times. Treatment is as described for early symptoms. In addition patients often learn on their own that the ingestion of something sweet will terminate an attack.

PREDOMINANT PAIN AND/OR VOMITING

Defined Causes

When pain or vomiting, or both, predominate, investigations must be made to exclude recurrent ulcers, mechanical obstructions at or near anastomoses, bezoars, and the afferent loop syndrome. The abdominal pain that these patients experience may be provoked by eating, may occur between meals, or, in the case of recurrent ulcer, may be partially relieved by eating. With obstruction at or near the anastomosis, the vomiting may occur during or shortly after meals. In the case of the afferent loop syndrome, distention of the loop occurs in response to feeding, and vomiting of bile-stained fluid may occur after a meal. Epigastric tenderness to palpation may be seen in those with recurrent ulcers. In the afferent loop syndrome, distention may be visible. However, physical examination is often not helpful in the differential diagnosis.

These patients should be referred for an evaluation, which must include barium x-ray and endoscopy. Barium x-ray is done to rule out obstruction and the endoscopy is performed primarily to rule out recurrent ulceration.

Recurrent ulcers often respond to cimetidine therapy. Antacids are ineffective because they empty too rapidly. If cimetidine is used, healing should be documented with follow-up endoscopy. Operation is often necessary if ulcers recur promptly after a course of cimetidine. The surgeon often finds that a purported previous vagotomy was incomplete. For the elderly and infirm, maintenance cimetidine may be the most useful option. Mechanical obstruction at or near the anastomosis and the rare afferent loop syndrome require reoperation. Bezoars usually respond to enzymatic dissolution and direct-vision "break up" at endoscopy.

Ill-Defined "Causes"

When no clearly defined cause as already outlined is found, nonobstructive delayed emptying is often invoked. This seems especially true for those with recurrent bezoars. These patients are advised to take a low-fiber diet and metoclopramide is used; this helps some patients.

In other patients, especially those with predominant abdominal pain, the term "reflux gastritis" is often applied. The presumption is that reflux of duodenal contents into the stomach results in the pain and vomiting. Unfortunately, there is no specific way to make the diagnosis of this syndrome. Gastritis is a misnomer here because most patients (asymptomatic) develop nonerosive gastritis in the gastric remnant after antrectomy and vagotomy. Furthermore, endoscopic color changes are no more abnormal in these patients than in asymptomatic patients who have had similar operations. Therefore, reflux gastropathy is a clinical diagnosis of exclusion and reflects our ignorance concerning the pathogenesis. Various empiric trials with antacids, bile salt binding agents such as Metamucil and cholestyramine, and metoclopramide are used with unpredictable and variable success. In desperate situations we sometimes recommend operation to divert the bile and pancreatic juice further downstream away from the gastric remnant (the Roux-en-Y procedure). As with medical therapy, the results are unpredictable. Some patients improve, some do not; we cannot predict who will respond.

DEPRESSION AND ANXIETY

When no remedy can be found for those with the severe symptoms already described, major psychiatric problems may develop. It is important to be aware of this and to refer the patients for evaluation and therapy before the reactive depression and anxiety become dominant in the patient's symptom complex. For those with less severe symptoms who are able to cope, common sense support usually suffices.

ANEMIA

Iron deficiency anemia is the most common type of anemia found in those with postgastrectomy syndromes, and the most common reason it occurs is failure to replenish iron stores after operation. Many of these patients have had surgery for bleeding from peptic ulcer and they leave the hospital with inadequate iron stores. Their problem is further compounded by the fact that iron absorption is probably reduced after operation for peptic ulcer. When a patient with iron deficiency is evaluated after ulcer surgery, one must bear in mind that the iron deficiency may be unrelated to the ulcer operation. Therefore, the patient should be investigated as would any other patient for iron deficiency anemia; then, if no cause is found, the iron deficiency anemia can be attributed to the ulcer surgery.

Vitamin B_{12} malabsorption is much less common after gastric surgery and is usually due to bacterial overgrowth. Folic acid deficiency is the least common type of anemia; when it occurs, it is usually in patients with Billroth II anastomoses. Vitamin B_{12} and folic acid deficiency are usually late developments after gastric surgery.

Therapy of the anemia is straightforward. It includes replacement and follow-up study to ensure that it has been corrected.

DIARRHEA/MALABSORPTION

As mentioned previously, many patients have more frequent and less-formed stools after operation for peptic ulcer. Sometimes severe diarrhea occurs immediately after surgery and persists; this has been referred to as "postvagotomy diarrhea." If the diarrhea is unaccompanied by malabsorption with weight loss, two therapeutic trials can be instituted before one makes a decision concerning referral for more detailed investigation. The first is to eliminate dairy products from the diet because relative lactase deficiency may have been unmasked by surgery. In other words, more rapid gastric emptying and transit through the proximal small bowel do not provide sufficient contact time to promote normal absorption of lactose. When this occurs, patients may have diarrhea and flatulence. A prolonged trial is not required; there should be a prompt improvement in symptoms within 24 to 48 hours if relative lactase deficiency is the main cause of the patient's diarrhea. If dairy product withdrawal fails, an empiric 10-day trial of a broad-spectrum antibiotic such as tetracycline can be employed as a diagnostic-therapeutic test for bacterial overgrowth.

Mild malabsorption with slightly elevated fecal fat output is common and goes unnoticed. However, if patients have diarrhea with continuing weight loss or marked hyperphagia, they should be referred for further evaluation. Investigations may reveal related causes such as severe bacterial overgrowth, or, more rarely, unmasked celiac sprue, or pancreatic enzyme maldigestion due to poor mixing. In some patients, an unrelated cause of the malabsorption syndrome may be detected.

If no cause is found after a thorough investigation, a trial with cholestyramine or an antidiarrheal agent may be recommended for the patient with diarrhea without significant fat malabsorption (steatorrhea). Nutritional deficiencies will require supplements. In the patient with severe steatorrhea, a low-fat diet may help to control symptoms.

OTHER PROBLEMS

Metabolic Bone Disease

Fortunately, the late complication of metabolic bone disease is rare. It may be detected incidentally, as a presentation with bone pain or fractures, or in the course of an investigation for malabsorption after gastric surgery. It should not be presumed that the bone disease is due to a previous ulcer operation performed many years ago. These patients require referral for a workup of their metabolic bone disease.

Gastric Cancer

There is a slight but definite increased risk of cancer in the gastric remnant, beginning 15 years after antrectomy and Billroth I or II anastomoses. As yet there is no simple way to identify the tiny subgroup of these patients in whom cancers will develop. At present, opinion is divided concerning how intense surveillance and follow-up study should be.

HOW SHOULD THE PATIENT BE FOLLOWED AFTER SURGERY FOR PEPTIC ULCER?

The importance of adequate nutrition should be stressed. Patients should be seen at one year to check for anemia. Thereafter the frequency of follow-up study may be every two to four years, depending on the patient's age. Patients should be told to report any unexplained weight loss or change in stool color, which are symptoms of malabsorption. They should not be burdened with a list of all of the possible late complications.

SUMMARY AND PERSPECTIVE

After conventional operation for peptic ulcer, a host of symptoms may develop. They are only troublesome in 5% to 10% of patients. The most common symptoms after gastric surgery can often be ameliorated with simple dietary maneuvers.

Those individuals with prominent pain and vomiting syndromes should have certain remediable conditions ruled out. A small subset of patients continue to have a myriad of postoperative complaints that are refractory to empiric therapy even after thorough investigation. One should be on the alert for signs of anemia or malabsorption because these are treatable.

In the United States the frequency of ulcer surgery is declining. This, coupled with the increasing use of the proximal gastric vagotomy, will hopefully result in many fewer patients with the symptoms and syndromes described here.

SELECTED READING

Herman RH: Postgastrectomy malnutrition syndromes. *Practical Gastroenterol* 4:45–49, 1980.

Meyer JH: Chronic morbidity after ulcer surgery, in Sleisenger MH, Fordtran JS (eds): *Gastrointestinal Disease*. Philadelphia, WB Saunders Co, 1978, pp 947–968.

Spiro HM: Postgastrectomy and postvagotomy syndromes, in Spiro HM (ed): *Clinical Gastroenterology*. New York, MacMillan Publishing Co, 1977, pp 369–391.

CLINICAL PROBLEMS

I. A 47-year-old man undergoes a truncal vagotomy, antrectomy, and Billroth I anastomosis for duodenal ulcer disease. He makes a seemingly uneventful recovery, but comes to the physician's office two weeks after the operation with complaints of postprandial dizziness and weakness. Ever since the operation, he has had to lie down immediately after the meal. He can resume his normal activities a half-hour later, but sweating and fatigue often develop one or two hours afterward. He is especially likely to have these problems if he eats sweet foods.

1. What problem is the patient experiencing?
2. What diagnostic tests should be pursued?
3. What therapeutic measures can be tried?

II. A 55-year-old woman with a history of recurrent ulcer disease undergoes an antrectomy, truncal vagotomy, and Billroth II anastomosis. One year later she comes to the physician with complaints of episodic epigastric abdominal pain that has been occurring for the past three months, often after eating. Although the pain is very similar to her ulcer pain, it is only minimally improved now with antacids.

1. What problem is the patient experiencing?
2. What diagnostic tests should be pursued?
3. What therapeutic measures can be tried?

III. A 72-year-old man is seen for a routine physical examination. He has been well all of his life except for a bleeding ulcer, for which he had part of his stomach removed 24 years ago. He has had no recent change in weight, although he weighs 10 pounds less than he did before his operation. His physical examination is unremarkable and his stool is negative for occult blood. His hemoglobin concentration is 9.7 gm%.

1. What problem is the patient experiencing?
2. What diagnostic tests should be pursued?
3. What therapeutic measures can be tried?

Discussion

I. 1. The patient is describing both early and late postprandial symptoms arising as a consequence of the altered emptying pattern of his stomach. These are common variants of the "dumping" syndrome. The early urge to lie down may be due to a relative hypovolemia from the intestinal release of vasodilatory substances and the intraluminal collection of fluid. The later diaphoresis and fatigue result from a reactive hypoglycemia.

2. Although one could perform glucose tolerance tests and measure blood pressures with the patient in the supine and

erect positions in the postprandial period, from a practical point of view the history establishes the diagnosis.

3. The patient should be advised to consume small frequent meals, separating his liquid and solid food ingestion by one to two hours. He should reduce his intake of high-carbohydrate foods and liquids. If he is unable to eat at work, care should be taken that an adequate diet is consumed over the day. He should be reassured that many of these symptoms will probably improve in the next year.

II. 1. Postgastrectomy pain may be due to a number of disorders, as previously discussed. The chief considerations are a recurrent ulcer, a mechanical obstruction (near the anastomosis), bezoars, and the afferent loop syndrome. The more ill-defined lesions of delayed emptying and reflux gastropathy should also be considered. Of course, the patient may have some nongastric source of the pain as well.

2. The diagnostic evaluation in these patients centers around endoscopic evaluation, although a barium upper gastrointestinal series is often also obtained before this more invasive procedure. Such patients will usually require gastroenterologic consultation.

3. The therapy clearly depends on the cause of the pain. Recurrent ulcers should be treated with cimetidine; failure to heal or prompt recurrence usually necessitates surgical intervention. The other "defined causes" will also require surgical or endoscopic therapy. Reflux gastropathy and delayed gastric emptying may or may not respond to the variety of measures described previously. These should be undertaken with gastroenterologic consultation and guidance.

III. 1. Postgastrectomy anemia is commonly seen many years after the operation. Most commonly it is due to iron deficiency, although vitamin B_{12}, and even folate, deficiencies are seen. Other causes for anemia should also be sought.

2. The patient should undergo the standard anemia workup, with special attention paid to the nutritional factors (iron, vitamin B_{12}, and folate). If iron deficiency is found, the patient should be evaluated carefully for the various causes.

3. If the anemia is in fact due to the lack of one or another of the various nutritional factors, it (they) should be replaced.

13

MARVIN DEREZIN

Inflammatory Bowel Disease

The term "inflammatory bowel disease" technically encompasses any disease of the intestinal tract in which an inflammatory response occurs. These disorders include infectious processes, ischemic enteritis, and damage due to toxins or physical agents in addition to the two diseases that gastroenterologists think of when the term is mentioned. Since the other conditions are either discussed elsewhere, or are beyond the scope of this book, this chapter will deal only with ulcerative colitis and Crohn's disease. In order to understand some of the aspects of diagnosis and management, differences in the pathophysiology of these two should be appreciated. The etiology of both diseases is unknown.

Ulcerative colitis is a mucosal disease of the colon with the inflammatory process beginning in the rectum and remaining within the superficial layers of the colon. The disease extends in continuity around the bowel, involving part or all of the colon. In some cases the terminal ileum may be involved by an ulcerative process similar to that of the colon. The term "backwash" ileitis has been used to describe this abnormality and seems to be a toxic manifestation of the diseased colon, since quieting of the inflamed colon or colectomy will result in healing of the ileum. Thus, for practical purposes ulcerative colitis can be considered a disease localized in the colon.

Crohn's disease is an indolent inflammatory process that begins in the submucosa of the intestine and extends both toward the lumen and the serosa. The microscopic findings include round-cell inflammation, scarring, and thickening with narrowing of the lumen and an inflammatory response extending to the local lymph nodes. Deep fissures can occur from mucosa to serosa. The fissures may then extend into other loops of uninvolved intestine to become fistulas or may extend locally forming irregular "Swiss cheese" abscesses. The fissures and ulcerations lead to cobblestoning of the mucosa. Granulomas may be present within the inflammatory response of the intestine and local lymph nodes. Extensive undermining perianal fistulas are common with Crohn's disease.

While ulcerative colitis is limited to the colon, Crohn's disease may involve many parts of the gastrointestinal tract from the mouth through to the anus. The most common areas involved are the terminal eight to 10 inches of ileum and the right colon. Other segments involved less frequently include the jejunum, duodenum, stomach, esophagus, and pharynx. Characteristics of this mysterious inflammatory disorder is the segmental involvement of intestine with normal areas of bowel between diseased portions. "Skip area" is the term used for these normal areas of bowel. Just as segments of bowel are involved, portions of the circumference of the bowel may also be diseased while the opposite wall may be spared, giving the eccentric appearance on x-ray that is one of the characteristics of this disease.

HOW DO I MAKE THE DIAGNOSIS?

There are two aspects to establishing the diagnosis. The first is to determine whether any inflammatory bowel disease is present. If so, then one must specifically identify the entity; in particular, for purposes of this chapter, one must differentiate ulcerative colitis and Crohn's disease.

The most common manifestation of these diseases is diarrhea. The earlier chapter on diarrhea discussed identifying these processes as a result of damaged mucosa (inflammatory bowel disease), and this material need not be repeated here.

Ulcerative colitis and Crohn's disease usually appear in patients between the ages of 20 and 40; some cases appear earlier or later. The symptoms and clinical presentation depend on the length of intestine involved and the severity of the inflammatory process. A patient with a 10-cm segment of ulcerative proctitis may have at most two to three loose stools a day with tenesmus and bleeding without any systemic symptoms. However, a patient with a severe inflammatory response involving large segments of intestine may complain of severe diarrhea associated with cramping abdominal pain, weight loss, anorexia, fever, and fatigue. The diarrhea in Crohn's disease is frequently mild, consisting of five to six soft bowel movements scattered throughout the day associated with cramping, periumbilical, or right lower quadrant pain. Blood in the stool is less frequent in the diarrhea of Crohn's disease than in ulcerative colitis. However, when the colon is primarily involved in either disease, the patient may be distressed by severe diarrhea consisting of 10 to 20 stools a day with cramping abdominal pain and tenesmus.

During the initial evaluation, the patient is qustioned about previous attacks of diarrhea. A family history of ulcerative colitis or Crohn's disease is present in many patients with these disorders. A valuable clue to the presence of inflammatory bowel disease is the existence of extraintestinal manifestations, which occur in two percent to five percent of patients. (See Table 1 and the section on complications.)

Physical findings will depend on the severity and the chronicity of the inflammatory response and may include evidence of weight loss, pallor, and the edema of hypoproteinemia. Aphthous ulcers may be present in the mouth. The abdomen is usually flat without distention. There is frequently tenderness along the colon without rebound tenderness. If diffuse tenderness with rebound is found, the patient may be in a phase of fulminating enteritis, which requires urgent attention.

External examination of the anal area may reveal indurated fistulas with reddened, thick overhanging edges and abscesses. Digital examination may be normal despite extensive mucosal disease. In some instances it may reveal a tender mass that was not felt on abdominal examination.

Hepatic
  Fatty liver
  Hepatitis
    Acute (posttransfusion)
    Chronic (chronic active hepatitis)
  Pericholangitis
  Sclerosing cholangitis
  Biliary tree carcinoma
  Gallstones
  Amyloidosis
Renal
  Pyelonephritis
  Renal calculi
Skin
  Erythema nodosum
  Pyoderma gangrenosum
Arthritis (including ankylosing spondylitis)
Ocular
  Uveitis
  Episcleritis
Others
  Anemia
  Thromboembolic disease

If the terminal ileum is specifically involved (Crohn's disease), abdominal examination will frequently reveal a sausage-shaped, very tender mass in the right lower quadrant. Sometimes it will be freely movable and sometimes, if involved by abscess or bound down, it will be fixed. If the inflammatory mass is involved with an abscess, there may be very high fever with reddening of the skin above the mass and exquisite tenderness. Findings of associated obstruction would include distention, tympany, and hyperactive bowel sounds.

Just as in the initial evaluation for any patient with prolonged diarrhea, sigmoidoscopy is performed with the collection of a fresh stool specimen for white cells, bacterial culture, and study for amoebas. Sigmoidoscopy is performed without preparation, since the diarrhea usually cleanses the rectum enough to see the mucosal process in its natural state. Enemas cause artifacts and increased friability, making the examination inaccurate.

The appearance of the acutely inflamed mucosa of ulcerative colitis and Crohn's disease is similar to the maternal side of the placenta, with redness, granularity, and friability separated by ulcerations and yellow exudate. Swabbing will result in profuse oozing. When the acute process subsides, the mucosa will look edematous or reddened with loss of normal vascularity; rubbing with a swab will cause multiple pinpoint areas of oozing.

Since Crohn's disease does not necessarily involve the rectum, sigmoidoscopy may be totally normal or reveal tiny, 1-mm to 2-mm red ulcers with surrounding erythema in an otherwise normal-appearing colon. Biopsy of these discrete isolated ulcerations frequently reveals inflammation and granulomas. When it does involve the rectum, the findings may be indistinguishable from ulcerative colitis with the mucosal lining appearing friable, oozing blood and purulent material.

The rectal response to all inflammatory diseases is often very similar and, therefore, very difficult to differentiate. Ulcerative colitis, Crohn's disease, amebiasis, and shigellosis all can appear similar. Thus, the differential diagnosis is made by culturing the stool for bacterial pathogens and aspiration of fresh stool and exudate for amoebas. Biopsies are helpful in the acute stage to search for amoebas but rarely differentiate Crohn's disease from ulcerative colitis. Rectal biopsy is helpful for patients who have mild diarrhea and normal sigmoidoscopy, since microscopic inflammation may sometimes suggest a more proximal inflammatory bowel disorder.

Colonoscopy is contraindicated in patients who have active bowel inflammation for fear of perforation, worsening the active disease, or stimulating toxic megacolon with air insufflation. During the quiescent phase, however, endoscopy will define the areas of involvement in the colon more precisely than does radiography. (At this point, however, the clinical implications of this more accurate assessment are unknown; knowledge of prognostic and therapeutic parameters have all been based on radiographic monitoring.)

Barium enema is contraindicated for the same reasons in patients with severe active disease. However, a barium enema performed when the patient is stable and not having severe diarrhea or

Table 2 Comparison of Crohn's Disease and Ulcerative Colitis

	Crohn's Disease	Ulcerative Colitis
Clinical manifestation		
Diarrhea	Present	Present
Hematochezia	Usually absent	Usually present
Extraintestinal complications	May be present	May be present
Perirectal disease	Complicated fistulas, abscesses in addition to fissures or hemorrhoids	Fissures, hemorrhoids
Rectal disease (sigmoidoscopic)	Often absent	Present
Radiographic		
Small intestine	Involved (bowel ulcerated, narrowed)	Not involved (except "backwash ileitis," in which ileum is dilated)
Continuity of involvement	Skip areas	Continuous
Ulceration	Deep with fissures, submucosal undermining	Superficial
Strictures	Present	Uncommon
Symmetry of involvement	Often asymmetrical	Usually symmetrical
Enteric fistula	Present	Absent
Pathologic		
Granuloma	Often present	Absent
Crypt abscesses	Present	Present
Transmural disease	Present	Absent
Pseudopolyps	Absent	Present

toxicity will be very helpful for diagnosis and therapeutic considerations. Areas of disease with skip areas of normal bowel and eccentric involvement of the lumen suggest Crohn's disease. Reflux into the terminal ileum frequently makes the diagnosis of ileal Crohn's disease.

Radiographic examinations of the upper gastrointestinal tract (stomach and small intestine) are also useful in these two inflammatory bowel diseases. With the exception of the previously described backwash ileitis, small-intestinal disease is not seen in ulcerative colitis. The radiographic demonstration of ulcerated, strictured jejunum or ileum excludes its diagnosis. Furthermore, the upper gastrointestinal series with small-bowel follow-through more precisely describes the total intestinal involvement in Crohn's disease than does the barium enema alone. During the active inflammation, a small-bowel series following the barium to the rectum may add information and not activate the disease. However, in most acute inflammatory bowel disease, this diagnostic step is not necessary.

Laboratory studies are usually nonspecific. They may reveal anemia (due to chronic disease and iron deficiency), hypoalbuminemia, and liver abnormalities. During acute exacerbations, leukocytosis and an elevated erythrocyte sedimentation rate are common.

Differentiating Crohn's disease and ulcerative colitis is usually not a problem. However, at times (especially when the Crohn's disease is limited only to the colon) this differentiation is more difficult. Since certain management decisions depend on which disease is present, this differentiation is important. The two diseases are compared in Table 2. (It should be noted that, in about 10% to 20% of patients with only colonic involvement, this differentiation cannot be made.)

WHAT ADDITIONAL WORKUP DOES THE PATIENT REQUIRE?

A number of processes can produce an acute colitis (Table 3). In particular, infectious diseases such as amebiasis, shigellosis, and *Campylobacter* must be considered. In these diseases the onset is abrupt and frequently friends or family will have had similar symptoms beginning at the same time in a less intense fashion. Thus, patients with acute flare-ups of their illnesses (especially those in whom

Table 3 Diagnostic Considerations in Patients With Acute Colitis

Ulcerative colitis

Crohn's disease

Infectious colitis (amebiasis, shigellosis, *Campylobacter*)

Pseudomembranous colitis (postantibiotic)

Radiation colitis

Ischemic colitis

a previous diagnosis of ulcerative colitis or Crohn's disease has not been established) should have stool examinations and cultures performed for these infectious agents. Serologic tests for amebiasis should also be obtained.

Postantibiotic diarrhea may also be associated with an inflammatory process (pseudomembranous colitis); the diarrhea may persist for weeks after the antibiotic has been stopped. The drug that produces this syndrome most commonly is clindamycin, although almost all of the broad-spectrum antibiotics taken orally have been implicated. The toxin of an anaerobic organism, *Clostridium difficile,* has been thought to be responsible for this process, and techniques are available to identify both the organism and the toxin in the stool.

Most commonly Crohn's disease is located in the terminal ileum and ascending colon. Other diseases can also be found in this anatomic distribution; they are listed in Table 4. The differentiation of Crohn's disease can usually be accomplished on clinical grounds.

HOW SHOULD I TREAT THE PATIENT?

The specific therapeutic approach to ulcerative colitis and Crohn's disease is different, and each disease will be discussed

Table 4 **Diseases Involving the Terminal Ileum and Ascending Colon**

Crohn's disease

Infectious
    Tuberculosis
    Fungi (especially actinomycosis)

Malignancy
    Cecal carcinoma
    Lymphoma
    Carcinoid

Radiation

Appendiceal abscess

Ischemic enteritis

separately. However, certain principles that are common to the management of both maladies should be touched upon briefly.

Analgesics, antidiarrheal agents, and anticholinergics are avoided if possible, since they mask response to therapy and, if used in high doses, may precipitate toxic megacolon. When used for prolonged periods of time, they become less effective. However, if the patient is improving and the diarrhea is annoying and interfering with rest, small doses of Lomotil or Imodium may be used sparingly.

Lactose intolerance is commonly seen in both diseases; milk products may be added to the diet if they do not cause an exacerbation of the diarrhea. Each patient should be specifically questioned about this potential problem.

The clinical course of Crohn's disease and ulcerative colitis is extremely variable, making prediction of recurrences and the need for operation impossible. Each patient must be approached as having a unique problem. In urban areas there are many patients with inflammatory bowel disease who can share their frustrations concerning the course and relative incurability of these diseases. The National Foundation for Ileitis and Colitis, Inc. (NFIC) has chapters in most populated areas and is helpful for those patients who would like to discuss their troubles with people who are similarly affected and to gather information about the diseases themselves.

Ulcerative Colitis

Exacerbation of ulcerative colitis has been classified, on the basis of clinical presentation, into categories of mild, moderate, and severe. The details of this classification are enumerated in Table 5. Prognostic and therapeutic decisions can be generalized from the severity of the attack.

In patients with ulcerative colitis, mild disease is the most common form seen. Such patients are usually bothered only by diarrhea (with or without blood) and do not require hospitalization. The disease can be treated with enteric-coated sulfasalazine (Azulfidine) as a dose of 1 to 2 gm four times a day with food. This drug is a combination of a poorly absorbed sulfa drug and aspirin. Common side effects include anorexia, nausea, headache, and abdominal pain. In susceptible individuals allergic reactions, hemolysis, and leukopenia may occur rarely. The side effects seem to be lessened

Table 5   Classification of Attacks of Ulcerative Colitis[a]

Symptom	Mild	Moderate	Severe
Fever	−	±	+
Tachycardia	−	±	+
Weight loss	−	±	+
Anorexia	−	±	+
Abdominal cramps	−	+	+
Frequency of stool	< 4	4–6	> 6
Hematochezia	±	+	+
Tenesmus	±	±	+
Anemia	−	±	+
Leukocytosis	−	±	+
Hypoalbuminemia	−	−	+

[a] −, absent; ±, sometimes present; +, usually seen.

if the drug is started with 0.5 gm four times a day with meals and is gradually increased to 8 gm a day or up to the level of intolerance. At least one to two weeks would seem to be the minimal time to wait for a response. Between attacks, a maintenance dose of 2 gm a day should be given in an attempt to reduce the frequency of disease relapse. Steroid therapy is usually not necessary.

In patients with ulcerative colitis, severe disease is the least common form seen, but it is the most dramatic clinically. These patients are seen with fulminant disease and obviously require hospitalization. They are usually treated initially with steroids and supportive measures. It is important to remember that, if such therapy does not have any effect after a few days, operation (total colectomy) should be undertaken. Delaying surgery will increase overall mortality.

The major therapeutic decisions therefore arise in the patients with moderate disease. The decision to hospitalize depends primarily on the patient's toxicity and debilitation. Often other considerations must also play a role (e.g., whether the home or hospital environment is more stressful).

If the patient is hospitalized, it is most important that there are toilet facilities in very close proximity. Accidents are common and morally devastating. Both physical and mental rest is essential and the hospital staff must make all attempts to keep visits by personnel and family to a minimum, as well as judiciously scheduling diagnostic studies.

Immediate relief usually follows the administration of intravenous fluids and discontinuance of oral intake. Corticosteroids are begun at an average dose of 100 mg of hydrocortisone intravenously every eight hours. Some believe that adrenocorticotropic hormone (ACTH) given intravenously is more effective than hydrocortisone. However, there does not seem to be any objective evidence to support that contention. Since these patients are often debilitated, it is better to rely on exogenous hydrocortisone than to depend on the adrenal response to ACTH.

Many physicians administer broad-spectrum antibiotics although there is no scientific evidence to support their use. It is postulated that the severely ulcerated colon becomes available for invasion by coliform bacteria that constantly bathe the denuded mucosa. Ampicillin, 1 gm every four hours, or one of the cephalosporin drugs may be used.

If the patient is very malnourished, peripheral hyperalimentation may be started. If the intravenous route is required for a long period of time, total parenteral nutrition through a central venous line may be very beneficial in some patients.

Signs of improvement include the return of a sense of well-being, a decrease in fatigue, and an increase in appetite with a decrease in number of diarrheal stools. There is a decrease in fever and tachycardia as dehydration is corrected and toxicity improves. The abdominal examination will reveal less tenderness. Improvement as seen through the sigmoidoscope takes a long period of time and, therefore, is of limited usefulness during the acute phase.

When the clinical findings of significant improvement occur, oral feedings are resumed with mild liquids such as broths and teas. The consistency and quantity of food are increased gradually if the symptoms do not worsen. As the diet is increased, milk and milk products are avoided, for some patients seem to do better without them. Until the patient has totally improved or has reached a plateau, residue is avoided in the diet and then is gradually increased to the patient's liking.

When the intravenous route is removed, antibiotics are usually discontinued and prednisone is begun at 40 to 60 mg as a single morning dose. Later, as the prednisone is tapered, sulfasalazine, 0.5 gm to 1 gm four times a day with food, may be initiated. Lomotil, 1 or 2 tablets four times a day, may be useful to diminish the diarrhea, but should be used cautiously.

If, instead of improving, the patient shows signs of deterioration (a rising fever, tachycardia, or a worsening of diarrhea or pain), repeated evaluations are necessary to detect the appearance of toxic megacolon. Abdominal examination in these patients will reveal distention with the appearance of diffuse and rebound tenderness. As atony develops in the paralyzed and thinned bowel wall, there may be a paradoxic decrease in the amount of diarrhea. Evidence of volume depletion resulting from third spacing in the colon will be reflected by tachycardia and decreasing blood pressure. Leukocytosis will worsen and abdominal flat films will show progressive distention of the transverse colon. Unless there is immediate and careful resuscitative medical therapy followed by early surgical intervention, the disease will lead to continued thinning of the bowel wall with microperforations, peritonitis, sepsis, and, most frequently, death.

The physician and surgeon working closely together will decide on an optimum time for operation, which preferably would include a total proctocolectomy and ileostomy. For those patients who are too severely ill for these procedures, segmental colostomies and ileostomy may be a temporary life-saving procedure. The choice of operation will rest on the surgeon's judgment during surgery.

During the hospitalization, conferences with the patient's family and friends are necessary to determine the emotional impact of the disease. Currently, there is no evidence that ulcerative colitis is caused by emotional unrest; however, when the patient's disease is active, emotional stresses can aggravate the symptoms. When the disease is quiescent, if it is appropriate, a psychiatrist familiar with inflammatory bowel disease may evaluate the patient for ongoing psychotherapy. During the acute illness, emotional support usually comes from the staff taking care of the patient and, if possible, from family and friends. If necessary, however, care by a gentle psychiatrist may be invaluable during the acute period. As the patient recovers it is essential that the treating physician evaluate with the patient stresses from the environment as well as internal problems that may contribute to activation of the disease. Continuing psychological care, if done carefully, may help not only the disease itself but the patient's adjustment to the illness.

As recovery continues at home, physical activity is increased and work is resumed in a gradual manner. The dosage of prednisone is then tapered by approximately 5 mg every four to seven days. The drug is totally discontinued or stopped at a level above which symptoms recur. Too rapid a withdrawal of steroids almost invariably results in a rebound of activity of the inflammatory disease. Many patients with ulcerative colitis will reach a dose of prednisone somewhere between 10 and 20 mg and seem to be unable to taper the drug any further, requiring long periods of low-dose therapy. Ideally, the drug is eventually discontinued totally since there is no evidence that steroids prevent either recurrences of activity or the need for operation. On the other hand, sulfasalazine (2 gm a day) taken chronically is of value in preventing recurrent attacks, and thus could be continued indefinitely if the drug is well tolerated.

The asymptomatic patient with ulcerative colitis is advised to report any exacerbation as soon as symptoms occur. (These are usually manifested as cramping abdominal pain and diarrhea with or without blood.) Frequently, outpatient management is possible. A short period of rest at home with high-dose steroids (approximately 40 to 60 mg of prednisone a day) may rapidly bring an attack under control. Some patients will respond to prednisone, 20 mg a day, with sulfasalazine, 2 gm a day. The type of response frequently helps predict what methods will be required to control the next attack. (A successful program may be reemployed in future exacerbations.) After the disease has diminished and stabilized, the drugs are again tapered slowly as previously described.

If the disease is localized to the left side of the colon, oral steroids sometimes may be avoided by the use of the cortisone enema preparations (Cortenema). These solutions contain 100 mg of hydrocortisone and are optimally administered gently and slowly at room temperature (so as not to induce cramps) with the patient in the left lateral position. After removal of the nozzle, the patient remains in a lying position and changes from side to side attempting not to expel the contents. Barium studies have shown that these preparations may rise as high as the left colon exerting the topical steroid effect. The instillation may be given twice a day. For the enemas to be optimally effective, the solution should be administered when the patient can stay in a flat position moving gently from side to side for at least 20 to 30 minutes.

A variable amount of systemic steroid effect may occur because of absorption of hydrocortisone through the inflamed mucosa. A nonabsorbable steroid preparation, methylprednisolone acetate (Medrol), which is administered at a dose of 40 mg twice a day, has the same topical effect as the hydrocortisone preparation but without systemic absorption. The expense of the topical steroid solutions can sometimes be offset by the preparation of large quantities of hydrocortisone acetate solution by hospital or local pharmacies.

Ulcerative proctitis is almost a separate disease entity from ulcerative colitis in that the distal 10 to 15 cm of the rectum is involved, with more proximal extension of disease occurring only rarely. The symptoms include cramps, tenesmus, and four to six stools a day that, for the most part, include small amounts of fecal material mixed with a varying amount of mucus, pus, and blood. If spasm from inflammation is severe, the stool will be narrowed. Proctoscopic examination demonstrates the usual changes of ulcerative colitis with a clear demarcation between diseased mucosa and normal mucosa. These patients are to avoid constipation with the use of residue and Metamucil if needed. Irritation by a hard firm stool will usually make the small rim of inflamed tissue bleed. Sulfasalazine, at the same dosages as for ulcerative colitis, frequently controls the illness. If not, patients do very well with steroid enemas or the foam preparations (Cortifoam and Proctocort), which supply hydrocortisone by aerosol spray into the distal 10 to 15 cm of rectum. If the involvement includes a thin rim 1 to 2 cm above the anal verge, hydrocortisone suppositories can be helpful. This is a local disease without complications.

A total colectomy and ileostomy are curative for ulcerative colitis. This operation is reserved for those patients whose lives are miserable, despite intensive and careful follow-up therapy. Early in the course of ulcerative colitis, this option should be referred to in a gentle manner, although most patients, by the time they reach the doctor's office, are quite aware of this "way out." The decision must be made by both the patient and the physician after extensive talks and visits from representatives of the local ostomy societies. The emotional consequences can be devastating unless the patients are prepared; if they are, the beneficial response is astounding. Besides the emotional complications, the other untoward side effect of the surgery is male impotence (related to sacral nerve dissection). This occurs only rarely, however.

Recently the Kock pouch, or continent ileostomy, has become available for patients with ulcerative colitis. The small bowel is fashioned into a pouch so that the contents are periodically emptied by placing a cannula into the pouch opening on the abdominal wall. Appliances are unnecessary. This new technique avoids many of the aesthetic and emotional objections of wearing a bag that is constantly filled with stool. However, even for those patients who have a standard ileostomy, the appliances are so well fitting and odor proof that normal daily activities (including sex) and even physical exertion and sports are possible.

Crohn's Disease

Crohn's disease manifests itself over a wide spectrum of clinical activity. The symptoms and signs may be due to the bowel inflammation per se or to one of a number of complications. In fact, the symptoms are sometimes due to a combination of both. This section will deal with the treatment of the inflammatory disease; the complications and their management will be discussed later in this chapter.

In the past few years it has become fashionable to attempt to quantitate the degree of activity of Crohn's disease. The best known of these scales, the Crohn's Disease Activity Index, is described in Table 6. This scale can be used to assess active inflammation, and serial quantitations can even be used to demonstrate response to therapy.

The same agents used in ulcerative colitis, sulfasalazine and steroids, are also used in exacerbations of Crohn's disease. Steroids may be particularly useful in small-intestinal disease, whereas sulfasalazine may be more efficacious when colonic disease is present.

Patients whose symptoms are not debilitating can frequently be managed as outpatients. Since the disease often produces narrowing of the intestinal lumen, high-residue foods, in addition to lactose-containing ones, should be withheld. Sulfasalazine can be used in the same regimen as described for ulcerative colitis. If an inadequate response occurs, prednisone can then be tried, beginning with 40 mg as a single morning dose. The sulfasalazine may be continued or, if there clearly was no response at all (and especially if only small-bowel disease exists), it may be stopped. The 30%

Table 6   **Crohn's Disease Activity Index (CDAI)**[a]

Clinical Item	Multiplication Factor
Number soft/liquid stools in preceding week	2
Sum of abdominal pain rating for each day in preceding week (0 = none, 1 = mild, 2 = moderate, 3 = severe)	5
Sum of rating for well being for each day in preceding week (0 = well, 1 = slightly below par, 2 = poor, 3 = very poor, 4 = terrible)	7
Complications of Crohn's disease present (count 1 for each of arthritis or arthralgia, skin or oral lesions, iritis or uveitis, active perirectal disease, fistula, fever > 100 F)	20
Use of opiate antidiarrheal agent (0 = no, 1 = yes)	30
Abdominal mass (0 = absent, 2 = questionable, 5 = present)	10
Hematocrit (males = 47-actual hematocrit, females = 42-actual hematocrit)	6
Body weight: $100 \left(1 - \dfrac{\text{body weight}}{\text{standard weight}}\right)$	1

[a] The CDAI is calculated by computing the number for each clinical item, multiplying it by the multiplication factor for that item, and then adding these eight products together. The higher the CDAI, the more active the disease. An index of greater than 150 indicates active inflammatory disease.

placebo effect that is seen with any type of treatment for many organic diseases must always be considered in evaluation of response to therapy. Prednisone should be held off as long as possible.

When there is objective improvement that stabilizes for a while, the dose of prednisone may then be tapered. Improvement includes the return of a sense of well-being; lessening of pain, diarrhea, and fever; and the return of appetite and weight gain. Physical examination will confirm the subjective symptoms while laboratory data will show an increase in the hemoglobin as well as the albumin if initially lowered.

The tapering of prednisone is best done slowly, with the dosage diminished by 2.5 or 5 mg every four to seven days. The goal is to eventually discontinue the prednisone entirely, for there is no current evidence that long-term steroid or sulfasalazine treatment will prevent either the natural recurrences of Crohn's disease or the need for operation. It is, however, a frequent clinical observation that, once steroids have been started, they can be withdrawn totally only with difficulty. It is often necessary to continue low dosages (in the range of 5 to 10 mg of prednisone per day) for long periods of time.

Patients with severe active disease manifested by fever and debilitation are treated with bowel rest and intravenous fluids. Steroids are administered intravenously at an equivalent dose of 40 to 60 mg of prednisone (hydrocortisone, 75 mg every eight hours) if there are no findings of sepsis. In patients with high fever, intravenous broad-spectrum antibiotics may also be started. When improvement is seen the antibiotics are discontinued and prednisone is begun by mouth; the patients are then managed as mentioned previously.

The surgical treatment of Crohn's disease is segmental resection when possible. Total colectomy and ileostomy are sometimes necessary for Crohn's disease involving the colon. In these cases, an ileostomy of a standard type is used. The Kock pouch is contraindicated in Crohn's disease at the present time.

There are a group of patients who have chronic activity of Crohn's disease despite all medical therapy and present special operative risks because of the extent of their disease. Some of these patients have been placed on home total parenteral nutrition and are able to live fruitful lives. This technique may have particular application in avoiding growth arrest in the adolescent patient with Crohn's disease. Only time will tell whether this therapy will remain in the armamentarium for Crohn's disease in general.

Recent studies have advocated the use of either 6-mercaptopurine or azathioprine in the long-term management of patients with Crohn's disease. These drugs have considerable toxicity in the doses recommended. Such treatment should only be considered after gastroenterologic consultation and with a strong commitment to close follow-up.

The medical-surgical management of patients with Crohn's disease is highly individual and requires a great deal of communication with the patient, the family, and the treating physician. Constant reevaluation is necessary for medical therapy, which is not curative but only palliative. Operation can remove diseased tissue, but recurrence is almost certain and no drug therapy can prevent this from occurring.

As an example of individualized care necessary in the management of Crohn's disease, consider the case of a 25-year-old woman who is in the midst of a budding career and is socially active. She may have her illness controlled with 40 mg of prednisone a day and a low-residue diet. However, the emotional turbulence caused by the steroids and the adverse cosmetic effects, as well as the frequent exacerbations of her disease, may make operation an early consideration despite a continuing "good therapeutic medical program." Another patient, the same age but in a different life pattern, may not want surgery with its risks and chance of recurrences, but would rather take azathioprine in order to tolerate a lower dose of steroid. For another similar patient, the long-term "neoplastic" side effects of azathioprine may be unacceptable and she would rather tolerate the disease as is. On the other hand, if the patient were 50 years old, azathioprine might be a viable alternative to high-dose steroid therapy despite its possible neoplastic side effects.

Since Crohn's disease is so variable in its manifestations, progression, and response to therapy, it is best to inform the patients of all the facts and to share with them the alternatives and their complications so that they may participate in all major decisions. Participation in the local chapter of the NFIC may add a great deal of emotional support. Generally it would seem that conservative

Table 7   **Side Effects of Steroids and Sulfasalazine**

Steroid related
   Sodium retention
   Hypokalemia
   Hypertension
   Cushingoid features
   Diabetes mellitus
   Osteoporosis
   Immunodeficiency (infections, ?neoplasms)
   ? Peptic ulcer disease

Sulfasalazine
   Anorexia, nausea, vomiting
   Leukopenia
   Headache
   Abdominal pain
   Skin rash

therapy should be pursued and operation only considered when the disease does not respond to management and when it interferes with the patient's quality of life.

WHAT SHOULD I EXPECT FROM SUCCESSFUL THERAPY?

Successful therapy should promote a reduction in the symptoms related to the acute exacerbation of the illness. Ideally all of the clinical manifestations should disappear, but unfortunately this is frequently not the case. Although the long-term course for any patient cannot be predicted, both ulcerative colitis and Crohn's disease are characterized by clinical exacerbations and remissions. Other than the prophylactic use of sulfasalazine in ulcerative colitis, nothing has yet been shown to alter the natural history of these illnesses.

WHAT MIGHT CAUSE A FAILURE OF TREATMENT?

Since we do not know precisely what causes inflammatory bowel diseases, we have no specific treatment directed against them. Rather, the treatment regimens previously described reduce inflammation in a nonspecific manner. For this reason, treatment failure occurs either when the inflammation is so severe that antiinflammatory measures are inadequate (e.g., in toxic megacolon) or, more commonly, when the symptoms are due to a complication that is not related to the acute inflammatory component (e.g., small-bowel obstruction secondary to chronic fibrosis rather than acute spasm and edema). These complications either have been or will be discussed. Interestingly, unlike many other chronic diseases, treatment failure in inflammatory bowel disease is not usually related to poor patient compliance.

WHAT ARE THE SIDE EFFECTS OF TREATMENT?

The toxicities of steroids and sulfasalazine are well known and are summarized in Table 7. A few of the postsurgical problems have been alluded to previously. The remainder will be discussed in the later sections.

HOW SHOULD THE PATIENT BE FOLLOWED?

Much of this material has already been discussed. Recommendations for screening of patients with ulcerative colitis for cancer can be found in the section on management of complications. Only a few general principles need to be emphasized here.

Patients with Crohn's disease or ulcerative colitis often blame all gastrointestinal symptoms on their chronic inflammatory bowel disease. In point of fact, they are just as likely to have other gastrointestinal disturbances (such as viral infections) as is the general population. These processes need to be considered before a particular symptom is attributed to "another flare-up of the inflammatory bowel disease."

WHAT COMPLICATIONS CAN OCCUR?

The various extraintestinal manifestations of both ulcerative colitis and Crohn's disease have been enumerated in Table 1. All of these have been seen in both diseases, although pyoderma gangrenosum is very rare in Crohn's disease. In addition, each of these diseases have other problems that are unique to one or the other, and these will be discussed separately.

Ulcerative Colitis

Local rectal disease can be seen in ulcerative colitis but it is usually limited to hemorrhoids or fissures. The complicated fistulas and abscesses that are often seen in Crohn's disease are encountered only rarely in patients with ulcerative colitis. This reflects the mucosal nature of ulcerative colitis as compared to the transmural involvement in Crohn's disease.

A dread, but rare, complication of ulcerative colitis is toxic megacolon, which was described previously. This may arise as a progression of the inflammatory process itself; it may also ensue as an iatrogenic complication, as from the injudicious use of anticholinergic medication or barium enema (or the cleansing preparation for this examination). In fact, it is appropriate to avoid laxative or enema preparation altogether in patients with inflammatory colonic disease of any cause and to use only several days of a clear-liquid diet. If this results in inadequate preparation, cathartics or enemas can then be added gradually.

Toxic megacolon appears when the inflammatory process becomes florid. The bowel wall, through and through, is overcome by acute inflammation. The muscular layer becomes paralyzed and progressive dilatation takes place with the appearance of micro-perforations through the serosa. The mortality rate approaches 50% unless careful combined medical and surgical care is provided rapidly.

The major concern in patients with ulcerative colitis is cancer. After eight to 10 years of active inflammation, an increasing chance of carcinoma appears. Cancer of the colon will develop in approximately 10% of patients after 10 years of the disease; the risk increases by one percent per year so that after 30 years of disease a 30% chance of cancer is present. Since this disease primarily affects young adults and adolescents, the cancer risk becomes a major consideration in the middle years. Unfortunately, there is no specific warning of early cancer. Rectal bleeding or exacerbation of the disease is the most common presentation and by the time it appears the cancer has already spread. The pattern of cancer does not follow the distribution of the normal population and all parts of the colon are involved.

The risk of cancer is also related to the extent of disease. Thus, it is greatest in patients in whom the entire colon is involved (pancolitis). Patients with ulcerative proctitis do not have an increased risk of malignancy.

Since ulcerative colitis is a mucosal disease, benign strictures are uncommon. When they are found, they are usually due to localized thickening of the muscularis mucosa. However, when a stricture is found carcinoma must be ruled out. Fistulas are uncommon and when they appear they involve the perineal area, sometimes extending to the bladder in the male or the vagina in the female.

Crohn's Disease

A number of complications related to the intestinal involvement of Crohn's disease are listed in Table 8. The first, perirectal disease, is often severe, complicated, and disabling; the fistulas and abscesses are multiple in location and sites of drainage. The cause of this severe disease is unclear, as colitis may be minimal or absent.

Intraabdominal abscesses may arise as a consequence of the transmural disease with leakage into the peritoneal cavity. On the other hand, the inflamed intestine may adhere to neighboring structures, and a fistula will form with other intestine (enteroenteric), bladder (enterovesical), skin (enterocutaneous), or vagina (enterovaginal). Bladder fistulas will cause sputtering of urination and recurrent urinary tract infections, while fistulas to the vagina will result in a foul or feculent vaginal discharge.

The transmural disease can produce transient bowel wall edema and spasm during the acute inflammation or chronic fibrosis and bowel narrowing may ensue. This latter condition persists after the acute inflammation subsides. Both states may produce intestinal obstruction (partial or, rarely, total).

Since Crohn's disease typically involves the terminal ileum, it can interfere with normal physiologic functions specific to that area, vitamin B_{12} and bile salt absorption in particular. Bile salts that reach the colon stimulate water secretion and thus can produce diarrhea on that basis.

Table 8 **Intestinal Complications of Crohn's Disease**

Perirectal disease (especially rectal fistulas, abscesses)
Intraabdominal abscess
Enteric fistula
Intestinal obstruction
Vitamin B_{12} and bile salt malabsorption
Malignancy
Toxic megacolon
Postoperative

There are some data that the rate of intestinal malignancy is also increased in Crohn's disease. The risk, however, is not nearly as high as is the case for ulcerative colitis.

Toxic megacolon occurs primarily in patients with ulcerative colitis. However, there have been several instances of this complication in patients with Crohn's colitis.

Several problems can arise after surgical resection for Crohn's disease. Recurrence can produce abscesses, fistulas, and luminal narrowing. Resection of the terminal ileum can produce vitamin B_{12} and bile salt malabsorption. When less than 100 cm is resected, diarrhea may occur as a result of the action of nonabsorbed bile salts on the colon. Extensive resection, with more than 100 cm removed, may produce steatorrhea and weight loss. This results from the extensive loss of bile salts into the colon; the liver is no longer able to synthesize enough to allow micelle formation. The malabsorbed dietary fats, no longer emulsified in the small bowel, pass into the colon, where they are broken down into hydroxy fatty acids that also act as cathartics.

HOW SHOULD THESE COMPLICATIONS BE MANAGED?

Most of the extraintestinal manifestations have their activity correlated with the activity of the bowel disease. Thus, they are managed by treating the intestinal process. (Occasionally, however, especially in ulcerative colitis, the extraintestinal disease may be so severe that surgical extirpation of the involved bowel may be necessary for control.) The biliary tract problems (including the pericholangitis) and the ankylosing spondylitis are exceptions to this rule, and may continue to progress even if the bowel disease is controlled.

Ulcerative Colitis

Toxic megacolon is usually managed with steroids, as described for severe ulcerative colitis. If no substantial response is seen in two to three days, operation should be undertaken as soon as medical resuscitation is completed. In the past prolonged trials of medical immunosuppression often resulted in disaster. It has become fashionable in recent years to treat both ulcerative colitis and Crohn's disease with bowel rest and parenteral nutrition. In the case of toxic megacolon, it is likely that prolonged courses of this therapy, in the absence of early improvement, are likely to have an unfavorable outcome.

There is no sure way of detecting those patients with ulcerative colitis who will develop cancer or of detecting the cancer early, that is, during a curable stage. Over the last several years, however, multiple biopsies from patients with ulcerative colitis have revealed dysplasia, a severe disorder of the normal mucosal pattern. Patients with dysplasia may have a very high risk of carcinoma coexisting in their colon or may be prone to develop carcinoma in the future. This predictive value of dysplasia is controversial; furthermore, the histologic differentiation requires an experienced pathologist. Thus, colectomy should not be recommended routinely solely on the basis of a biopsy report of dysplasia.

How should a patient with long-standing (more than 10 years) ulcerative colitis be followed? Since no method can surely predict the occurrence of carcinoma, my personal preference at this time is to share the facts and findings with patients, objectively presenting the statistics for carcinoma and the limitations of screening. I recommend that, after 10 years of disease, they have a prophylactic total colectomy and ileostomy. If they decide not to, I place them in a screening program in which total colonoscopy and double contrast barium enemas are alternatively obtained every six months.

Crohn's Disease

Patients with severe perirectal disease must be managed very carefully with the consultation of a surgical colleague. Extensive debridement and drainage are necessary. Some dramatic responses have been reported with total parenteral nutrition. The limiting factors are the long periods of time required and the expense as well as the recurrence of the perineal disease once the parenteral nutrition is discontinued and oral intake begins. However, for patients debilitated with fistula and abscesses, a period of parenteral nutrition may allow for reconstitution of nutritional status and improvement of the inflammation around the fistula; it may make the extent of surgery and the risk of operation considerably less.

If the patient has a very tender mass, high fever, and leukocytosis, studies are done to determine if an abscess is present. Flat films of the abdomen may show air outside of the bowel wall. An ultrasound or CAT scan may show extraluminal collections. Should the situation then worsen, despite therapy, with more severe pain and erythema of the overlying skin, operation is necessary. If left alone a Crohn's disease abscess will perforate through the skin resulting in an enterocutaneous fistula. The goal of surgery is to drain the abscess and, if possible, to resect the diseased tissue.

Enteroenteric fistulas may or may not require therapy. However, fistulas to the skin, bladder, or vagina usually do. Bowel rest and total parenteral nutrition may be successful in a small proportion of patients, but surgical therapy is usually required if the fistula is to close permanently.

Small-bowel obstruction that occurs during a period of active Crohn's disease usually responds to nasogastric decompression, intravenous antibiotics, and steroids. Obstruction during asymptomatic periods is frequently caused by dietary residue blocking the narrow lumen. These patients also do very well with decompression but repeated bouts of obstruction that interfere with living may require operation.

The diarrhea that results from faulty absorption of bile acid in the terminal ileum (due to disease or operation) can be managed nicely with cholestyramine (Questran) resin, 4 gm in a glass of juice one to four times a day. (In patients with luminal narrowing, the cholestyramine may exacerbate obstructive symptoms.) Vitamin B_{12} malabsorption can be treated with periodic injections.

Whereas total colectomy and ileostomy are curative for ulcerative colitis, operation for Crohn's disease often results in recurrence of disease at the line of anastomosis. The incidence is as high as 50% at two years after surgery even though the two segments of bowel that were anastomosed were free of disease by microscopic examination. As time progresses, the incidence of recurrence increases. Therefore, the decision for surgical intervention in Crohn's disease must be considered carefully since recurrent disease is almost inevitable. However, for those patients with very complicated debilitating disease the recurrence after operation may be more manageable than the original disease.

The problem of fat malabsorption after extensive ileal resection is a difficult one. Some symptomatic relief may be provided by the strict dietary restriction of long-chain fats, which require micelle formation for absorption, and the substitution of medium-chain triglycerides, which can be assimilated without bile salts.

SELECTED READING

Inflammatory bowel disease. *Clin Gastroenterol* 9(2):229–481, May 1980.

National Cooperative Crohn's Disease Study. *Gastroenterology* 77:825–944, 1979.

Cello JP, Meyer JH: Ulcerative Colitis, in Sleisenger MH, Fordtran JS (eds.): *Gastrointestinal Disease*. Philadelphia, WB Saunders Co, 1978, pp 1597–1653.

CLINICAL PROBLEMS

I. A 28-year-old man complains of a three-week history of lower abdominal cramps and bloody diarrhea. He is having low-grade fevers and has lost five pounds during this time. Upon further questioning he states that he has had several episodes of bloody diarrhea over the past three years, but has never sought medical advice. There is no family history of any bowel problems. His physical examination demonstrates a temperature of 100 F, a pulse rate of 120, and some generalized lower abdominal tenderness.

Sigmoidoscopic examination demonstrates friable, erythematous mucosa up to and beyond 18 cm, the point where the examination is terminated because of patient discomfort. The liquid stool is overtly bloody and the smear demonstrates many white blood cells. No amoebic trophozoites are seen. Stool cultures for bacteria grow out only normal enteric organisms. Subsequent stools do not demonstrate any ova or parasites.

Laboratory data are as follows:

    Hemoglobin: 11.8 gm%

    White blood cell count: 13,800/mm^3 (73% Polymorphonuclear leukocytes—PMNs)

    Serum albumin: 3.8 gm%

SGOT, SGPT, bilirubin, alkaline phosphatase: all
normal
Amoebic serology: negative

1. What further diagnostic evaluation should the patient undergo?
2. How should the patient be treated?
3. What is his course likely to be?

II. A 32-year-old man complains of occasional bouts of bloody
diarrhea that last one to two days and are associated with
marked tenesmus. He has had these every few months for a year.
There is no associated fever, weight loss, or other systemic
symptoms. The family history is negative for any bowel disorder. His physical examination is entirely normal.

Sigmoidoscopic examination demonstrates inflamed mucosa
to 10 cm, beyond which point the mucosal appearance is normal.
No perirectal disease is present. The stool contains white and
red blood cells but no parasites are seen.

His laboratory data are as follows:
Hemoglobin: 14.8 gm%
White blood cell count: 8,300/mm³ (52% PMNs)
Serum albumin: 4.2 gm%
SGOT, SGPT, bilirubin, alkaline phosphatase: all
normal

1. What further diagnostic evaluation should the patient undergo?
2. How should the patient be treated?
3. What is his course likely to be?

III. A 25-year-old girl complains of midabdominal, moderate to
severe cramping pain and diarrhea (four to five stools a day)
for two weeks. She has noted an associated fever and she has
lost 12 pounds. Although she has never had this problem before,
her mother also used to have diarrhea and pain. The patient is
unaware what disease her mother had, as she died of a pulmonary embolus when the patient was a young girl. The physical
examination is positive for fever (101.8 F), evidence of recent

weight loss, tachycardia (pulse, 115), mild hypotension (blood pressure, 96/50), and a right lower quadrant abdominal mass.

Anoscopy reveals a few internal hemorrhoids and a small rectal fissure. Sigmoidoscopy to 12 cm shows normal mucosa. The stool is watery and positive for occult blood. A stool smear demonstrates red and white blood cells.

Preliminary laboratory data are the following:

Hemoglobin: 10.1 gm%
White blood cell count: 12,300/mm³ (85% PMNs)
Serum albumin: 3.2 gm%
SGOT: 54 IU (normal, < 40 IU)
SGPT: 61 IU (normal, < 45 IU)
Alkaline phosphatase: 110 IU (normal, < 85 IU)
Total bilirubin: 0.9 mg%

1. What further diagnostic evaluation should the patient undergo?
2. How should the patient be treated?
3. What is her course likely to be?

Discussion

I. 1. The patient appears to have some form of colitis, and the workup to this point has failed to reveal an infectious cause. An abdominal flat plate (x-ray) should be obtained, because the ulcerated mucosa can often be seen in this manner and an estimation of the extent of the disease can be made. The diameter of the colon can also be assessed. Serum electrolytes and red blood cell indices (as well as iron studies) can be obtained because of the coexistent problems of diarrhea and anemia. A barium enema (or colonoscopy), which will ultimately be used to define the extent of the process, should be deferred during this acute phase of the illness because of the danger of precipitating a toxic megacolon.

2. At this point a presumptive diagnosis of ulcerative colitis would be reasonable. By the usual criteria, this is of moderate severity. The decision as to whether or not to hospitalize in this case will depend on a multitude of factors.

The patient as described is not very toxic. An attempt to manage him as an outpatient could be undertaken if his home environment is supportive. Although he may respond to sulfasalazine, corticosteroid therapy would usually be required. Broad-spectrum antibiotics and parenteral nutrition are not likely to be needed. As noted, analgesics and other anticholinergics should not be used. The dietary recommendations can be limited to the temporary avoidance of milk products (unless it is clear that lactase deficiency is not present).

3. The patient will continue to have exacerbations of his disease. He should be given maintenance sulfasalazine after his acute flare-up enters remission, as this reduces the frequency of exacerbations. During a quiescent period he should undergo radiographic evaluation of his entire gastrointestinal tract to assess the extent of the colonic process and to exclude the presence of small-bowel disease. If he has pancolitis, he will be at especial risk of developing cancer in the decades to come. Often these patients come to colectomy for the activity of the disease.

II. 1. This patient appears to have a localized proctitis in contradistinction to the more diffuse colitis in the previous case. The important diagnoses to exclude in such patients are infectious processes (less likely here with the recurrent history), especially venereal diseases. He should be specifically asked about homosexual activity and cultures should be obtained for gonorrhea in addition to the more routine infectious disease evaluations previously described.

2. Patients with ulcerative proctitis usually do well with sulfasalazine with or without the intermittent use of steroid enemas. Systemic steroids are usually not required. Constipation should be avoided with bulk agents.

3. Although patients with ulcerative proctitis also have periodic exacerbations, they do not appear to be at any higher risk of developing cancer than the general population.

III. 1. The patient appears to have an intraabdominal inflammatory condition that needs to be evaluated. Although it would be tempting, in the context of this chapter, to diagnose Crohn's disease (involving perhaps the right side of the colon and terminal ileum), other processes must be considered, an abdominal abscess in particular. The patient should be admitted and evaluated for this latter possibility with blood cultures, abdominal flat plate (x-ray), ultrasound, and so forth. There is no apparent evidence of colitis and, if the diagnosis is in question, even contrast x-rays of the lower and upper gastrointestinal tracts can be performed. (Remember that the abscess need not be from Crohn's disease, but may be due to other factors such as a perforated appendix.)

2. It would not be inappropriate, until and unless the diagnosis of Crohn's disease is established, to treat such a patient with broad-spectrum antibiotics and intravenous fluids. If she has Crohn's disease, it is clearly active. (From the information available, the Crohn's Disease Activity Index appears to be approximately 400.) Steroids would probably be the first agent of choice in this case.

3. If she has Crohn's disease, it will probably pursue an unpredictable course of exacerbations and remissions. She may or may not develop the various problems described in this chapter, but she will require medical follow-up for the rest of her life.

14

ARTHUR D. SCHWABE

Functional Bowel Syndrome

The gastrointestinal tract may react to nonspecific stress with a variety of disturbances in motor and sphincteric function. The symptoms, which may be either perceived throughout the entire GI tract or localized to a specific area, consist of anorexia, belching, dyspepsia, nausea, vomiting, abdominal pain, distention, constipation, or diarrhea. The more severely affected patients usually have coexistent signs of anxiety, depression, aggressiveness, hysteria, phobias, tension, rigidity, or obsessive-compulsive behavior. Collectively these clinical manifestations are usually referred to as the functional, or irritable, bowel syndrome, but many other terms, too often focusing on a particular segment of the GI tract, have appeared in the literature (Table 1).

The functional bowel syndrome (FBS) is the most common gastrointestinal disorder in developed countries and accounts for approximately 50% of all digestive disease conditions seen in private practice. It is responsible for almost as much absenteeism in industry as the common cold. Physicians often experience difficulty in wading

219

Table 1 Functional Bowel Syndrome: Synonyms

Dysfunctional bowel syndrome
Functional bowel disease
Irritable bowel syndrome
Irritable colon syndrome
Dyssynergia of the colon
Adaptive colitis
Mucous colitis
Spastic colitis
Nervous colon
Spastic colon
Unstable colon

through a maze of symptomatology before arriving at the correct diagnosis.

It is important to remember that the common denominator of all of the various manifestations of FBS is an abnormality associated with intestinal smooth-muscle contractions. Thus, the gastrointestinal symptoms that the patient reports are actually occurring within the abdominal cavity. Virtually every individual in our society has the capacity to develop some of these "functional" symptoms, especially when subjected to emotional stress. Who among us has not had "butterflies in the stomach" before a public appearance? How many develop constipation when traveling in a strange city? Patients who bring symptoms of FBS to their physicians are merely undergoing a quantitative increase either in the activity of these smooth-muscle contractions or in their sensitivity to the same degree of contraction.

HOW DO I MAKE THE DIAGNOSIS?

The diagnosis of FBS is based on carefully elicited historical features. Characteristically, the symptoms are of long duration, intermittent, variable in location and intensity, and precipitated or exacerbated during periods of stress. It is not necessary to rule out every other known disease before the diagnosis of FBS can be established.

DISEASE ENTITIES

In fact, in most cases the diagnosis is made on the basis of the history and physical examination. In some patients one or more symptoms predominate and have led to some arbitrary subdivisions and recognition of clinical variants (Table 2).

Functional Dyspepsia

Chronic epigastric discomfort, often accompanied by nausea, anorexia, excessive belching, and occasionally by bilious vomiting, are the hallmarks of functional dyspepsia. The symptoms may simulate those of peptic ulcer, although they tend to be more chronic, unrelated to meals, and not relieved by antacids. Afflicted patients are often depressed. Endoscopic and radiographic examinations of the upper gastrointestinal tract are negative.

All patients with functional dyspepsia should have a complete blood count, serum electrolytes, serum calcium, and urinalysis. The diagnosis is best confirmed by a normal upper gastrointestinal endoscopy.

Functional Nausea

Episodic nausea may be the predominant symptom of FBS. It is believed to be related to abnormal motility of the tranverse colon, but may also be due to impaired sphincteric activity. Patients usually

Table 2 **Functional Bowel Syndrome: Clinical Variants**

Functional dyspepsia
Functional nausea
Functional (psychogenic) duodenal ileus
Functional abdominal pain
Functional constipation
Functional diarrhea
Gaseous distention
Splenic flexure syndrome
Proctalgia fugax

complain of nausea soon after arising, generally before breakfast. On gastroscopy increased bile reflux through the pylorus may be observed but no other structural abnormalities are noted. The nausea tends to occur more frequently during periods of stress and at these times may be accompanied by vomiting. Such patients should be evaluated for alcoholism and drug ingestion; where appropriate, a blood sugar or serum calcium, or both, should be obtained. In women the possibility of pregnancy should also be considered.

Functional Duodenal Ileus

Nausea, vomiting, weight loss, and progressive dilatation of the duodenum characterize functional, or psychogenic, duodenal ileus. It is a very unusual manifestation of FBS that occurs almost exclusively in young, hyposthenic, lordotic women who have suffered sudden or severe emotional stress. The upper gastrointestinal x-rays reveal a markedly dilated duodenum with little or no peristaltic activity and narrowing at the level of the ligament of Treitz. Many of these patients were once presumed to have mechanical obstruction due to compromising of the intestinal lumen by the superior mesenteric artery. However, it is now clear that functional dilatation of the duodenum occurs far more often than dilatation from all the mechanical causes put together.

Functional Abdominal Pain

Abdominal pain is one of the cardinal presentations of the FBS and is usually accompanied by disturbances in stool frequency and consistency. The pain may be diffuse or localized to any quadrant but most often is experienced in the lower half of the abdomen. It is often intermittent, cramping, or pinching and is usually relieved by a bowel movement or the passage of gas. It may prevent patients from falling asleep but amazingly almost never awakens them from sound sleep. The pain, which can be experimentally reproduced by balloon distention of the distal colon, has been shown to be a manifestation of disordered motility in the colon.

Occasionally the pain is perceived predominately in the left upper quadrant near the left costal margin and may radiate to the substernal region, the left shoulder, and down the left arm. Afflicted patients often have high, redundant splenic flexures of the colon. This variant of FBS, often referred to as the splenic flexure syndrome, may simulate the pain of coronary artery disease or diffuse esophageal spasm. Balloon distention of the splenic flexure, a research technique, has reproduced this pain pattern in these patients. Abdominal pain was discussed in a previous chapter. Specific tests to be ordered depend on the specific clinical situation.

Gaseous Distention

Fullness or bloating that is relieved by the passage of gas is a common complaint of patients with the FBS. It is usually not detectable by the examining physician. For further details, see the chapter on gas.

Functional Constipation

Many patients with FBS consult a physician because of constipation, which in a few may even be intolerable. They may have used multiple available laxatives and cathartics and even resorted to enemas for relief. On careful questioning it becomes apparent that the constipation may sometimes alternate with periods of diarrhea. Abdominal pain, flatulence, and distention accompany the constipation in most patients.

The stools are described by patients as hard, dry, pellet-like, or sticky. Some stools have the appearance of goat or rabbit pellets (scybala), but others are very large in diameter and can be expelled only with great difficulty. Usually the rectum is empty on digital examination but occasionally fecal impactions are encountered. The frequency of stool passage may vary from one to two times a day to once a week. Barium x-rays of the colon may be normal. (Chronic laxative abusers may have the "cathartic colon," which is void of haustrations and dilated.) Sigmoidoscopy is usually normal; if anthraquinone laxatives (e.g., senna or cascara) have been used for a prolonged time, brown or black mucosal mottling, known as melanosis coli, may be seen. When constipation is the only sign or symptom, drug ingestion, hypercalcemia, and hypothyroidism should be excluded by the appropriate history, physical examination, and laboratory tests.

Functional Diarrhea

Diarrhea may be the predominant symptom in FBS, although it may alternate with periods of constipation or normal stools as stated previously. The stools, which are usually mushy or creamy in consistency, may be small in volume. A copious amount of mucus may be present. Although many stools may be passed during the day, the diarrhea rarely awakens the patients at night. Diagnostic studies should include a complete blood count, stool examinations for blood and for ova and parasites, sigmoidoscopy, and barium enema. As a rule, all of the studies will be within normal limits. However, marked irritability, localized spasm, luminal narrowing, and increased pseudohaustrations may be visible on barium enema, lending support to the diagnosis of FBS.

Proctalgia Fugax

Sudden, recurring attacks of excruciating pain in the anorectal area characterize proctalgia fugax. The pain, which may be described as tearing, boring, burning, expanding, or cramping, usually begins abruptly and lasts from one to 15 minutes. Proctalgia fugax occurs most commonly in men between the ages of 25 and 50, particularly in professionals, such as doctors, lawyers, and teachers. Concomitant symptoms may be tachycardia, profuse perspiration, pallor, priapism, and occasionally loss of consciousness. The pain may be due to spasm of the perirectal muscles or contractions of the sigmoid colon. Intervals between the attacks range from a few days to several months. The diagnosis is based entirely on the history of self-limited, recurring attacks of excruciating rectal pain. Sigmoidoscopic examinations reveal no abnormalities in these patients.

WHAT ADDITIONAL WORKUP DOES THE PATIENT REQUIRE?

A number of other gastrointestinal disorders share many of the symptoms of the FBS and must be ruled out by appropriate studies to confirm the diagnostic impression, to reassure the patient, and to provide the physician with adequate support to institute appropriate therapy. These tests have been considered under the various syndromes listed previously.

A major diagnostic pitfall in patients with FBS is ordering too many studies. This is a clinical diagnosis and cannot be established positively by any laboratory test. (The various motility tests described previously are not available outside the university setting.) The ordering (and reordering) of multiple blood, urine, sonographic, endoscopic, or radiographic studies only convinces the patient that the physician is not sure that the proffered diagnosis (FBS) is correct. Thus, if the symptoms have not changed and the reasonable studies have been performed, the appropriate course of action is not to order more laboratory tests and procedures.

On the other hand, if the symptoms are of recent onset or change in character, especially in patients over the age of 40, many of these studies may be indicated. Similarly, certain symptoms or signs should point the physician toward some diagnosis other than FBS. These include gastrointestinal bleeding, fever, weight loss, dehydration, or electrolyte imbalance. In the case of the latter, consideration should be given to laxative abuse.

HOW SHOULD I TREAT THE PATIENT?

Most patients with FBS will respond to reassurance, an explanation of the cause of the symptoms, and gentle symptomatic therapy. If anxiety, tension, and insomnia are prominent features, a mild tranquilizer may be added. If severe emotional disturbances exist, a psychiatric evaluation and appropriate psychiatric treatment should be obtained. Patients with cancerophobia require clear reassurance that the workup has excluded the presence of cancer. All previously used drugs should be discontinued. A balanced and attractive diet containing adequate amounts of high-residue foods should be instituted.

When the symptoms are directly referable to the colon, we have found that bulk agents, such as psyllium hydrophilic mucilloid (Metamucil) or plantago ovata (Konsyl) are beneficial for most patients. In long-standing functional constipation normal toilet habits have usually been abandoned. Such patients require a prolonged period of reeducation, emphasizing exercise, regular visits to the bathroom, proper positioning, a high-residue diet supplemented with bulk agents, and discontinuation of all laxatives and enemas. Initially, stimulation and lubrication for the passage of stool by the insertion of a glycerin suppository 15 minutes before attempting defecation may be a useful adjunct in some patients. The use of anticholinergic drugs has not been shown to be effective in controlled trials for relief of functional diarrhea.

FBS is a ubiquitous condition. Therefore, it is not unusual to encounter patients with coexistent gastrointestinal illness such as peptic ulcer disease or gallstones. Often the symptom complexes are distinguishable, but, especially with regard to pain, it may not be clear where one illness separates from the other. Very successful therapy of one process (e.g., healing of an ulcer or removal of the gallbladder) may not produce alleviation of the symptoms. By appreciating the presence of both processes, the expectations of both the physician and the patient to the outcome of treatment can be tempered appropriately.

WHAT SHOULD I EXPECT FROM SUCCESSFUL TREATMENT?

FBS is characterized by remissions and exacerbations. The great numbers of pharmacologic agents, dietary regimens, and psychiatric approaches presently in use are proof of the difficulty encountered in sustaining permanent remissions in most patients. Therapy is most successful if maintained for a long time and if periodically reinforced by one physician who understands the patient's needs, reactions, and problems.

WHAT MIGHT CAUSE FAILURE OF TREATMENT?

Treatment failures in the FBS are caused by changing reactions to stress and by a patient's inability to adapt to new life situations. The physician must take time to review all matters important to the patient, to provide renewed reassurance, and to make necessary adjustments in therapy. Patients with functional constipation may feel that they have become refractory to bulk agents and revert to old patterns of extensive laxative and enema use. A change in the dose of hydrophilic colloid or the substitution of another similar agent may reestablish normal evacuation. Patients with abdominal pain do not require strong analgesics but rather reassurance that cancer has not developed in their gastrointestinal tracts. An open dialogue between patient and physician is usually more beneficial than a myriad of drugs. In fact, the long-term use in FBS of any agent with potential anticholinergic effects leads to the induction of superimposed motility abnormalities, followed by adaptation and, finally, exacerbation of the original symptoms when the drug is withdrawn. Thus, the chronic use of these agents should never be instituted in FBS.

HOW SHOULD THE PATIENT BE FOLLOWED?

During the initial period of treatment, patients should be seen every one to two weeks to receive reassurance, to air new problems, and to obtain adjustments in therapy. Gradually the intervals between visits may be extended. The physician must be available, however, to deal quickly with new or changing symptoms. If major emotional disturbances are present, the patient should be followed regularly by a competent psychiatrist.

WHAT COMPLICATIONS CAN OCCUR?

Complications from FBS itself are rare. Some patients with functional vomiting or severe diarrhea may become dehydrated and electrolyte disturbances may develop. (Again, the possibility of laxative abuse must be considered in this situation.) Because of an intrinsic disorder of bowel motility, diverticulosis, with consequent diverticulitis and diverticular abscesses, is more likely to develop.

A few patients and physicians are convinced that the problem can be solved by exploratory laparotomy. A scarred abdomen from multiple previous operations with negative or equivocal results attests to the futility of this approach. It is not unusual to see patients in whom various organs deemed to be the source of symptoms have been removed with little or no improvement in symptomatology.

Complications can also occur from inappropriate treatment.

Many patients with abdominal pain are given narcotics for relief by well-meaning physicians. Addiction to opiates constitutes the major complication in patients with FBS. If anticholinergics are prescribed, the physician must be alert to such side effects as worsening constipation, urinary retention, blurring of vision, and cardiac arrhythmias. Caution should also be exercised if tranquilizers or sedatives are prescribed, not only because of their side effects, but also because of the risk of overdosage. Complications are avoided by limiting the number of medications and by close follow-up during the initial period of treatment. The management of the FBS requires the utmost in skill and patience on the part of the physician.

SELECTED READING

Cimmino CV: Arteriomesenteric occlusion of the duodenum: an entity? Radiology 76:828–829, 1961.

Connell AM, Jones FA, Rowlands EN: Motility of the pelvic colon. IV. Abdominal pain associated with colonic hypermotility after meals. *Gut* 6:105–112, 1965.

Harvey RF: Colonic motility in proctalgia fugax. *Lancet* 2:713–714, 1979.

Karras JD, Angelo G: Proctalgia fugax. Clinical observations and a new diagnostic aid. *Dis Colon Rectum* 6:130–134, 1963.

Ritchie JA, Ardran GM, Truelove SC: Motor activity of the sigmoid colon of humans: a combined study by intraluminal pressure recording and cineradiography. *Gastroenterology* 43:642–662, 1962.

Sullivan MA, Cohen S, Snape WJ Jr: Colonic myoelectrical activity in irritable bowel syndrome. *N Engl J Med* 298:878–883, 1978.

Swanson DW, Swenson WM, Huizenga KA, et al: Persistent nausea without organic cause. *Mayo Clin Proc* 51:257–262, 1976.

Young SJ, Alpers DH, Norland CC, et al: Psychiatric illness and the irritable bowel syndrome. Practical implications for the primary physician. *Gastroenterology* 70:162–166, 1976.

CLINICAL PROBLEMS

I. A 27-year-old man is being evaluated for intermittent diarrhea. He states that he has had bouts of this on and off for at least

10 years. The episodes last one to two weeks and occur several times a year. While in college he was evaluated by the student health service; these records reveal a normal barium enema, sigmoidoscopy, and stool examination for cells, ova, and parasites. He has no associated fever and there has been no change in his weight. He has not noted any relationship of the diarrhea to milk, which he drinks "all the time." He denies the use of any medication, alcohol, or illicit drugs. The diarrheal stools are characterized as "frothy," nonbloody, about 50 to 100 ml in volume, and occurring three to four times a day. He denies any abdominal pain except mild, low abdominal cramps that are relieved by the passing of the diarrheal stool. His symptoms have recently exacerbated again, and he wants to be checked out "to make sure nothing is wrong" before he gets married next week. Upon closer questioning, he notes that the symptoms occur when he is under severe stress. The physical examination is completely normal. A diarrheal stool is negative for occult blood.

1. What disorder does the patient have?
2. What further tests should be performed?
3. How should he be treated?

II. A 42-year-old man complains of intermittent episodes of epigastric pain. These episodes occur every one to two months; intermittent pain is then present for up to a week. Between episodes he feels well. There is a decided tendency for the symptom to arise when he is under stress. The pain may come on at any time but especially after meals. However, he has pain at times when he awakens in the morning. There is no associated fever, alteration in bowel habits, or weight change. He has been taking antacids for this discomfort ever since they first began 15 to 20 years ago; sometimes the antacids help but at other times they do not. His friend has an ulcer and the patient wants to know whether he does also. An evaluation five years earlier, including upper gastrointestinal x-ray, was entirely normal. His physical examination is normal except for some minimal epigastric tenderness. His stool is negative for occult blood.

1. What disorder does the patient have?
2. What further tests should be performed?
3. How should he be treated?

III. A 72-year-old woman has had constipation and low abdominal cramping pains "all of her life." She has just moved to a new city and is seeing the physician for the first time. She states that she had regular examinations by her previous physicians as well as a number of barium enemas and sigmoidoscopies; the last one was three years ago. She was told that she had "nervous constipation" and "diverticulosis." She recognizes that the symptoms become worse when she is under stress, and, in fact, for the past three months they have again done so in association with her preparations for moving. She has lost 10 to 15 pounds during this time because she "isn't hungry," but attributes this also to her anxiety. She does note, however, that weight loss has never occurred before with these symptoms. She denies any fever or hematochezia. Her physical examination demonstrates evidence of weight loss but is otherwise normal. The rectal examination reveals the presence of hard stool, which is positive when tested for occult blood.

1. What disorder does the patient have?
2. What further tests should be performed?
3. How should she be treated?

Discussion

I. 1. The patient is describing a very typical history of functional diarrhea. Its important elements are chronicity, the lack of systemic symptoms, small-volume stools with mucus ("frothy"), absent blood, a relationship of the exacerbation to stress, and, finally, a previous negative diagnostic evaluation.

2. No other tests need to be performed.

3. The patient should be reassured. The relationship between emotional stress and abnormal motility should be explained to him. Lactose intolerance is not present and no dietary restrictions need be imposed.

II. 1. Many aspects of the history are compatible with peptic ulcer disease. The disconcerting notes, however, are the negative diagnostic evaluations, the variable response to antacids, and the presence of pain in the morning on awakening. The differential diagnosis at this time, therefore, includes acid-peptic disease and functional bowel syndrome. Remember that he may have both.

2. Peptic disease needs to be excluded, and the most sensitive tool for accomplishing this is upper gastrointestinal endoscopy. (See the chapter on peptic ulcer disease.)

3. If an ulcer crater is demonstrated, it should be treated as discussed previously. If no evidence of acid-peptic disease is found, the patient can still be given antacids for their placebo effect, but he should understand that no actual hole in the mucosa is present. Anticholinergics, analgesics, and cimetidine should not be offered. The occasional use of tranquilizers may be appropriate but, more importantly, emotional support should be employed. Because of the frequency of his symptoms, this patient would probably do well with regularly scheduled visits to allow him the opportunity to vent some of his anxieties.

III. 1. Superficially this patient would appear to have another exacerbation of her functional bowel syndrome. Two disquieting features should be noted, however. They are the weight loss and the blood in the stool. Both of these represent recent changes in her presentation and they should be further investigated to rule in or out the presence of a primary colonic constricting lesion (carcinoma in particular but also even benign processes as a postinflammatory stricture) or even other systemic disease.

2. The patient should have a complete blood count, urinalysis, sigmoidoscopy (with careful attention to the perirectal area to look for local causes of bleeding), and barium enema. If no source for the blood is found, the upper gastrointestinal tract should be examined with a barium study as well. (If no source is found, the evaluation should proceed as described in the chapter on gastrointestinal bleeding.)

3. If any other disease is found, it should be dealt with. If not the patient can be treated with bulk compounds. (The danger of giving bulk compounds to an individual with an already existent colonic constrictive lesion is obvious.) The other measures described in the chapter should also be employed.

ARTHUR D. SCHWABE

Gastrointestinal Polyps

Polyps are best defined as masses of tissue that protrude into the lumen of hollow viscera. They may be found in any part of the gastrointestinal tract from the esophagus to the rectum and may be pedunculated or sessile. Polyps are usually classified according to the tissue of origin into epithelial, nonepithelial, and hamartomatous. There are five types of distinct epithelial polyps: (1) hyperplastic, (2) adenomatous (tubular or glandular), (3) villous adenomas, (4) villoglandular types and (5) polypoid carcinomas (Table 1). Nonepithelial polyps are lipomas, leiomyomas, neurofibromas, cysts, and hemangiomas. Hamartomas are mixtures of tissue native to the segment of gut involved, such as juvenile and Peutz-Jeghers polyps.

HOW DO I MAKE THE DIAGNOSIS?

Polyps may be asymptomatic and discovered only incidentally during barium or endoscopic examinations of the gastrointestinal tract. They may ulcerate and cause an iron deficiency anemia or

1. *Hyperplastic (metaplastic)* polyps represent simple proliferations of normal mucosal glands. They are very common, usually only 1 to 5 mm in diameter, and rarely cause clinical symptoms. They are not neoplastic and have no malignant potential.
2. *Adenomatous (tubular, glandular)* polyps are localized neoplastic tumors of mucosal glands, representing failure of normal differentiation and maturation. They may range up to 6 cm in size, appear pink to deep red in color, and have a smooth or nodular contour. Those of more than 1 cm in diameter carry a significant risk of malignant change.
3. *Villous* adenomas are tumors of surface epithelium. They are more often sessile than pedunculated and may range up to 15 cm in diameter. They are soft and velvety, have the color of the normal mucosa, and exhibit multiple, finger-like processes. Very large villous adenomas have the capacity to secrete copious amounts of fluid. These tumors have a high propensity to undergo malignant change and therefore should be totally resected when discovered.
4. *Villoglandular (papillary, tubulovillous, adenovillous)* polyps contain both adenomatous and villous components. They are likely to contain foci of dysplasia or frank carcinomas and require total removal.
5. *Polypoid carcinomas* are usually sessile. They may arise de novo or become superimposed on preexisting villous or adenomatous polyps. An aggressive surgical approach is indicated.

gross gastrointestinal bleeding. They may cause intussusception and give rise to the signs and symptoms of intestinal obstruction. Epithelial polyps have a significant potential for undergoing malignant change, particularly if they occur in the colon. Massive intestinal polyposis may present with diarrhea.

All polypoid lesions greater than 1 cm in diameter in the esophagus, stomach, and colon should be visualized endoscopically and, unless they are clearly submucosal, should be biopsied. Patients in whom large numbers of polyps are found may have one of the inherited polyposis syndromes, which may require special attention (Table 2). Two of these, familial polyposis coli and Gardner's syndrome, are characterized by adenomatous polyps and thus carry a high risk of malignancy. Their main features are discussed in the following paragraphs.

Familial Polyposis Coli

Familial polyposis coli (FPC), the most common polyposis syndrome, is transmitted as an autosomal dominant trait and is esti-

Table 2 Major Clinical Features of Three Polyposis Syndromes

Feature	FPC[a]	GS[b]	P-JS[c]
Inheritance	Dominant	Dominant	Dominant
Distribution of polyps			
Stomach	Very rare	Rare	Common
Small intestine	Very rare	Rare	Predominant
Colon	Predominant	Predominant	Common
Skin lesions	None	Cysts, fibromas, lipomas	Melanin spots
Bone lesions	None	Osteomas, exostoses	Clubbing, exostoses
Other tumors	None	Desmoids, fibrosarcomas, leiomyomas, adrenal tumors, ampullary tumors, thyroid carcinomas	Ovarian cysts, ovarian tumors
Malignant potential	Yes	Yes	No
Major complications	Cancer	Cancer	Bleeding, obstruction
Colectomy	Yes	Yes	No

[a] FPC, familial polyposis coli.
[b] GS, Gardner's syndrome.
[c] P-JS, Peutz-Jeghers syndrome.

mated to occur once in 8,300 births. The number of colonic polyps may vary from a few scattered groups to many thousands. In its most florid form, myriads of tiny, sessile mamillations carpet the entire colon and rectum. The location of the polyps is confined almost exclusively to the large intestine. The polyps are usually not present at birth, but appear after the age of 10 years (average, 25 years) and then rapidly increase in size and number. Carcinoma develops almost invariably in one or more sites in the colon. The average age of diagnosis of cancer in these patients is 40 years but it may occur as early as the second decade.

Gardner's Syndrome

The association of adenomatous polyps of the large intestine with soft-tissue tumors and osseous abnormalities characterizes Gardner's syndrome (GS). The disorder, which is also transmitted as an autosomal dominant trait, has an estimated incidence of 1 in 14,025 births. The diagnosis may be first suggested by the appearance of a variety of cutaneous and subcutaneous tumors, such as epidermoid cysts, fibromas and lipomas; dental abnormalities, such as supernumerary or unerupted teeth; or bony lesions, such as exostoses or osteomas. These extraintestinal manifestations may be present years before the gastrointestinal polyps become apparent. The polyps, which tend to be more discrete, scattered, and fewer in number than those in FPC, occur predominantly in the colon, but rarely are also seen in the small intestine and stomach. This syndrome is associated with a high incidence of colonic cancer as well as with carcinomas of the thyroid, adrenal, and periampullary region.

Peutz-Jeghers Syndrome

Other polyposis syndromes are characterized by hamartomatous polyps, which are not neoplastic. While the clinical and therapeutic implications are quite different, one in particular must be considered in the differential diagnosis.

The Peutz-Jeghers syndrome (P-JS) is characterized by mucocutaneous pigmentation (melanin spots) and hamartomatous polyps. Like the previous two syndromes, it is inherited as an autosomal dominant trait, but unlike them it does not carry the high risk of malignancy. The melanin spots may be found on the face, lips, buccal mucosa, forearms, palms, soles, digits, and the perianal region. Polyps of varying size may be present throughout the entire gastrointestinal tract, but are most common and numerous in the small bowel. They are susceptible to torsion with infarction, hemorrhage, and intussusception. Other associated findings include digital clubbing, exostoses, ovarian cysts, and ovarian tumors.

WHAT ADDITIONAL WORKUP DOES
THE PATIENT REQUIRE?

Once a polyp is found on routine sigmoidoscopy or barium enema examination, a careful search for additional polyps should be undertaken. An air-contrast barium enema will usually identify lesions missed on regular barium enema. If air-contrast x-rays are not available or prove to be inconclusive, a colonoscopy should be performed. If multiple adenomatous polyps are found, family history is reviewed in detail, in order to rule out one of the previously mentioned inherited adenomatous polyposis syndromes.

Juvenile polyps, even if present in large numbers, require no further workup. They occur most commonly in childhood and tend to disappear spontaneously. Although entirely benign, juvenile polyps also are liable to volvulus, secondary purulent inflammation, venous congestion, infarction, and autoamputation.

HOW SHOULD I TREAT THE PATIENT?

The treatment of gastrointestinal polyps depends on the histologic type on biopsy, on location, on size and growth rate, and on pattern of inheritance.

Histologic Type

Pedunculated epithelial polyps in accessible areas should be removed endoscopically. Large (> 2 cm) sessile adenomatous polyps, flat villous adenomas, and all polypoid carcinomas require surgical resection. Although some adenomatous polyps appear sessile on x-ray, a stalk can often be identified at endoscopy. Hyperplastic polyps, hamartomas, and nonulcerated submucosal polyps require no therapy.

Location

The following rules apply to epithelial gastric polyps, which are known to have a low potential for malignant transformation: (1) single pedunculated gastric polyps are removed endoscopically; (2) single, sessile adenomatous gastric polyps, 2 cm or greater in diameter, are removed surgically; (3) multiple, small gastric polyps, less than 2 cm in diameter, in asymptomatic patients do not require operation, but should be followed with exfoliative cytology and x-ray every six months for two years. If the cytology remains negative and if there is no increase in size during this period, only yearly cytologic examination is necessary thereafter.

Polyps in the small intestine are almost always of hamartomatous or nonepithelial origin. Surgical intervention is warranted
only for the complications of bleeding and obstruction. Colonic and
rectal polyps are treated more aggressively, as previously outlined.

Size and Growth Rate

In general, all epithelial polyps 2 cm or more in diameter in
the stomach and colon should be removed. A polyp of any size in
any location that doubles in diameter in six months or less is potentially malignant and should be removed surgically.

Pattern of Inheritance

Patients with multiple polyps and an established history of FPC
or Gardner's syndrome require a total colectomy. If involved, the
rectum is removed also. If the rectum is spared, an ileorectal anastomosis may be carried out. If this latter procedure is adopted, semi-
annual follow-up study and removal of any new rectal polyps by
fulguration or excision are mandatory.

HOW SHOULD THE PATIENT BE FOLLOWED?

No follow-up study is necessary for patients with obvious, nonulcerated, nonepithelial polyps or for those with histologically proven
hyperplastic, juvenile, or Peutz-Jeghers polyps in any location. The
management and surveillance of gastric polyps have already been
outlined. Patients over 40 years of age with adenomatous or villous
polyps of the colon or colonic cancer, or both, are at increased
risk for developing new neoplastic lesions. They should be followed
with air-contrast barium enema examinations alternating with colonoscopy each year for five years. If no new lesions are detected during
this period, the interval between reexaminations can be increased
to three years. Patients with more than 10 polyps, especially if there
is a family history of colonic cancer, should have yearly examinations.

Periodic testing of stools for occult blood is a useful adjunct to
the follow-up study of patients with gastrointestinal neoplasia. The

presence of occult blood in the stool may signal the development of new lesions and would warrant earlier reexamination.

SELECTED READING

Bussey HJR: *Familial Polyposis Coli.* Baltimore, Johns Hopkins University Press, 1975.

Dormandy TL: Gastrointestinal polyposis with mucocutaneous pigmentation (Peutz-Jeghers syndrome). *N Engl J Med* 256:1093–1102, 1141–1146, 1186–1190, 1957.

Moertel CG, Hill JR, Adson MA: Management of multiple polyposis of the large bowel. *Cancer* 28:160–164, 1971.

Muto T, Bussey HJR, Morson BC: The evolution of cancer of the colon and rectum. *Cancer* 36:2251–2270, 1975.

Shatney CH, Lorber PH, Gilbertsen VA, et al: The treatment of pedunculated adenomatous colorectal polyps with focal cancer. *Surg Gynecol Obstet* 139:845–850, 1974.

Welch CE, Hedberg SE: *Polypoid Lesions of the Gastrointestinal Tract,* vol. II. *Major Problems in Clinical Surgery,* ed 2. Philadelphia, WB Saunders Co, 1975.

Wennstrom J, Pierce ER, McKusick VA: Hereditary benign and malignant lesions of the large bowel. *Cancer* 34 (Suppl):850–857, 1974.

CLINICAL PROBLEMS

I. A 48-year-old man is found to have a single 2-cm polyp in the sigmoid colon during an evaluation of occult blood in the stool. He has a family history for colonic carcinoma in both his father and paternal uncle.

   1. What familial polyp syndrome does he have?

   2. How should he be managed?

   3. How should he be followed?

II. A 31-year-old man, also with a family history of colonic carcinoma (in his father and his father's only brother), undergoes evaluation for occult blood in the stool. His physical examination is normal. Both barium enema and sigmoidoscopy reveal polyps carpeting the mucosa.

1. What familial polyp syndrome does he have?
2. How should he be managed?
3. How should he be followed?

III. A 15-year-old boy is seen for a bout of colicky abdominal pain. He is noted to have melanin deposits on his buccal mucosa, lips, and perioral skin. An abdominal flat plate reveals a small-intestinal intussusception that resolves spontaneously. A subsequent barium x-ray of his small intestine demonstrates a polyp in the distal jejunum.

1. What familial polyp syndrome does he have?
2. How should he be managed?
3. How should he be followed?

Discussion

I. 1. Although the patient has a family history of colonic carcinoma, the presence of a single polyp is not consistent with either familial polyposis or Gardner's syndrome.

2. A polyp of this size should be excised.

3. The patient should be followed at yearly intervals with air-contrast barium enemas alternating with colonoscopy for five years. After that he can be followed with periodic testing of his stools for occult blood; if negative, the x-ray and colonoscopic examinations can be spaced more widely.

II. 1. These are typical findings for familial polyposis.

2. Because of the high risk of malignancy, the patient should undergo total colectomy.

3. With the colon removed, the disease process is "cured." However, other family members should be contacted and evaluated.

III. 1. This patient has a common presentation for Peutz-Jeghers syndrome.

2. At this point, the problem has resolved and the patient can

be followed conservatively. These polyps have no malignant potential.

3. The patient should be seen periodically and evaluated for recurrent pain or bleeding. If either becomes a significant problem, surgical excision of the polyp can be undertaken.

MARVIN DEREZIN

Perirectal Disease

Perianal diseases are not one of the more glamorous topics in the field of medicine. However, they linger and cause a great deal of discomfort in vast numbers of people. The popularity of over-the-counter hemorrhoid remedies attests to the enormity of this problem. (It has been estimated that 50% of the population past the age of 50 has hemorrhoids.) In large urban areas, perianal disease due to homosexuality is rapidly on the rise.

This chapter will discuss a number of these disorders: hemorrhoids, anal fissures, anorectal abscesses, perianal fistulas, pruritus ani, perianal venereal disease, proctalgia fugax, and rectal prolapse. Although these maladies are chronically discomforting, relatively few people consult their physician about them. Yet there are many simple common-sense approaches that may greatly alleviate the symptoms of these diseases.

HEMORRHOIDS

Hemorrhoids are the result of dilatation of the superficial veins that drain the anal canal and rectum. These veins anastomose

Table 1   Classification of Hemorrhoids

First degree:	Small, protrude into anal canal
Second degree:	Prolapse through anal orifice with defecation, but spontaneously reduce
Third degree:	Prolapse through anal orifice, require manual replacement
Fourth degree:	Chronically prolapsed and not reducible

with one another to form the inferior hemorrhoidal plexus, which gives rise to external hemorrhoids; internal hemorrhoids develop from dilatation of the superior hemorrhoidal plexus. Both networks communicate submucosally in the anal canal and lower rectum forming redundant erectile-like tissue.

Hemorrhoids may result from the upright posture of humans and the increased gravitational pressure in a valveless system. Additionally, a low-residue diet leads to forceful expulsion of hard stool and the increased intraabdominal pressure further dilates the anorectal veins. It may be that initially in the development of hemorrhoids the erectile hemorrhoidal tissue protrudes through the anus (e.g., during defecation); as the tissue becomes redundant and prolapsed, the tight anal sphincter strangulates the prolapsed hemorrhoids making them engorged and still more redundant.

Hemorrhoids may be graded by their size and redundancy; a useful classification is shown in Table 1. The stepwise progression from the first-degree hemorrhoid to the fourth-degree one represents the continuation of a repetitive injurious process.

Symptoms

The three cardinal symptoms of hemorrhoids are bleeding, prolapse, and pain. Pruritus, which will be discussed elsewhere in this chapter, is not a symptom of hemorrhoids per se, but may be due to associated low-grade chronic inflammation.

Hemorrhoids are the most common cause of rectal bleeding. This is frequently intermittent and asymptomatic, lasting for days at a time and disappearing for months on end, only to return at the most unexpected time. It is common for hemorrhoids to bleed with diarrhea or severe constipation. Hemorrhoidal bleeding may manifest itself with a stool streaked by bright-red blood, blood on the toilet paper, blood in the toilet water, or blood droplets sprayed on the toilet bowl. Occasionally patients will experience a frightening gush of blood during or immediately after defecation. Since blood is such an excellent pigment, relatively small amounts mixed in the water of the toilet bowl will appear as a large volume of blood loss. Most of the time, hemorrhoidal bleeding is minimal; iron deficiency anemia is only a very rare complication.

Chronic prolapse causes a great deal of discomfort; if the prolapsed tissue is not replaced, it becomes engorged, inflamed, and ulcerated. This may produce the sensation of something caught in the anal canal and an aching pain. It may also result in a mucoid discharge. Prolapse with incarceration leads to thrombosis.

Pain most frequently arises from acute thrombosis of the dilated hemorrhoidal veins and the resulting inflammation of the sensitive anal mucosa or perianal skin. The pain is most severe during the time of defecation and immediately thereafter. The thrombosis feels to the patient like a painful swelling within the anus and hurts especially with prolonged sitting or activity.

Diagnosis

Physical examination will usually reveal soft bulging hemorrhoids internally as well as externally. During bleeding episodes the insertion of an anoscope may stimulate oozing from the hemorrhoids so that the source of bleeding is documented as originating from the hemorrhoids. In the event of thrombosis, physical examination will reveal a blue, tense, shiny hemorrhoid with surrounding erythematous tissue that is exquisitely tender to touch. If not visualized externally, it may be felt on gentle digital examination. Usually a great deal of anal spasm is present.

Since rectal bleeding may also be the symptom of rectosigmoid carcinoma and ulcerative proctitis, an initial thorough evaluation is essential. Sigmoidoscopy followed by barium enema will dispel any question of tumor or proctitis. Patients with rectal bleeding who have a negative sigmoidoscopy (no hemorrhoids) and barium enema should be watched closely and repeated examinations should be performed to rule out missed lesions.

There is no evidence that over-the-counter remedies have any use in the acute management or prevention of hemorrhoids and their complications. Rather, the patient is placed on a high-residue diet with bran, or one of the psyllium mucilloids (Metamucil, Konsyl) is added so that the stool becomes soft, requiring less abdominal pressure to empty the bowels. Stool softeners (Colace, Surfak) may be used as well. Immediately after defecation, the patient is told how to use a lubricated little finger to gently push the hemorrhoids back into the anal canal and then to tighten the external sphincter voluntarily and remain standing for a short while for the sphincter to stay closed. Since there are no medical measures to reverse hemorrhoids, recurrent problems are to be expected.

At the time of the first hemorrhoidal bleeding, patients require a great deal of reassurance that the volume of blood they are passing is relatively small and that there are no long-term complications of hemorrhoids such as malignancy. They are warned that remissions and exacerbations are frequent. Surgical therapies are reserved for those patients whose bleeding results in anemia or who emotionally cannot tolerate the sight of their blood spilled repeatedly with bowel movements.

Should thrombosis occur, bed rest may relieve some of the pain by reducing the effects of gravity. Hot compresses (50% water and 50% witch hazel) on a cloth that is gently placed between the buttocks in contact with the hemorrhoids act as a very soothing remedy. Sitz baths are another alternative. The patient is placed on a high-residue diet with a stool softener (Colace or Surfak) and psyllium mucilloids (Metamucil or Konsyl) or bran is added. Oral pain medication may be necessary. If the patient is seen within the first day of thrombosis, the clot may be extracted with a simple incision with the patient under local anesthesia, shortening the convalescence that may otherwise take a week or longer. If recurrent thrombosis interferes with the patient's normal life pattern, one of the surgical procedures may be considered. Once an acute hemorrhoidal complication such as bleeding is resolved, patients frequently fall back into their old habits and pay very little attention to preventive measures such as keeping the stool soft and reinserting prolapsed hemorrhoids.

Surgical Treatment

Although hemorrhoids are very common and at times protrude extensively through the anal canal on a chronic basis, complications are relatively unusual; when they do occur they are usually treated adequately with the general measures previously outlined. Surgical intervention is necessary for those patients who have chronic and persistent bleeding or whose hemorrhoids are recurrently painful and interfere with life. The newer surgical techniques afford a high degree of success and a small incidence of complications with little discomfort, especially when compared to standard hemorrhoid surgery of the past.

One approach is to cause sclerosis and scarring at the base of the hemorrhoid within the rectum. This fixes the erectile tissue by scar so that it cannot prolapse during defecation and become engorged and thrombosed. Early methods used an injection of caustic solutions and cryosurgery using a freezing metal probe. There was profuse drainage after cryosurgery and the technique is no longer used very often. The current method of sclerosis consists of rubber band ligation at the base of the hemorrhoids resulting in sloughing and necrosis. Experienced physicians perform the procedure relatively painlessly and morbidity is almost nonexistent. It is successful in the majority of patients.

Another approach takes the view that the spastic external anal sphincter causes chronic engorgement and dilatation of hemorrhoidal tissue. The technique involves placing the patient under general anesthesia and dilating the sphincter forcibly. This simple technique has a very high permanent success rate with minimal complications. It may lead to incontinence in elderly people, however.

Surgical hemorrhoidectomy has been almost totally replaced by these newer techniques. Resective surgery is extremely painful and requires a hospital stay and a convalescent period.

ANAL FISSURE

Anal fissures are tears in the anal canal. They usually arise acutely as a result of trauma, probably related to the passage of a hard stool. They usually heal promptly; when they do not (possibly because of internal sphincteric spasm), chronic fissures ensue.

The symptoms of both acute and chronic fissures are the same, namely pain and bleeding. The bleeding is usually minimal and may only be appreciated as blood on the toilet paper. The pain is described as excruciating, tearing or burning, occurring with defecation, and lasting well after the bowel movement. It is sometimes replaced by a severe aching pain most likely due to muscle spasm. (The extraordinary pain will frequently discourage patients from moving their bowels.)

Fissures occur on the posterior wall in the midline in over 90% of the cases. Less often, they are found on the anterior midline. Multiple fissures or fissures located elsewhere should raise the question of underlying inflammatory bowel disease. Above chronic fissures there is a hypertrophied anal papilla and below there is an edematous sentinel skin tag.

External examination of the perianal area may reveal nothing unless the buttocks are spread widely and the anal ectoderm is visualized carefully. The sentinel skin tag may be seen in chronic fissures. Occasionally, the spasm and pain are so severe that digital examination is impossible unless liberal amounts of local anesthetic ointment are used. By gently separating the anal verge, the elliptical longitudinal fissure may be seen above the sentinel tag. A gentle digital examination with the little finger well lubricated may reveal the induration and thickness of the fissure. Anoscopy and sigmoidoscopy are very difficult because of the severe pain and spasm and may be postponed until treatment has successfully diminished the symptoms.

For both acute and chronic fissures, treatment consists of bulk agents and stool softeners. Sitz baths are used liberally and local anesthetic suppositories or ointment are instilled as often as necessary. Oral analgesics are sometimes required.

Most acute fissures will heal rapidly over a period of one to two weeks. Chronic fissures, on the other hand, do not, and surgical therapy is required. The principle of surgical therapy is to rupture the internal sphincter. (As previously noted, spasm may have a pathogenetic role in chronic fissures.) The most promising treatment available is dilatation of the anus under general anesthesia. This simple procedure is extremely effective, making resection of the fissure itself unnecessary. Another procedure performed under anesthesia is a lateral sphincterotomy, which severs the superficial layer of the internal sphincter along the anal canal. The success rate with this procedure is also extremely high. The choice of the surgical procedure lies in the hands of the surgeon who is treating the patient. The two approaches offer the advantage of no surgical resection of tissue and a very high success rate. However, incontinence is an occasional complication.

ANORECTAL ABSCESS

Anorectal abscesses occur in the soft-tissue spaces adjacent to the anus and rectum. The common areas for abscess collection are underneath the skin of the anus and in the ischiorectal space between the ischium and the external sphincter. They arise from perianal disease (anal cryptitis, fissures) or may be the presenting symptom of Crohn's disease or diseases of altered immunity.

The patient will frequently complain of pain and discomfort in the anorectal area with distress on sitting or walking. As the abscess becomes larger and more extensive, fever and even sepsis may appear. The higher up in the rectum the abscess occurs, the more likely that there will be lower abdominal discomfort without perianal distress.

The diagnosis is made by the presence of erythema, edema, and induration around the anus if the abscess is superficial. Digital examination will reveal tenderness and induration if deeper abscesses are present. It must be stressed that, although induration is felt without fluctuation, pus is almost invariably present and drainage should not be delayed. Delay will result in spreading of the abscess beyond the local tissue confines. Surgical or spontaneous drainage will result in an anorectal fistula in at least two-thirds of patients. Treatment is always surgical (drainage of the abscess). Antibiotics are usually required. The wound will have to drain from below and, if the tract is not kept open, abscesses may recur.

PERIANAL FISTULAS

Anal fistulas are tracts that extend from an anal crypt or an opening higher in the rectum to anywhere in the perianal area. These primary tracts may have secondary paths that open separately onto the perianal skin. They usually arise from an abscess in the wall of the rectum or crypt that has burrowed its way out to the perianal area. The tract remains after the abscess has ruptured or been drained surgically. Besides perianal disease, fistulas may arise from Crohn's disease, uncommon infections (tuberculosis, syphilis, or lymphogranuloma venereum), trauma, carcinoma, or radiation.

The patient complains of the drainage of pus and sometimes fecal material and blood from a tender opening somewhere alongside the anus. The area of drainage will intermittently become painful, red, tender, and edematous when free drainage has been blocked. Because of the extensive soft tissues in the area, fistular openings may occur at a good distance away from the anal orifice.

The diagnosis is made by finding an opening alongside the anus that is draining. It may be red and tender if drainage has not been complete. Digital examination will frequently reveal the thickened cord that extends from the crypt or lower rectum to the perianal area and fistula. The extent of the tract can be determined by passing a small probe through the fistula or by performing a fistulogram.

The differential diagnosis includes a draining pilonidal sinus, infected sebaceous cysts, hidradenitis suppurativa, or bartholin abscesses. These are local cutaneous lesions and do not communicate with an anal crypt.

Patients with anal fistula should be evaluated carefully for the presence of underlying inflammatory bowel disease. This is crucial and is done by sigmoidoscopy with biopsy and barium studies of the small and large intestine. Ideally these studies are accomplished before operation since such therapy in patients with Crohn's disease may result in extension and worsening of the perianal disease. Unfortunately, for many patients the diagnosis of Crohn's disease is first made when a simple fistulotomy is followed by the appearance of extensive fissuring, ulceration, and destruction of the perineum by the idiopathic inflammatory process. Thus, when the convalescent patient has continued difficulty with fistulas, sigmoidoscopic and barium x-ray examinations for underlying Crohn's disease or other types of infections should be undertaken.

The treatment for fistulas uncomplicated by inflammatory bowel disease is surgical (to establish adequate drainage by unroofing the tract, cleaning it out, and allowing it to heal by filling in from the base). The results of fistulotomy for uncomplicated fistulas are excellent. Complex ones are more difficult to treat and are associated with incontinence resulting from distortion of the anorectal area and interference with the sphincters.

PRURITUS ANI

Pruritus ani is an extremely common complaint that is frequently resistant to therapy. However, there are many known etiologic factors that, if corrected, can result in cure. It is therefore extremely important to be very familiar with all of the known causes of pruritus ani. These are listed in Table 2.

Pruritus is present at all times and characteristically is relieved only transiently by scratching. At night, when distracting stimuli of the day are absent, the itching seems to be worse. Patients with severe pruritus ani may scratch during their sleep and find blood on their fingers and in the perianal area on awakening in the morning.

Table 2 Causes of Pruritus Ani

Perianal disease
  Fistula (anal)
  Fissures
  Neoplasms
  Draining sinuses, cysts
  Dermatopathies
    Psoriasis
    Seborrhea
    Atopy
    Lichen planus
    Neurodermatitis
    Contact dermatitis
Infections
  Candidiasis
  Pinworms
  Trichomonas
  Pediculosis
  Scabies
  Condylomata acuminata
Systemic processes
  Diabetes mellitus
  Liver disease
  Oral antibiotics
Hygiene problems
  Increased moisture accumulation (hot climate, tight clothing, obesity, exercise)
  Poor general hygiene
Psychogenic

During the examination, evidence of systemic dermatologic disease is sought. External examination of a patient with a recent onset of symptoms may reveal erythema and excoriations with shiny exudative perianal skin; patients with chronic disease will have thickened, pigmented skin.

Evidence of acute disease should prompt a search for an infectious etiology. Scabies and pediculosis are self evident on examination. Pinworm ova can be sought by touching the perianal area with a piece of transparent tape and examining it under the microscope. Candidiasis may develop in diabetics and patients who are debilitated; the typical fungal appearance can be seen by adding 10% potassium hydroxide to skin scrapings and examining these microscopically.

The finding of chronic pruritus ani is more likely due to dermatologic disorders, a local anatomic problem (such as drainage of fecal material from prolapsed hemorrhoids), perianal irritations due to chronic diarrhea, or psychogenic disorders. The erogenous nature of the perianal skin may be one factor accounting for the difficulty in treating pruritus ani.

If underlying causes cannot be found, a general program is frequently helpful. If the stool is liquid or soft, a bulk agent in the form of psyllium mucilloid (Metamucil, Konsyl) or bran is added to the diet. If hemorrhoids are prolapsing, they are reinserted after each bowel movement. If there is any evidence of fecal stain, after each bowel movement gentle wiping is done with toilet tissue, followed by cotton or toilet paper moistened with warm water, and any remaining stool or secretion around the anus is dabbed off. The anal area is then patted dry and the patient is encouraged to wait before putting clothing back on to allow the moisture to evaporate. Tight clothing and snug underclothing are avoided. Soaps and detergents are changed. The area is not rubbed a great deal; the new soaps are used sparingly, as vigorous cleansing irritates the inflamed skin and perpetuates the cycle. Patients who scratch themselves during the night are advised to wear white cotton gloves. In the evening, or whenever possible, patients with severe skin changes may lie in bed without underclothing with their knees up; the involved skin is exposed to a lamp or heating source to dry the area.

Patients who have a severe exudative dermatitis from itching do well after the cleansing with an application of either zinc oxide ointment or talcum powder; the choice is made by the patient depending on the response. If there are still problems, 1% hydrocortisone cream can be applied in the morning and in the evening and the diet can be altered. Some believe that *Lactobacillus acidophilus* may make the stool acid and less irritating to the perianal area. Those patients whose disease remains refractory after all of these modalities have been tried often have an emotional disorder similar to neurodermatitis.

PERIANAL VENEREAL DISEASE

Perhaps due to increased sexual promiscuity, venereal diseases of the perianal area are becoming more common. These diseases include condylomata acuminata, gonorrhea, syphilis, lymphogranuloma venereum, chancroid, granuloma inguinale, and herpes.

Condylomata acuminata are venereal warts. In the beginning they are very small, but as they become larger they result in leakage of fecal material and itching. For small lesions in the perianal area, 10% podophyllin in benzoin may be used for fulguration. It must be applied carefully, avoiding the adjoining skin. For large lesions in the anal canal or in the perianal skin, surgical removal is required.

The diagnosis of rectal gonorrhea should be suspected when there is a history of anal intercourse. The symptoms are very much like those of ulcerative proctitis in that the lower rectum and upper anal canal are involved, with a purulent ulcerated mucosa. The symptoms are pain on defecation with profuse purulent discharge. The diagnosis is usually made by smear or culture. The disease responds to the usual treatment for gonorrhea. Lymphogranuloma venereum, in the acute stage, also presents as proctitis. Syphilis of the anus presents as an anorectal ulcer, chancroid as anorectal papules that ulcerate, granuloma inguinale as papulovesicles, and herpes simplex as vesicles or ulcers in the anal canal.

PROCTALGIA FUGAX

Proctalgia fugax is severe anal pain that occurs suddenly and lasts for 30 to 40 minutes. It is quite severe and disabling. The pain is probably due to spasm of the coccygeus and levator ani muscles. Most patients with this disease are extremely tense and the symptom complex may be emotionally stimulated. Usually there are no perianal lesions to explain the spasm. Treatment modalities include sedation, Sitz baths, and periodic massage of the tense muscles.

RECTAL PROLAPSE

Rectal prolapse occurs when the rectal mucosa itself prolapses through the anal orifice. Although it has been associated with cystic fibrosis, it commonly occurs in normal infants as well. It is rare in youngsters and young adults but again becomes more common in people over the age of 40.

Symptoms are related to the presence of the mass (initially only with defecation but eventually even with standing) and to the chronic irritation of the exposed mucosal lining (mucus discharge and bleeding). Patients with large prolapses have lax anal sphincters and they often have incontinence.

The diagnosis is made by inspection and palpation. If the prolapse is not readily apparent, the patient should be examined in the squatting position.

Treatment in young children is conservative. Measures designed to relieve constipation and straining are usually adequate. In adults, surgical therapy is often necessary, especially in severe cases.

SELECTED READING

Burkitt DP: Diet and its relation to hemorrhoids. *Coloproctology* 2:315–316, 1980.

Kaufman, HD: Hemorrhoids. Presentation and management. *Practical Gastroenterol* 4:51–57, 1980.

Muller CA: Internal hemorrhoidectomy by rubber band ligation. *Coloproctology* 2:317–319, 1980.

Schrock, TR: Diseases of the anorectum, in Sleisenger MH, Fordtran JS: *Gastrointestinal Disease.* Philadelphia, WB Saunders Co, 1978, pp 1875–1889.

CLINICAL PROBLEMS

I. A 45-year-old man complains of occasional episodes of red blood in his stool or on the toilet paper. He has noted this for the past four months. He denies any associated abdominal or rectal pain, weight loss, or fever. He has had no change in his bowel habits but he has been constipated "ever since I was a boy." He notes that the bleeding is most likely to occur if he passes a hard stool. He has no history or symptoms of any gastrointestinal disease. His physical examination is normal and a stool specimen is negative for occult blood.

A diagnostic evaluation is undertaken. A blood count and urinalysis are both normal. Sigmoidoscopy and anoscopy reveal internal hemorrhoids. A barium enema is normal except for two early diverticula.

1. What is causing the bleeding?
2. How should he be treated?
3. What problems might arise in the future?

II. A 38-year-old man complains of rectal bleeding, which is only noted as blood on the stool or toilet paper. This has been present for three to four months, and it is associated with a severe pain in the rectum associated with defecation. The pain persists, although less severe, for 15 to 30 minutes after the bowel movement. He denies fever, weight loss, or any previous gastrointestinal disease. He has tended to be constipated and this has become more of a problem in the past few months. The physical examination is unremarkable except for an edematous skin tag in the posterior anal orifice and increased anal sphincter tone. The stool does not contain occult blood.

Anoscopy is performed with difficulty; it demonstrates a 1- to 2-cm fissure in the posterior midline with a hypertrophied anal papilla above. The patient refuses sigmoidoscopy or barium enema because of the discomfort the anoscopy produced.

1. What is causing the bleeding?
2. How should it be treated?
3. What complication could arise from the disease or the treatment?

III. A 32-year-old man has noticed blood on the toilet paper after a bowel movement for the past month. He denies any blood in the stool, but he occasionally notes bloodstains on his pajama bottoms in the morning. He denies any real pain with the bowel movement, but notes that, if he has diarrhea, he has a burning sensation over the perianal skin. He has had no fever, weight loss, or any change in bowel habits. He denies previous gastrointestinal illness. His physical examination is remarkable for excoriated, thickened perianal skin. There is no other evidence of any skin disease elsewhere. The stool is negative for occult blood. When the perianal skin is observed and discussed with the patient, he states that the area has been itching on and off for years. This has been a problem especially in the past four to six weeks.

A diagnostic evaluation is undertaken. Anoscopy and sigmoidoscopy are both normal. Routine laboratory tests, including a blood count, urinalysis, liver tests, blood sugar, serum cholesterol, renal tests, electrolytes, and calcium, are also all normal.

1. What is the source of the bleeding?
2. Should any other tests be performed?
3. How should he be treated?

Discussion

I. 1. The presence of red blood would indicate that the bleeding is originating in the distal large intestine. The absence of blood in the stool or an anemia would argue against more proximal bleeding. The only lesions demonstrated are hemorrhoids and diverticula; the latter would not present in this fashion. Thus, the patient is bleeding from hemorrhoids.

  2. The patient should be advised to take a high-residue diet and bulk additives. There is no evidence that the hemorrhoids are prolapsing, so no therapy need be considered in this regard. The symptoms are minimal and operation would not be indicated.

  3. The major complications of hemorrhoids are thrombosis and more severe bleeding. In addition the hemorrhoids may enlarge and prolapse.

II. 1. The history and physical findings are typical of a chronic anal fissure, which was demonstrated on anoscopy. Although other lesions could coexist (carcinoma, proctitis) this is unlikely. Diagnostic sigmoidoscopy can be obtained after the fissure is healed if symptoms persist.

2. Bulk agents, stool softeners, Sitz baths, and local anesthetics may be tried, along with oral analgesics as necessary. It is likely, however, that medical therapy will be unsuccessful and that a surgical approach will be required (rectal dilatation or sphincterotomy).

3. Potential complications of the fissure are the development of a rectal abscess and subsequent fistula. Incontinence is a rare complication of the surgical therapy.

III. 1. In this case the source of the blood is the excoriated perianal skin. The patient has pruritus ani.

2. The patient can have the perianal skin examined for ova (the previously described tape test) and fungi (skin scrapings). The etiology of the pruritus ani is, however, likely either idiopathic or secondary to a neurodermatitis. (It may be that some patients in this former category suffer from skin irritation secondary to alkaline stool.)

3. In the absence of a demonstrable underlying etiology for the pruritus, the program previously described should be employed. This includes bulk agents if the stool is liquid or soft, gentle cleansing of the perianal area after each bowel movement, the avoidance of moisture collection in the perianal region (loose clothes, periods of air exposure of the skin), and changing soaps and detergents (to eliminate any possible contact allergens). If nocturnal scratching is occurring, the patient should wear soft gloves while sleeping. If these measures fail, a trial of hydrocortisone ointment or *Lactobacillus acidophilus,* or both, can be undertaken. If all of these measures fail, the symptoms continue to be substantial, and anxiety appears to be present, formal or informal psychotherapy may be undertaken.

17

RONALD L. KORETZ

Hepatitis

HOW DO I MAKE THE DIAGNOSIS?

A 25-year-old man comes to your office after having been at home for five days with nausea, vomiting, anorexia, lassitude, mild right upper quadrant discomfort, and jaundice. He denies the use of alcohol, illicit drugs, or medication. His past medical history is completely unremarkable. Jaundice and a slightly enlarged and tender liver are found on physical examination. Laboratory tests obtained that day reveal the following:

SGPT:	1,150 IU	(normal, 5–45 IU)
SGOT:	985 IU	(normal, 10–40 IU)
Bilirubin:	6.1 mg%	(normal, 0.1–1.2 mg%)
Alkaline phosphatase:	117 IU	(normal, 15–85 IU)

Acknowledgment: The author is most grateful for Sally Clement's patience and perseverance in the preparation of this manuscript.

Viral hepatitis is usually diagnosed on the basis of a typical clinical picture accompanied by biochemical parameters of hepatocyte necrosis. However, most hepatitis viral infections pass completely unnoticed by human hosts and their physicians, and thus this symptomatic, icteric case represents only the tip of the iceberg. Diagnosing this tip is important because these are the patients who seek medical attention.

The serologic identification of both hepatitis A and B has now enabled us to make etiospecific diagnoses, which in turn bear on immunoprophylaxis and prognosis. For this reason it is important to consider these serologic tests in more detail.

Hepatitis B is diagnosed by demonstrating the presence of the virus in the blood stream, and is one of the few instances of viral illness in which the agent itself (rather than a host antibody response) is sought. Hepatitis B surface antigen (HBsAg), previously referred to as the hepatitis-associated (HAA) or the Australia antigen, is a protein component of the outer shell or coat of the viral particle.

In some commercial laboratories, serologic panels of hepatitis B tests, which also include two host-derived antibodies, are being offered. Antibody to surface antigen, anti-HBs, represents the classic convalescent immune response. Anti-HBs is first found in the circulation weeks or months after HBsAg has cleared, remains for years, and quickly reappears or rises in titer if hepatitis B reexposure occurs (anamnestic response). The demonstration of endogenous anti-HBs in an individual implies immunity, at least against a "low-dose" exposure. (A low dose would be a few cubic centimeters or less of infected material, in contrast to a "high dose" such as a unit of blood.)

The second antibody system is a little more complex. Just as HBsAg represents a component of the outer shell of the viral agent, an antigen locus on the inner nucleoprotein core has also been identified. This is referred to as hepatitis B core antigen, or HBcAg. In the circulation the nucleoprotein center is surrounded by the surface material, and it cannot be demonstrated directly by an antigen-antibody reaction. However, HBcAg appears to be able to elicit a host antibody (possibly because it is exposed to the reticuloendothelial system in the liver), which is referred to as anti-core antibody, or anti-HBc. Anti-HBc arises early in the course of hepatitis B infection and can be found in the circulation shortly after HBsAg appears.

Usually HBsAg-positive blood is also positive for anti-HBc. However, anti-HBc may persist for years after hepatitis B infection has resolved by all other criteria. Unlike anti-HBs, anamnestic responses of anti-HBc are not seen.

Since anti-HBc is present during the entire course and recovery of hepatitis B, of what use is it? (Its demonstration does not differentiate recent from past infection.) Since it arises early in the course of disease, the absence of anti-HBc in a patient with clinical hepatitis virtually excludes the diagnosis of hepatitis B.

The various combinations of these three tests—HBsAg, anti-HBs, and anti-HBc—are displayed in Table 1. Although there are eight possible combinations of results, only five are likely to be encountered. HBsAg is usually seen with anti-HBc except if serum has been obtained in the few days before anti-HBc development. It is unusual to see both HBsAg and anti-HBs circulating together, as one or the other would exist in excess. (In those rare instances where both are seen together, subtype differences between the HBsAg and the anti-HBs are invariably found.) The most perplexing situation will arise when anti-HBc alone is found. This may indicate active hepatitis B or a residual convalescent marker.

Table 1 Serologic Combinations in Hepatitis B

HBsAg	Anti-HBs	Anti-HBc	Interpretation
−	−	−	No hepatitis B infection
−	−	+	Active or convalescent hepatitis B infection (see text)
−	+	−	Convalescent hepatitis B
−	+	+	Convalescent hepatitis B
+	−	−	Very early hepatitis B infection (rare situation)
+	−	+	Active hepatitis B infection
+	+	−	Very early hepatitis B infection with antibody of different subtype (extremely rare situation)
+	+	+	Active hepatitis B infection with antibody of different subtype (rare situation)

Adapted with permission from Koretz RL: Acute and chronic hepatitis, in Gitnick GL (ed): *Current Gastroenterology and Hepatology.* Boston, Houghton Mifflin Professional Publishers, 1979, pp. 234–275.

No commercial test is available for identifying the specific agent of hepatitis A, and, in any event, the viremic phase is likely to be short lived. Antibody to heptitis A, anti-HA, arises shortly after the onset of clinical illness and is often present when the patient is first seen. Thus, while a negative anti-HA test (especially if it is still negative several days later) would argue against the diagnosis of hepatitis A, the presence of the antibody may only reflect prior sub-clinical infection.

The problem of interpreting a positive anti-HA test has been surmounted. The early antibody arising in hepatitis A is of a specific immunoglobulin class, IgM. Techniques are commercially available that will selectively identify IgM-specific anti-HA. Thus, the acute infection can be differentiated from the convalescent state, in which the anti-HA is composed of IgG antibodies.

Other viruses besides the two classic agents, A and B, produce hepatitis (Table 2). Some of these (there are at least two) have been unrecognized previously, but appear to be important causes of disease in the posttransfusion and dialysis situations. Until such time that specific tests are developed for their identification, they will be known as "non-A, non-B hepatitis." Besides A, B, the non-A, non-B agents, cytomegalovirus, and the Ebstein-Barr agent, other viruses are only very rare causes of hepatitis.

Table 2 Hepatitis Viruses

Common agents
    Hepatitis A
    Hepatitis B
    Cytomegalovirus (relatively common)
    Ebstein-Barr virus (relatively common)
    Non-A, non-B hepatitis (at least two agents)

Rare agents
    Adenovirus
    Coxsackie
    Herpes simplex
    Mumps
    Reovirus
    Rubella
    Rubeola
    Yellow fever

WHAT ADDITIONAL WORKUP DOES
THE PATIENT REQUIRE?

In the usual situation the diagnosis of hepatitis is obvious and the history, physical examination, and battery of liver and serologic tests already noted are sufficient to make the diagnosis. Occasionally acute hepatitis pursues a virulent course, so-called fulminant hepatic failure or acute yellow atrophy. The process usually begins as typical viral hepatitis, but, over the next few days or weeks, obvious hepatic failure with deepening jaundice, encephalopathy, coagulopathy, and a variety of metabolic abnormalities ensue. Although there is no way to predict with certainty who is likely to develop this syndrome, patients who are first seen with more severe clinical or biochemical parameters of disease are at increased risk. Further biochemical evaluation of liver function (and closer observation, as will be discussed later) should be obtained, and a prolonged prothrombin time is an important indicator in this regard.

Serum bile acids are sensitive indicators of minimal liver dysfunction. However, in the setting of acute hepatitis there is no reason to measure them. Similarly no reason exists for performing a sulfobromophthalein (BSP) retention test. Examination of serum protein levels is also usually of little benefit.

Occasionally the differential diagnosis of jaundice is a problem. This may especially be the case in the small fraction of patients in whom a cholestatic phase of hepatitis develops. [The serum bilirubin begins to climb (> 10 mg%), the alkaline phosphatase elevation becomes more and more prominent while the transaminase levels return toward more normal values, and pruritus becomes a significant clinical problem.] In this subgroup of patients, other procedures that establish the presence or absence of biliary obstruction may need to be employed.

HOW SHOULD I TREAT THE PATIENT?

Treatment of the Patient

No specific therapy exists for hepatitis viral infections analogous to antibiotic treatment of bacterial diseases. Hence, the major therapeutic measures are designed to support the patient and to prevent the spread of illness.

Bed rest has been long advocated for patients with acute hepatitis. Many of the patients are significantly fatigued, so that they are incapable of conducting some or all of their usual daily activity anyway. On the other hand, other patients feel reasonably well and their question to the physician is usually how much activity they can undertake safely.

Several prospective controlled trials have been conducted in the past and none has shown any deleterious effect from exercise. It would seem reasonable, therefore, to allow the patient to perform as much of his or her daily routine as can be done comfortably, using fatigue as the end point.

Similarly a variety of diets have been proposed, most commonly one high in protein and low in fat. Again no evidence exists demonstrating any benefit for any particular dietary regimen. Since such patients often have problems with nausea and anorexia, the diet should be designed around whatever the patient can tolerate and will eat. Although an occasional drink is not likely to be detrimental, alcohol consumption should be discouraged during the acute stage of illness. There is no evidence that the use of vitamin supplementation is of any real benefit in a reasonably well-nourished patient. However, a daily multivitamin tablet is unlikely to do harm, is relatively inexpensive, and provides the patient (and the physician?) with the impression that an active therapeutic regimen is being undertaken.

Therapy with corticosteroids has been advocated for many years. It is possible that their use may be associated with an early, more rapid fall in the serum bilirubin. However, they do not have any long-term effect on the illness. Furthermore, like other agents used in clinical medicine, they have a large number of associated side effects, and their usage may be associated with a higher relapse rate. As such, steroids should not be employed in the usual case of viral hepatitis, and, in fact, recent studies have indicated that they are not effective even in severe cases of acute disease.

As a general rule the use of all drugs should be discouraged. Antibiotics do not appear to have any effect. Sedatives and tranquilizers, which are normally metabolized in the liver, may have significantly prolonged half-lives. The nausea and vomiting usually last only a few days. Antiemetics have been advocated, but, if the symptoms are particularly severe, thought should be given to hospitalization for intravenous fluid therapy as an alternative.

When should patients with viral hepatitis be hospitalized (Table 3)? When they can no longer be cared for or care for themselves at home, hospitalization becomes the only viable alternative. Thus, the indication may be a function of the social situation; patients who

Table 3 Indications for Hospitalization in Acute Hepatitis

Inability to be cared for at home
Observation for development of fulminant course
Liver biopsy
Prolonged course
Severe or progressive disease
Cholestasis
Diagnostic dilemma
Rule out underlying chronic hepatitis

live by themselves may require hospital support that patients with a spouse could find at home. Hospitalization also needs to be accomplished when, as noted previously, intravenous hydration is necessary. Severely ill patients should be hospitalized for observation if there is concern over the development of fulminant hepatitis. An abnormal prothrombin time may be a clue in this regard. Some physicians have also selected arbitrary biochemical criteria [e.g., a serum aminotransferase (transaminase) greater than 2,000 IU], but these guidelines must be tempered by the clinical appearance of the patient. (Occasionally such individuals are encountered who have virtually no symptoms!) Finally patients are admitted when there is diagnostic confusion and/or a liver biopsy is to be performed. For the usual clinical situation, a liver biopsy is unnecessary. The indications for liver biopsy in acute disease are included in Table 3.

Treatment of the Contacts

Epidemiologic Information

A major consideration in management is to prevent others from becoming infected with the virus. Some aspects of the epidemiology of the viruses should be considered in this regard.

The old epidemiologic assumption that all nonparenteral hepatitis represents hepatitis A is wrong. Sporadic disease may be due to A, B, or one of the non-A, non-B viruses. Nonetheless the major route of hepatitis A spread in the community is via fecal-oral contamination. For an individual with acute disease, fecal shedding begins before the serum aminotransferase rises. By the time the jaundice and biochemical tests of liver disease peak, fecal shedding is no longer demonstrable.

A great deal of information is known about the spread of hepatitis B largely because of the availability of a marker of the viral particle itself. The identification of the marker, HBsAg, came about because of the interesting biologic property of this virus to produce the carrier state. Chronic HBsAg carriers are individuals who, at any point in time, demonstrate HBsAg in their serum. They may or may not have underlying liver disease. The DNA hepatitis B virus appears to establish some type of symbiotic relationship with the host. (Hepatitis A, an RNA virus, does not produce a carrier state.) It is estimated that 0.1% to 0.5% of the population in the United States is a carrier, and the rate is 10 to 100 times higher in other, less developed, areas of the world.

When considering the epidemiology of hepatitis B, the hepatitis B e antigen (HBeAg) must also be reviewed. This is yet another of the hepatitis B antigen systems. (We have previously covered the surface and core antigens.) HBeAg would appear to be another nucleoprotein component of the virus, but it is less firmly bound to the viral core and can be found floating in the circulation. Its important clinical value is that HBsAg-positive material which also contains HBeAg is more infectious than HBsAG-positive material that contains the host-derived antibody (anti-HBe) or neither e marker. Unfortunately this is not a black and white relationship; HBeAg-positive exposures will not always result in hepatitis B transmissions and anti-HBe–positive material may still be infectious. (Remember that HBsAg-positive fluids may contain HBeAg, anti-HBe, or neither, but HBeAg positivity is only seen when HBsAg is present.) Thus, although HBeAg testing is likely to become commercially available in the near future, its utility for any given clinical situation will be limited. For purposes of immunoprophylaxis, any HBsAg-positive exposure must be considered as potentially infectious, regardless of the e status of the exposing agent.

In the setting of acute hepatitis B, the duration of HBsAg positivity (and presumed infectivity?) is variable, lasting from days to weeks. (Anything lasting longer would fall into the realm of chronic hepatitis, which will be discussed separately.) During this time all fluids, not just blood, are potentially infectious. In spite of this, it has been shown that hepatitis B is not effectively transmitted throughout the household,′ and, in fact, only the spouse is at significant risk of infection. However, between 25% and 50% of anti-HBs–negative spouses will acquire at least serologic evidence of hepatitis B exposure.

This observation about selective spouse susceptibility has added support to the notion that hepatitis B is a sexually transmitted disease. Other lines of evidence are that serologic evidence of past or present hepatitis B is more common among individuals with broad sexual experiences (e.g., prostitutes, male homosexuals), that semen and vaginal secretions are HBsAg positive, and that hepatitis B has been produced experimentally when HBsAg-positive semen was injected into chimpanzees. All of this evidence is indirect and does not imply that the virus actually crosses the genital mucosa. It is probably fair to consider hepatitis B a disease of intimacy, but no evidence yet exists establishing it as a venereal disease in the sense that syphilis or gonorrhea are sexually transmitted.

Certain other populations are at increased risk of hepatitis B exposure. These include residents and staff of institutions, patients and workers in hemodialysis units, health care workers in general, and neonates of mothers positive for HBsAg in the third trimester (especially if the mother has acute hepatitis rather than being a chronic carrier). On the other hand, although a few epidemics of hepatitis B have been traced back to HBsAg-positive health care workers, such individuals as a general rule do not represent a risk to their patients. Prospective follow-up examinations of 558 contacts of 10 such health care workers (with both acute and chronic disease) have failed to demonstrate any hepatitis transmission.

Since at least two non-A, non-B agents appear to exist, and since specific serologic tests are unavailable, statements about epidemiologic patterns are difficult to make. However, non-A, non-B disease appears to account for some (10% to 25%) of the sporadic hepatitis seen in the community. It is the most common cause of posttransfusion hepatitis and it may be becoming a significant problem in the dialysis unit. Finally, at least one of these agents also produces the chronic carrier state.

Prophylaxis Information

What is reasonable advice to give the hepatitis patient with regard to protecting his or her family and the community in general? It is likely that the virus is present in all body fluids and these should be isolated as much as possible. The patient who lives in a residence with two bathrooms should use one and the rest of the family should use the other. If separate facilities are not available, care should be taken to isolate urine and feces, employing such measures as double flushing and the washing of retained particulate matter off the toilet bowl after a bowel movement. Meticulous hand washing should also be stressed. The patient should make sure other bathroom implements such as combs, razor blades, and toothbrushes are not shared with other family members. The patient should not prepare food for others and should use disposable plates and utensils for eating. (These restrictions may be excessive in cases of hepatitis A and they may be relaxed after immunoprophylaxis has been provided.)

What about sexual activity? If the patient is having significant symptoms, he or she usually will avoid sex anyway. However, if the patient is feeling reasonably well, one of the first questions asked is whether he or she may indulge in sex. It is appropriate to present the concept to the patient that the possibility for transmission is there and, in general, it is also appropriate to advocate abstention. It is problematical, however, whether such advice is always heeded.

One situation that must be considered is the question of immunoprophylaxis. Who gets gamma globulin? When should it be given? What type should be provided? The answers to these questions depend on the exact agent causing the disease.

In hepatitis A, standard immunoglobulin (SIG) is effective. It should be given to all household contacts at a dosage of 0.02 ml/ kg within seven days of exposure. (Some evidence exists that SIG given in the second week after exposure will produce attenuation of the disease.) Any individual with preexistent anti-HA is already immune and requires no prophylaxis.

Passive immunoprophylaxis for hepatitis B is another problem entirely. Because it has generally been believed that SIG is ineffective against hepatitis B, a special immunoglobulin (hepatitis B immune globulin, or HBIG) was produced with a high titer of anti-HBs. This material has been shown to be effective in several clinical situations, but it is quite expensive ($\cong$ \$150 per injection). If it is to be used, 0.06 ml/kg should be given, within seven days of exposure, and a second injection should be given four weeks after the first.

HBIG has been shown to prevent disease in anti-HBs–negative health care workers who were inadvertently exposed to HBsAg-positive material, either through percutaneous or mucosal routes. It likewise protects susceptible spouses of patients with acute hepatitis B. The third area where it is likely to be of benefit is in neonates of mothers with acute hepatitis B in the third trimester.

HBIG prophylaxis has also been shown to be effective in hemodialysis units when it is used in an ongoing program of injections every few months. However, the cost of such a program is staggering and other cheaper methods of infection control are probably equally effective.

Similarly HBIG may be effective in protecting the spouses and neonates of chronic carriers, but again the cost is immense, as lifelong treatment may be required. Spouses of carriers usually develop their own natural immunity and only infrequently develop clinically apparent acute or chronic disease.

Theoretically some benefit might accrue to neonates by offering passive immunoprophylaxis until their own immune system matures to the point that there is less risk of their developing the chronic carrier state and chronic hepatitis. (Neonates of mothers who have acute third-trimester disease often develop anicteric chronic hepatitis and the HBsAg carrier state.) However, with the exception of Oriental families, most neonates of chronic carriers fail to develop chronic disease themselves and the exact role of HBIG immunoprophylaxis is unclear. One injection of HBIG at birth does not provide significant long-term protection to the neonates of chronic carriers.

In conclusion, HBIG immunoprophylaxis should be given to potentially susceptible (anti-HBs–negative) individuals if they have been inoculated accidentally with material containing HBsAg or if they are spouses or neonates of individuals with acute hepatitis B (Table 4).

Work is currently under way to develop vaccines against both hepatitis A and B. Neither vaccine, however, is commercially available at the present time, although one for hepatitis B will probably be released in the near future.

No specific recommendations can be made concerning passive immunoprophylaxis for non-A, non-B disease. Some evidence suggests that SIG may be effective, and it should be provided in those situations which are analogous to the use of HBIG in hepatitis B.

WHAT SHOULD I EXPECT FROM SUCCESSFUL TREATMENT?

The long-term prognosis of hepatitis A is excellent once the patient recovers. The chronic carrier state or chronic hepatitis, or both, are unrecognized in this illness.

Table 4 Indications for the use of Hepatitis B Immune Globulin

Prophylaxis should be provided to:
  Susceptible[a] victims of mucocutaneous exposures to HBsAg
    ("needlestick")
  Susceptible[a] spouses of patients with acute hepatitis B
  Neonates of mothers with acute third-trimester hepatitis B
Prophylaxis may be effective, but is economically unfeasible, in:
  Spouses of chronic carriers
  Health care workers employed in high-risk areas (e.g., dialysis units)
  Neonates of chronic carriers

[a] "Susceptible" refers to those patients who do not have serologic evidence of past or present hepatitis B infection.

The situation for both hepatitis B and non-A, non-B hepatitis is different than for hepatitis A. Both diseases produce chronic hepatitis and the chronic carrier state in a certain percentage of people. For icteric hepatitis B the number often quoted is 10%, but this may be inaccurate. Most chronic carriers are and have been anicteric. After chronic disease is established, a small number may have an acute exacerbation (or even some other viral or nonviral cause for an acute illness). This episode may be identified inappropriately as being "acute icteric hepatitis B" with subsequent "chronic disease."

At least one of the non-A, non-B viral infections also appears to result in chronic hepatitis in a significant number of cases. In the posttransfusion situation (where the dose of virus is huge) some 20% to 70% of patients develop prolonged periods of transaminase elevations, and liver biopsies have revealed both chronic active and chronic persistent hepatitis. Chronic hepatitis has also been seen in non-A, non-B disease resulting from low-dose exposures, but its frequency of occurrence is not established.

Therefore, most of the time one can anticipate a successful resolution of the illness. The serum aminotransferases will gradually return to normal, usually over a period of weeks to months. For unexplained reasons, fatigue and malaise may be noted by the patient for some time after biochemical resolution has occurred. This "post-hepatitis syndrome" also usually clears up over time.

The management of chronic hepatitis will be discussed in subsequent sections.

WHAT MIGHT CAUSE A FAILURE
OF TREATMENT?

As there is no specific treatment for viral hepatitis, it is not appropriate to consider therapeutic failures. However, progression to fulminant hepatitis represents a failure of the disease process to resolve without serious acute sequelae. Fulminant hepatitis carries a grave prognosis, with mortality rates ranging between 60% and 95%. A number of specific therapeutic modalities have been attempted but they are currently either thought not to be efficacious or still experimental (Table 5). The management program consists of intensive supportive care, with close attention to fluid and electrolyte balance and acid/base defects as well as correction of

Table 5   **Proposed Treatments for Fulminant Hepatitis**

Corticosteroids[a]
Exchange transfusions[a]
Plasmapheresis
Heparin[a]
Cross circulation (human, baboon)
Extracorporeal isolated liver
Liver transplant
Hemodialysis
Hyperbaric oxygen
Antacids/cimetidine[a]
Anti-HBs globulin (for hepatitis B)[a]
Total body washout
Exchange resins[b]
Absorbent hemoperfusion[b]
Insulin and glucagon[b]

[a] Shown not to improve survival in controlled, prospective, randomized trials (heparin trial to acetaminophen-induced, not viral, fulminant hepatic failure).
[b] Experimental technique.

coagulopathies (using available clotting factors such as fresh frozen plasma) and hypovolemia. Antiencephalopathic measures (lactulose or neomycin) are also appropriate. Prophylactic acid reduction (using antacids or cimetidine) reduces the incidence of bleeding, and should be used even though no improvement in survival has been shown to result.

Occasionally patients are advertently or inadvertently exposed to nonviral hepatotoxins, which may make the disease worse or may even be responsible for the hepatitis. It is imperative that careful drug histories be elicited, including substances that can be obtained without prescription, such as analgesics or laxatives. The issue of alcohol use (or abuse) is also important in some patients.

In the event of continuing jaundice, the question of other disease processes invariably arises. This subject has already been covered extensively. It should be pointed out that gallstones traversing the common bile duct have been known to transiently raise the aminotransferase levels, even into the thousands. Unlike hepatitis, however, the aminotransferase quickly returns to normal (usually within a few days), while the bilirubin and alkaline phosphatase continue to rise if ductal obstruction supervenes.

WHAT ARE THE SIDE EFFECTS OF TREATMENT?

Since there is no specific therapy for viral hepatitis, there are no side effects either.

HOW SHOULD THE PATIENT BE FOLLOWED?

Since there is no primary therapy for disease, the major short-term goals are to protect the contacts and to rule out the development of fulminant hepatitis. The former topic has already been considered. With regard to the latter, a fulminant course is seen only in patients with identifiable severe disease at some point. Therefore, the patients at risk (with regard to developing this problem in the follow-up period) are those who have markedly symptomatic (usually icteric) disease, especially those whose prothrombin times are prolonged (> 2 seconds over that of control).

Such patients, if they are not hospitalized, should be seen a few days after their initial visit, when repeat biochemistries are obtained, including a prothrombin time. If there has been no clinical or biochemical deterioration, visits can be lengthened to every week and then, when clinical and biochemical improvement is seen, further follow-up study can be accomplished as described in the next paragraph. At the time of the initial visit, careful instructions should be given to other household members to watch for changes in behavior in the patient.

The patients in whom progression to fulminant disease is not a consideration can be seen at biweekly intervals for the first month; then routine follow-up study should consist of monthly or bimonthly biochemical (and serologic in cases of hepatitis B) determinations until the liver tests have returned to normal. (For hepatitis B, the HBsAg should disappear as well.)

In the usual case, the aminotransferases will return to normal, the jaundice will disappear, and the patient will become asymptomatic. If the aminotransferases do not return to normal (or if the HBsAg remains positive), consideration should be given to the development of chronic hepatitis.

WHAT COMPLICATIONS OF THE DISEASE CAN OCCUR?

The problem of fulminant hepatitis has already been discussed. A small percentage of patients will develop a cholestatic phase of disease, which has also been discussed previously. In these patients problems in the differential diagnosis of jaundice arise, and may need to be resolved by means of the techniques described in the chapter on jaundice.

Acute viral hepatitis has been associated with a large number of complications. Many of these are itemized in Table 6. Arthritis or skin rashes, or both, are common prodromal phenomena in acute hepatitis B. The other complications are rare; many of them are believed to be due to the circulation and deposition of antigen-antibody immune complexes.

The major sequela that needs to be mentioned, and which will occupy the remainder of this chapter, is the question of chronic hepatitis. Before embarking on this discussion, certain concepts need to be defined.

Hematologic
    Anemia of varying causes, including aplastic
    Reticulocytopenia
    Leukopenia
    Thrombocytopenia
    Coagulopathies
Rheumatologic
    Arthritis and arthralgia
    Dermatomyositis
    Glomerulonephritis
    Tenosynovitis
    Myopathy
Dermatologic
    Urticaria
    Maculopapular rashes
    Papular acrodermatitis of childhood
Miscellaneous
    Pancreatitis
    Labyrinthitis
    Pericarditis
    Renal failure
Chronic hepatitis

The term chronic hepatitis (CH) stirs up different images in different minds. For the purposes of this chapter, only a very general interpretation will be employed. Chronic hepatitis will refer to the presence of inflammation in the liver that has lasted for at least six months. It is to be emphasized that the term will not refer to a date of onset (which may or not be known), etiology, prognosis, histology, or symptoms. The terms chronic active hepatitis (CAH) and chronic persistent hepatitis (CPH) will refer to specific histologic appearances, and again will not implicate considerations of clinical presentation and prognosis. CAH is characterized by piecemeal necrosis, inflammation, increased fibrosis, and hepatocytolysis. The necrosis may extend only into the hepatic lobule, or it may extend across one lobule (bridging necrosis) or several lobules (multilobular necrosis). CPH, on the other hand, has the inflammatory infiltrate confined to the portal tract and may or may not have associated intralobular hepatocytolysis.

Unfortunately the term CAH has become identified in many people's minds with a progressive clinical syndrome characterized by severe symptoms and the ultimate development of cirrhosis and liver failure. It is becoming clear that most of the patients who demonstrate CAH on liver biopsy do not have this rapidly progressive disease, and in fact many are asymptomatic. Why has this happened?

The initial descriptions of CAH were confined to a clinical illness usually appreciated in young women who also had a multitude of clinical and biochemical autoimmune features; this disease came to be known as "lupoid" hepatitis. If untreated a large number of these patients developed cirrhosis and died of liver failure. As will be discussed further in the next section, treatment with corticosteroids significantly improved the morbidity and mortality.

In the past 10 to 15 years, the advent of multichannel autoanalyzers has resulted in the identification of large numbers of asymptomatic individuals with abnormal aminotransferases. It would have been predicted that such people would demonstrate CPH on biopsy, since the clinical correlation of this lesion is an asymptomatic patient with nonprogressive liver disease (i.e., disease that does not produce cirrhosis). However, when these patients underwent biopsy, some displayed the histologic features of CAH.

In a similar vein, HBsAg screening of units of blood has identified asymptomatic chronic carriers. Some of these people also are shown to have CAH when liver biopsy is performed.

The natural history of asymptomatic CAH is unknown. It is clear that, if cirrhosis and liver failure occur, the process takes years, possibly even decades. On the other hand, nonalcoholic patients are occasionally seen who first present with problems related to end-stage liver disease, and histologic examination of their livers often reveals CAH in addition to the cirrhosis ("postnecrotic cirrhosis").

As has been mentioned before, both hepatitis B and at least one of the non-A, non-B agents pursue chronic courses. It is often difficult to determine when the disease began and to answer the question of whether acute has become chronic. Some information is available, however, especially in the posttransfusion situation. As an outgrowth of studies of posttransfusion hepatitis, patients have been followed from the time of exposure (before they have acute infection) through the acute stage into long-term follow-up. If inflammation is measured by elevations in aminotransferase, a sizeable proportion of patients with non-A, non-B disease are shown to maintain their hepatitis for more than six months. (The figure has been reported to be as high as 70%!) Some of these patients have undergone liver biopsy, and both CPH and CAH have been found, providing histologic confirmation of the observed biochemical chronicity. Some suggestive evidence is beginning to accumulate that non-A, non-B viral disease pursues a chronic course in the nontransfusion situation as well.

Among HBsAg chronic carriers with abnormal aminotransferases, the incidence of CAH is 10% to 20%. (Interestingly among carriers with normal aminotransferases this frequency is only 1% to 2%.) Presumably hepatitis B is etiologically related to their histologic abnormalities, and at one time these individuals probably become infected with the virus (the acute phase of the illness).

Since acute becomes chronic, what is the long-term prognosis of such patients? It is clear that such people do not pursue a rapid downhill course. On the other hand, HBsAg-positive patients with clinically end-stage postnecrotic cirrhosis are found. How did these patients get to this point? Did they have previously unrecognized CAH? Similarly if one peruses the reports of the long-term follow-up studies in non-A, non-B posttransfusion hepatitis, occasional patients are described with histologic evidence of cirrhosis or clinical or biochemical findings of portal hypertension and liver failure. Will more of these patients also ultimately progress to end-stage liver disease? The answers to all of these questions are unknown at this time.

HOW SHOULD CHRONIC HEPATITIS BE MANAGED?

It has been established that immunosuppressive agents are effective in the autoimmune variant of CAH in which the patients have symptoms, high-grade aminotransferase activity, and liver biopsies that reveal bridging or multilobular necrosis or cirrhosis. The doses used are either: (1) prednisone, 20 mg a day or (2) prednisone, 10 mg a day and azathioprine, 50 mg a day. The situation is not as clear for the less severe variant, which is frequently seen in patients whose illness appears to have a viral etiology. In fact no evidence is currently available to indicate whether immunosuppressives are effective at all in this situation. One could even argue that they are contraindicated in an illness caused by a chronic infection. (At this time experimental protocols are in existence testing antiviral agents directly, but these materials are not currently available and they are not likely to become available in the near future.) On the other hand, if the progressive nature of the illness is due not to the viral infection per se but to the host inflammatory process, it is conceivable that such agents as corticosteroids may be effective in preventing the progressive inflammation, with consequent fibrosis.

Since no rational answer is available based on hard data, it has become necessary to make one up until the appropriate trials are done. In fact, every hepatologist has made his answer up, so there are virtually as many answers as there are hepatologists. The following scheme, although rational, may not be correct and represents only one possible approach. The management scheme is detailed in Figure 1. As can be seen, we pick the story up at the point in time when a patient has been identified as having an abnormal aminotransferase. The patient may or may not be symptomatic or icteric.

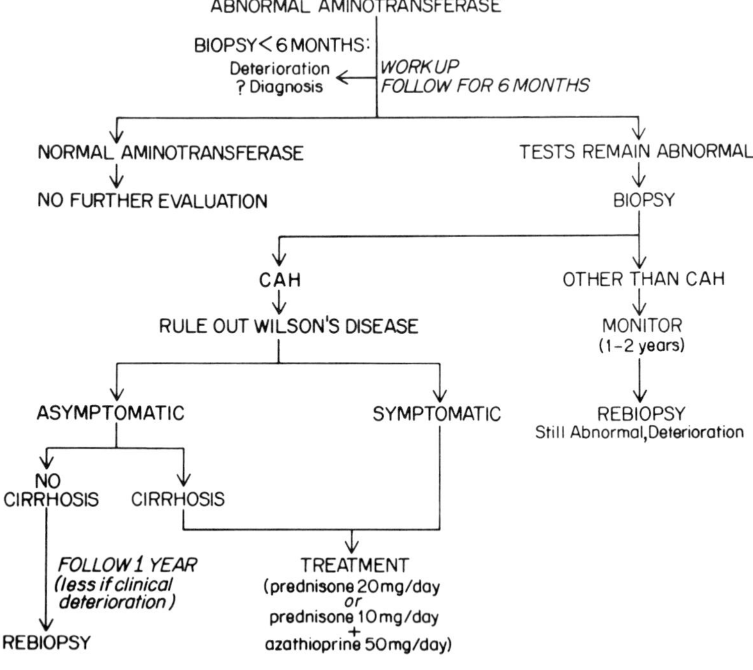

Figure 1 Algorithm outlining the management of chronic hepatitis.

The enzyme abnormality has existed for an indeterminate period. At the time of the first visit, a workup is undertaken to determine the cause of the elevated aminotransferase. (In the context of this chapter, the patient presents with acute hepatitis.) Follow-up study is obtained for the next six months, during which time the aminotransferase either returns to normal or does not. If it is abnormal at the end of this period, liver biopsy is performed to determine the nature of the biochemical CH. If during the six-month period the patient deteriorates (and steroid therapy is planned) or some diagnostic question exists, biopsy may be obtained earlier.

The biopsy may or may not demonstrate CAH. If a less severe lesion is encountered, the patient can be reassured and followed with biochemical determinations every few months. If these tests remain abnormal, a repeat biopsy may be performed one to two years later to make sure a more severe lesion was not missed. If the tests return to normal, no further workup need be performed.

If the biopsy reveals CAH, a serum ceruloplasmin should be obtained to rule out Wilson's disease. If the patient is symptomatic and has CAH, even if the enzyme levels are low grade, immunosuppressive therapy may be offered in an attempt to eradicate the symptoms. If the patient is asymptomatic and does not demonstrate cirrhosis, it would seem reasonable to follow him or her for one year and then to rebiopsy, looking for histologic progression (to cirrhosis).

If the patient is asymptomatic, but has cirrhosis, the issue is less clear. However, in the absence of other cirrhotogenic processes (e.g., alcohol), the biopsy is demonstrating irreversible disease. As such it is not unreasonable to offer the patient a course of steroids (with or without azathioprine) in an attempt to prevent more irreversible damage. It is debatable at this time whether or not such treatment is helpful, but no other treatment program is currently available.

What about the asymptomatic HBsAg carrier? If aminotransferase levels are abnormal, the previously mentioned scheme would be applicable. If, however, the levels are normal, the incidence of significant coexistent histologic disease (CAH and/or cirrhosis) is very small, and it does not appear justified to even perform a liver biopsy. Such patients should be followed with serial aminotransferases every few months and only undergo biopsy if these enzymes become abnormal. This situation is not unusual—approximately 50% of carriers have normal aminotransferases.

Once again it must be stressed that the scheme described here
is unsubstantiated by any data, as no real data concerning the treatment of asymptomatic CAH exist at the current time. Such patients
should be managed in conjunction with gastroenterologic consultation.

SELECTED READING

Czaja AJ, Summerskill WHJ: Chronic hepatitis. To treat or not to treat.
Med Clin North Am 62:71–85, 1978.

Dunnick JK, Galasso GJ: Clinical trials with exogenous interferon: summary of a meeting. *J Infect Dis* 139:109–123, 1979.

Gust ID: Recent developments in hepatitis A. *Pathology* 10:229–306,
1978.

Koretz RL: Current concepts of acute and chronic hepatitis, in Gitnick
GL (ed): *Current Gastroenterology and Hepatology*. Boston,
Houghton Mifflin Professional Publishers, 1979, pp. 234–275.

Koretz RL, Lewin KJ, Rebhun DJ, et al: Hepatitis B surface antigen
carriers—to biopsy or not to biopsy. *Gastroenterology* 75:860–863,
1978.

Krugman S, Overby LR, Mushahwar IK, et al: Viral hepatitis, type B.
Studies on natural history and prevention re-examined. *N Engl J
Med* 300:101–106, 1979.

Norkans G, Frosner G, Hermodsson S, et al: The epidemiological pattern
of hepatitis A, B, and non-A, non-B in Sweden. *Scand J Gastroenterol* 13:873–877, 1978.

Parry HF, Brown AE, Dobbs LG, et al: The epidemiology of hepatitis B
infection in housestaff. *Infection* 6:204–206, 1978.

Seeff LB, Hoofnagle JH: Immunoprophylaxis of viral hepatitis. *Gastroenterology* 77:161–182, 1979.

Vyas GN, Cohen SN, Schmid R: *Viral Hepatitis*. Philadelphia, Franklin
Institute Press, 1978.

CLINICAL PROBLEMS

I. Consider the patient described in the opening paragraph of this
chapter. Additional serologic data reveal that HBsAg and anti-
HBc tests are positive and anti-HBs is negative.

1. What recommendations would you make concerning bed rest, home care, diet, and sexual activity?
2. What globulin prophylaxis would you offer to the patient's contacts?
3. What possible courses might the patient follow?

II. Again consider the patient described in the opening paragraph, but instead the serologic data are as follows:

Anti-HA:	positive
IgM–anti HA:	positive
HBsAg:	negative
Anti-HBc:	positive
Anti-HBs:	positive

1. What recommendations would you make concerning the parameters of bed rest, home care, diet, and sexual activity?
2. What globulin prophylaxis would you offer the patient's contacts?
3. What possible courses might the patient follow?

III. Once again consider the clinical situation described in the opening paragraph. In this cases, the patient was transfused two months earlier. His serologic studies reveal:

Anti-HA:	positive
IgM–anti-HA:	negative
HBsAg:	negative
Anti-HBc:	negative
Anti-HBs:	positive

1. What recommendations would now be appropriate concerning bed rest, home care, diet, and sexual activity?
2. What globulin prophylaxis would you offer to the patient's contacts?
3. What possible courses might the patient follow?

Discussion

I. 1. Assuming the patient's nausea and vomiting can be handled
       at home, he should be advised to undertake only those activi-
       ties that do not tire him further. If possible, he should use a
       separate bathroom than other members of his household. If
       not, care should be taken to avoid sharing implements such
       as combs, toothbrushes, or razor blades. The toilet should
       be cleaned meticulously. The patient should not prepare food
       and should use disposable plates and utensils. He should be
       cautioned that sexual activity may spread the disease. No
       dietary restrictions need be imposed.

    2. The only contact who is at significant risk is a recent sex-
       ual one. This individual (or individuals) should ideally be
       screened for prior hepatitis B exposure; those who have no
       serologic evidence of past or present hepatitis B infection are
       then given HBIG prophylaxis. The time constraints may not
       allow these contacts to have their serology tests performed
       within seven days of contact. In this case a dose of HBIG can
       be given after the blood is drawn. (Those who have already
       had hepatitis B exposure can at least be spared the second
       injection.)

    3. Most of these patients will clear their infection without se-
       quelae. (Some will, during the course of their recovery,
       develop some evidence of a cholestatic phase.) A few (1%)
       will develop fulminant hepatitis. Approximately 10% will
       develop the chronic carrier state and chronic hepatitis.

II. 1. The recommendations would remain basically the same.
       Once the disease has peaked clinically and biochemically,
       and once household contacts have been provided prophy-
       laxis, the danger of household spread is small.

    2. For hepatitis A, SIG provides adequate protection. Only
       close contacts need be given prophylaxis (e.g., household
       contacts). Theoretically only those without anti-HA would
       require globulin, but it is cheaper to provide prophylaxis to
       all than to spend the time and money screening all of the
       contacts.

    3. Hepatitis A may produce fulminant hepatitis in occasional
       patients. The rest recover uneventfully.

III. 1. The various recommendations would be the same as for hepatitis B (see case I).

2. No serologic tests are available for non-A, non-B hepatitis, so it is impossible to determine who has had prior exposure. The epidemiology of this virus (these viruses) is also unknown, but there are similarities clinically between the non-A, non-B disease seen in the posttransfusion situation and hepatitis B. Thus, presumably the sexual contact is the only person at risk; protection should be provided within seven days of contact. SIG should be used.

3. As was true for hepatitis B, the infection may rarely pursue a fulminant course. More likely the disease will resolve or develop into a chronic hepatitis. This latter event (chronic hepatitis) appears to occur more often than the 10% quoted for acute hepatitis B.

18

NEIL KAPLOWITZ

Cholelithiasis

Approximately 16 to 20 million Americans have gallstones and many hundreds of thousands of new cases are discovered annually. Of people over age 65, 30% have stones. More than one million cholecystectomies are performed each year. Therefore, cholelithiasis is a major public health problem.

HOW DO I MAKE THE DIAGNOSIS?

What Factors Predispose to Cholelithiasis?

In clinical practice two types of chemically distinct stones are seen. Pigment stones, composed mostly of calcium bilirubinate, are found with increased frequency in patients with chronic hemolysis, chronic bacterial infection of the bile, or cirrhosis (one-third of such

Acknowledgment: I wish to thank Nick Onstott for his superb administrative assistance.

patients). Stones composed predominantly of cholesterol are associated with the female sex (three times more common than in men and more common in multiparous than in nulliparous women); obesity; certain ethnic groups, especially American Indians; disease (e.g., Crohn's) or resection of the terminal ileum; and the long-term use of oral contraceptives and clofibrate. The pathophysiology of the formation of both pigment and cholesterol stones remains poorly understood. However, it seems clear that the sine qua non for formation of the latter type of stone is excessive cholesterol secretion in bile relative to the ability to keep it soluble.

What Are the Symptoms of Cholelithiasis?

Generally speaking a diagnosis of gallstones is sought in patients who have symptoms of an abdominal origin. Occasionally, gallstones are found fortuitously in the evaluation of another organ system. The major symptom that reflects gallstones is recurrent right upper quadrant or epigastric abdominal pain. This symptom is referred to as biliary colic, a misnomer in that the pain is persistent rather than colicky in nature. The symptom begins suddenly and often the patient can recall the precise instant of onset; it progresses rapidly to its maximum intensity and then persists for one to several hours, after which it subsides somewhat more slowly than it started. Pain of longer duration and associated with fever, tenderness, jaundice, or clearcut pancreatitis points to a complication.

In biliary colic the patient may be nauseated and even vomit, although this is often not a prominent feature. On physical examination there is generally little to be found and the laboratory data are usually unremarkable. The pathophysiology of this condition is simply related to the impaction of stones in the cystic duct or the biliary tree. Considering the frequency of this phenomenon, the relative infrequency of the complications is truly remarkable.

There are two common misconceptions about the symptomatology of gallstones and chronic cholecystitis. One is that fatty food intolerance reflects disease of the gallbladder. The other is that symptoms of a chronic, vague abdominal nature, particularly in the upper abdomen, reflect chronic cholecystitis. Neither of these statements is true. These vague symptoms seen in some patients with gallstones have been inappropriately attributed to stones when the symptoms are often related to functional bowel disease, reflux esophagitis, or ulcer disease. Labeling a patient with gallstones as having symptomatic disease is only justified if recurrent symptoms typical of biliary colic have been experienced.

How Do You Establish the Presence of Gallstones Objectively?

When gallstone disease is suspected, diagnostic confirmation can be sought with several modalities (Table 1). Clearly the most useful are oral cholecystography and ultrasonography. (See Figure 1 for the diagnostic sequence.)

Oral Cholecystography

Oral cholecystography (OCG) requires the ingestion of iodinated contrast agent on one or two consecutive evenings. The agent is slowly absorbed, taken up, and metabolized by the liver and excreted in bile. Within the gallbladder it becomes concentrated, enabling visualization of the accumulated and concentrated dye. There is a trend to perform the x-rays on the morning after two consecutive evening doses rather than after each individual dose, thereby maximizing the efficiency of the test.

The most straightforward findings are radiopaque (calcified) stones seen on the scout film or demonstration of lucencies in the visualized dye-loaded gallbladder that move with positioning of the patient. Nonvisualization or faint visualization is more difficult to interpret. Although this most often means that there is a poorly functioning, diseased gallbladder, one must be certain the oral con-

Table 1 **Diagnostic Methods for Cholelithiasis**

Plain film of abdomen
Oral cholecystography
Ultrasonography
Intravenous cholangiography
Endoscopic retrograde cholangiopancreatography
Duodenal drainage for cholesterol crystals
Recovery of stones in feces

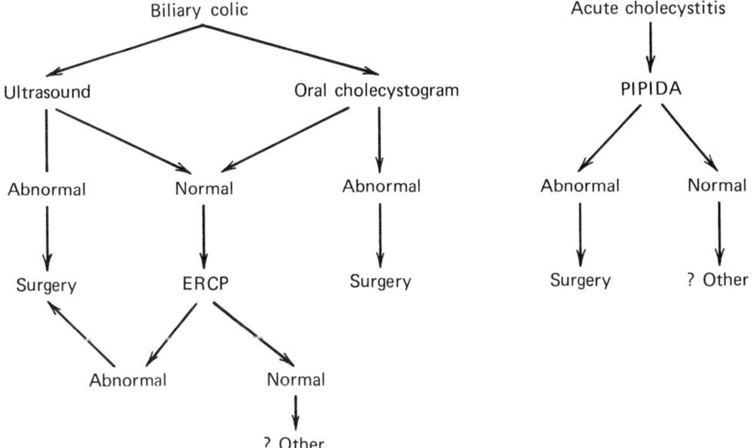

Figure 1 Diagnostic approach to cholelithiasis with biliary colic (left) and acute cholecystitis (right). If biliary colic is suspected and either ultrasound or oral cholecystogram is normal, the other should be performed. "Other" refers to exploratory surgery for strong clinical suspicion despite normal tests; this is rarely necessary.

trast agent was truly ingested, then absorbed, taken up by the liver, and excreted in the bile. Therefore, gastric outlet obstruction, small-intestinal mucosal disease, and liver disease could result in a false-positive result. There is no point in attempting this study in the face of hyperbilirubinemia.

The oral cholecystogram, performed in a setting in which factors that yield false positives are excluded (such as delayed gastric emptying, malabsorption, and liver disease), has an accuracy of 95%. There is some suggestion that nonvisualization with double-dose oral cholecystogram indicates more severe disease with a poorer prognosis (in terms of frequency of complications) than visualization with gallstones present.

Ultrasonography

In recent years the ultrasound examination has been rapidly gaining popularity, so that it may soon become the procedure of choice, alone or in combination with the oral cholecystogram. Ultrasound also has approximately a 95% accuracy in diagnosing stone disease as well as other distinct advantages: no preparation or ingestion of dye with all the attendant pitfalls and no x-irradiation. The examination does not assess "function" of the gallbladder in the fashion of a cholecystogram with dye-concentrating ability. However, stones in the gallbladder are the sine qua non for chronic cholecystitis, and the additional information concerning concentrating ability is of limited clinical value when stones are seen.

The characteristic feature of stones on ultrasound are: echogenic foci in the gallbladder (discrete dark areas); movement of calculi with positioning of the patient; and, most importantly, an acoustical shadow behind the stone (Fig. 2). Another feature that suggests chronic cholecystitis is the lack of ability to locate the gallbladder on two consecutive studies with the patient fasting. Since the gallbladder lies anteriorly in the abdomen, difficulties with gas are not encountered in obtaining a good examination; this is in contrast to deeper organs, in which gas poses frequent problems.

Other Tests

Other less frequently employed means for diagnosis of gallstone disease include intravenous cholangiography (IVC) and endoscopic retrograde cholangiopancreatography (ERCP). These should not be used for simple cholelithiasis but are employed when patency of the duct system must be evaluated (e.g., in choledocholithiasis).

ERCP may occasionally be employed in a patient with classic symptoms of gallbladder disease (recurrent biliary colic) in whom oral cholecystogram or ultrasound, or both, are normal. This will occur in a few patients with symptomatic stones. In this setting introduction of dye by ERCP leads to sharp contrast in the gallbladder, allowing for excellent conditions for visualization of gallstones. IVC is usually inadequate in this setting because of the less sharp contrast obtained. This approach may avoid unnecessary operation in the patient who has no stones. It is probably valuable when symptoms are equivocal and less clearly necessary when symptoms are classic.

There are a few other less often employed techniques to diagnose stones. One is biliary drainage for cholesterol crystals. Again, in ambiguous circumstances finding cholesterol crystals in gallbladder bile, collected from the duodenum after stimulated gallbladder emptying, may be helpful. However, one needs to resort to this test only when the other studies are normal and the symptoms are equivocal. One should be aware that false positives will occur frequently in pan-

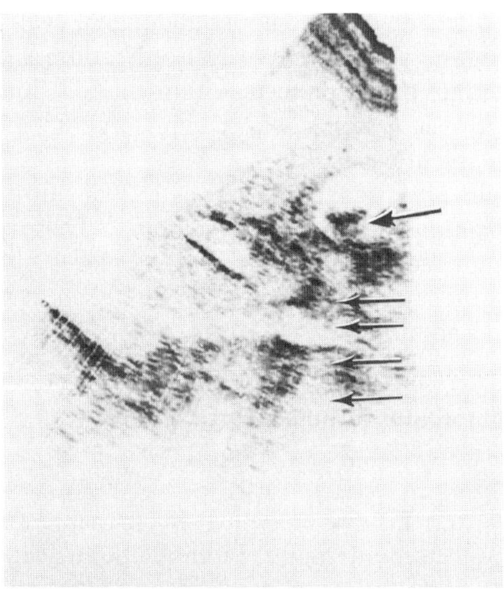

Figure 2 Ultrasound showing cross section of abdomen. A calculus (large arrow) is seen in the gallbladder with an acoustical shadow behind (small arrows).

creatic and liver disease, and therefore the test should not be performed under these circumstances.

Finally, an approach that I have found useful in an outpatient setting is the recovery of stones in feces. The patient is instructed to collect and strain feces through a standard spaghetti strainer attached to a toilet seat at home. Stools are collected for three to four days immediately after an attack of biliary colic. What could be more gratifying to the patient than participating in the diagnosis? This approach has been particularly useful in patients who develop recurrent pancreatitis and gallstones that have not been demonstrated with the usual techniques.

HOW SHOULD I TREAT THE PATIENT?

What Is the Natural History of Cholelithiasis?

Gallstones are discovered in somewhat more than half the instances because of colic or other typical symptoms. However, sometimes they are discovered in the upper abdominal evaluation of other organs or in routine screening. We can only address ourselves with accuracy to the fate of the patients with identified stones and not to the millions with silent stones who comprise perhaps half of all individuals with cholelithiasis.

Once stones are discovered there is a 20% to 40% chance of serious complications ultimately developing. These complications relate to the impaction of calculi in various places outside the gallbladder during their travels, and will be discussed in more detail in a later section (Table 2).

How Is Symptomatic Cholelithiasis Treated?

Patients with a history of typical biliary colic should undergo elective cholecystectomy. Usually the cholelithiasis can be confirmed by oral cholecystography or ultrasound but occasionally these are normal. In these instances I prefer to seek confirmation of cholelithiasis with biliary drainage (for crystals) or ERCP, or both. In the rare case in which all of the tests are negative and the symptoms are classic, cholecystectomy may still be performed. The reason for cholecystectomy for symptomatic cholelithiasis rests on the fact that colic will be recurrent in many and the risk of complications and the

Table 2 **Complications of Cholelithiasis**

Acute cholecystitis
    Ruptured gallbladder
    Empyema of the gallbladder
Bile ducts
    Obstructive jaundice
        Ascending cholangitis
        Liver abscess
        Secondary biliary cirrhosis
    Stricture of ampulla of Vater
Pancreatitis
Carcinoma of the gallbladder
Gallstone ileus

resultant mortality, including that from emergency surgery, far outweigh the risk of an elective cholecystectomy. The key is that operation is aimed at relieving recurrent symptoms and preventing serious complications. The complications of elective surgery with simple cholecystectomy are rare: death occurs in less then 0.5% and postoperative stictures and abscess are very infrequent.

At the time of operation, it has become routine to perform operative cholangiography. This allows a good look at the bile ducts and therefore selects individuals in whom duct exploration for stone removal, a higher-risk procedure, is required. With this standard approach the incidence of postoperative retained stones has been drastically reduced from 10% to less than 1%.

What Should Be Done With Asymptomatic Cholelithiasis?

The approach to the truly asymptomatic case is much more controversial. Over 90% of serious complications of gallstone disease are preceded by symptoms of biliary colic. Therefore, this generally serves as a useful warning and allows for a somewhat more conservative approach to the truly asymptomatic case. There is no scientific answer as to how to treat these asymptomatic patients. In patients under the ages of 40 to 50, many physicians recommend elective cholecystectomy simply because the chance of a serious complication over several decades is probably greater than the risk of operation in a "young" person (Table 3).

Certain other factors may enter into a decision. For example since diabetics appear to have a higher mortality with acute cholecystitis, they probably should be treated with cholecystectomy when stones are identified. There is some suggestion that the nonfunctioning gallbladder (nonvisualization on oral cholecystography) or the presence of a large stone (> 2.5 cm) may be associated with higher complication rates and weigh toward definitive surgery. On the other hand, the middle-aged individual with calculi on oral cholecystogram but no symptoms should probably be instructed to report the development of symptoms and simply be followed medically. The medical facilities and budget of the United States could not handle the definitive treatment of the millions of cases of asymptomatic stones. If the entire adult population were screened and those with asymp-

Symptom	Cholecystectomy		
	Yes	No	Maybe
Biliary colic at any age	+	−	−
Choledocholithiasis	+	−	−
Acute cholecystitis (past or present)	+	−	−
Gallstone pancreatitis	+	−	−
Asymptomatic cholelithiasis with:			
Nonvisualized oral cholecystogram			
< Age 40–50[a]	+	−	−
> Age 40–50	−	−	+
Functioning gallbladder with calculi			
< Age 40–50	−	−	+
> Age 40–50	−	+	−

[a] Age cut-off in consideration of general health of patient and surgical risk factors.

tomatic stones were treated surgically, the operative mortality would be 10 times the current annual death rate from cholelithiasis.

When Should Gallstones Be Dissolved?

Another therapeutic approach on the near horizon is treatment with chenodeoxycholic acid (or perhaps ursodeoxycholic acid) in order to dissolve gallstones of the cholesterol type. I believe that this therapeutic modality will have very limited application because of the expense and the long-term requirement for therapy. Symptomatic disease should still be treated surgically mainly because of the long delay in complete dissolution by medical means (at least six months to one year). Furthermore, radiopaque (calcified) stones will not dissolve. Nonvisualization of the gallbladder on oral cholecystogram implies cystic duct obstruction, therefore predicting that medical therapy will not work. At best one-half to two-thirds of selected cases (without radiopaque stones and with functioning gall-bladders) can be treated effectively in this way.

The only significant side effect of dissolution therapy appears to be diarrhea. Intermittently abnormal serum transaminases have been noted in experimental trials, but significant liver toxicity has not been observed. Therefore, gallstone dissolution should be reserved for patients who have other serious medical problems that contraindicate operation. Also, there may be a prophylactic role for chenodeoxycholate in certain settings (e.g., in American Indians, who have an 80% gallstone incidence, and in patients taking clofibrate).

WHAT COMPLICATIONS OF THE DISEASE CAN OCCUR?

Acute Cholecystitis: Diagnosis and Treatment

Acute cholecystitis refers to acute inflammation of the gallbladder wall. The process appears to be initiated by a calculus obstructing the cystic duct. The symptoms consist of abdominal pain and vomiting as in colic. However, the pain persists for many hours to days and takes on a localized peritoneal character. Therefore, in contrast to the restless, moving, diaphoretic patient with "colic" the patient with acute cholecystitis generally lies quietly. The pain is often referred to the back, right costal margin, scapula, or right shoulder.

Physical examination usually reveals fever and right upper quadrant tenderness with localized peritoneal findings. This is the so-called Murphy's sign: tenderness in the right midclavicular line or more laterally, below the liver edge, that is accentuated by deep inspiration.

Laboratory tests generally reveal a leukocytosis. An elevated serum amylase may be seen despite the absence of pancreatitis.

Acalculous acute cholecystitis is a rare condition that can result from vascular insufficiency in fasting postoperative patients or in patients with polyarteritis nodosa.

The differential diagnosis of acute cholecystitis may present the physician with quite a dilemma. The entities to be considered in the patient with right abdominal pain, tenderness, and fever are listed in Table 4. Urinalysis and chest x-ray will help in evaluating renal or pulmonary disease and should be performed in this setting.

Table 4 **Differential Diagnosis of Acute Cholecystitis**

Acute pancreatitis
Appendicitis
Pyelonephritis
Renal calculus
Peptic ulcer disease
Acute hepatitis
Pneumonia
Pulmonary infarction
Hepatic abscess
Hepatic neoplasm

Hepatitis, viral or alcoholic, will be associated with diffuse liver tenderness and hepatomegaly rather than the more localized gallbladder tenderness. Hepatic abscess, or even tumor, may be very difficult to distinguish on clinical grounds. These should always be thought of and, if the setting is appropriate, excluded by liver scan.

Often pancreatitis and appendicitis can be difficult to distinguish from acute cholecystitis. For this reason it is helpful to confirm the latter diagnosis in some noninvasive way. Observing gallstones on the plain film of the abdomen or ultrasound is indirect and not very helpful. The prevalence of calculi in the general population is great enough to allow for the frequent coincidence of cholelithiasis and another form of pathology. Therefore, studies directed at examining the patency of the cystic duct are more useful in directing attention to the pathophysiologic key in acute cholecystitis.

There are two ways to evaluate the patency of the cystic duct: intravenous cholangiography and cholescintigraphy (with technitium-labeled HIDA or PIPIDA). In both cases, an agent is administered that is taken up by the liver and excreted in bile, thereby flowing into the gallbladder. The radioisotopic approach appears to be preferable in that visualization of bile ducts occurs even in moderate jaundice. Therefore, the demonstration of isotope accumulation in the gallbladder testifies to the patency of the cystic duct, and, for practical purposes, excludes acute cholecystitis (Fig. 3).

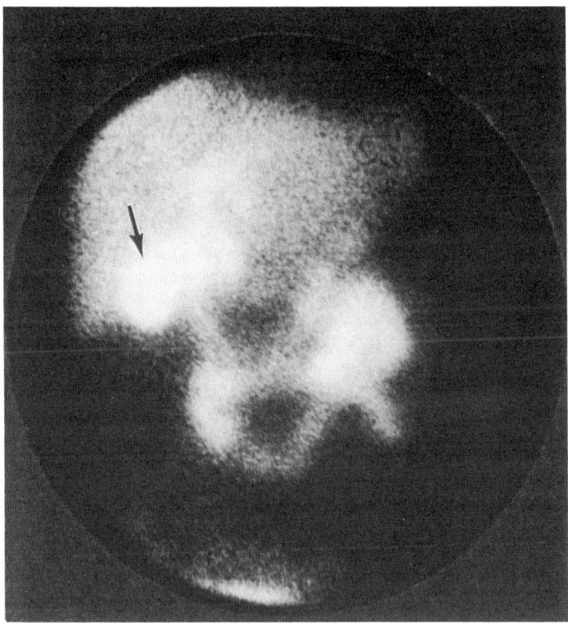

Figure 3 PIPIDA cholescintigraphy of the hepatobiliary system showing the accumulation of radioisotope in the gallbladder (arrow) and bile ducts after parenchymal hepatic uptake and excretion in bile. This is a normal study.

Conversely, nonvisualization of the gallbladder when the ducts and, later, the intestine are seen, favors the diagnosis of acute cholecystitis (Fig. 4). We routinely perform this simple, valuable study early in the course of disease in patients with suspected acute cholecystitis. If the study is normal, we direct our attention to other possibilities, such as liver abscess or acute pancreatitis.

Acute cholecystitis is associated with jaundice about 20% of the time. It is useful to consider two types of jaundice in this setting. If the bilirubin is mildly elevated (less than 5 mg/dl), there is usually no apparent cause for jaundice, that is, no stones in the bile duct. Usually if the bilirubin is greater than 5 mg/dl, and certainly if it is greater than 10 mg/dl, there is associated choledocholithiasis.

Acute cholecystitis is attended by several life-threatening complications that emphasize the need for appropriate diagnostic efforts

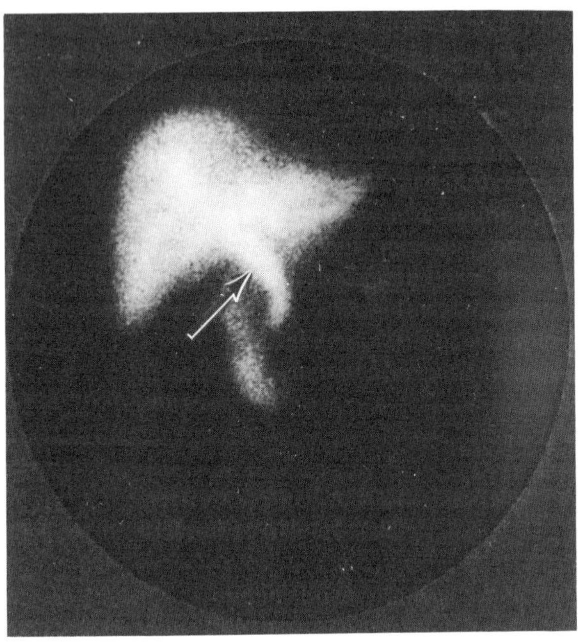

Figure 4 PIPIDA scan showing absence of accumulation of technitium in the gallbladder. However, the bile duct is seen (arrow). Therefore, cystic duct obstruction is implied and there is objective support for the diagnosis of acute cholecystitis.

and definitive therapy. Perforation of the gallbladder is the most serious complication. This may be localized (resulting in a pericholecystic abscess), free, or into the intestine (cholecystenteric fistula). If the latter is associated with a large stone, gallstone ileus may supervene. It is because of the potential for these complications that definitive early operation has become a popular approach. The early diagnosis of rupture of the gallbladder can be very difficult because the patient often feels improvement as a result of the decompressive perforation of the gallbladder. Sepsis and abscess will make the diagnosis more obvious, but these are delayed manifestations.

The patient with acute cholecystitis should be admitted to the hospital and placed on nasogastric suction and intravenous hydration. Antibiotics are reserved for signs of clear-cut sepsis, such as worsening fever, chills, or the development of an abdominal mass. Operation is indicated once the diagnosis is firmly established. We prefer early surgery (within a few days of admission) if the illness is subsiding and emergency operation if sepsis or impending perforation seems evident. Early elective surgery seems to reduce the length of hospital stay and minimizes the development of complications. However, many physicians prefer to wait a month or so after the patient recovers before performing elective cholecystectomy.

Choledocholithiasis and Its Complications

About 15% of patients operated on for cholelithiasis have concomitant choledocholithiasis. The complications of choledocholithiasis include cholangitis, hepatic abscess, secondary biliary cirrhosis, and pancreatitis.

Obstruction of the Bile Duct by Stones

Stones may impact in the bile duct acutely or chronically. When acute, the patient develops sudden biliary colic that may be followed by jaundice and septic cholangitis. The diagnostic evaluation in this setting is described in the chapter on jaundice.

Once the diagnosis is established, operation is generally performed on a semielective but expeditious basis unless sepsis cannot be controlled with antibiotics, in which case emergency surgery is indicated. The surgical approach often involves simple removal of the calculi and a cholecystectomy. However, if there is difficulty or uncertainty about the removal of all the stones or if the duct system is dilated, a definitive biliary drainage by sphincteroplasty or choledochoenterostomy should be performed. I prefer the latter because of its definitive drainage but the skill and experience of the surgeon often dictate which is performed.

Since the surgical mortality for complicated choledocholithiasis may be high (5% to 15%), especially in the elderly, nonsurgical approaches are sometimes useful. Currently there is enthusiasm for endoscopic retrograde sphincterotomy. A cautery wire introduced through an endoscope essentially slices the sphincter of Oddi, effecting drainage and passage of impacted stones. This procedure is indicated most clearly in the postcholecystectomy setting with choledo-cholithiasis and increased risk for operation and in the patient with common duct stone(s) in whom surgery is contraindicated.

When retained stones are seen in a patient with a T tube in place, extraction of the calculus with a basket (Dormia) inserted through the tube into the duct works well. Alternatively cholangial infusions of various solutions, such as saline, heparin, cholic acid, or mono-octanoin, have been used through the T tube with reasonable success.

Chronic choledocholithiasis may not be associated with prominent pain symptoms. However, chronic partial obstruction of the bile ducts will promote stasis, induce proliferation of bacteria, and result in recurrent cholangitis. This may be complicated by single or multiple pyogenic hepatic abscesses. Long-standing obstruction, particularly in association with recurrent cholangitis, may produce secondary biliary cirrhosis with eventual hepatic failure and portal hypertension. The key clinical clue to the chronic presence of stones in the bile duct is recurrent fever and rigors; the biochemical clue is a persistently elevated serum alkaline phosphatase. Treatment of choledocholithiasis in this setting is the same as was described previously.

Pancreatitis

Another important complication of the passage of stones through the biliary tree is pancreatitis. This may be in the form of single or recurrent acute attacks. Gallstone pancreatitis is the most common form of the disease. The diagnosis of a gallstone etiology in a patient with clear-cut pancreatitis is strongly suggested by chole-lithiasis on ultrasound or the recovery of stones passed in the feces, or both. Pancreatitis may result in a number of serious complications, including hemorrhagic, life-threatening pancreatic necrosis; pseudocyst; and pancreatic abscess, all of which are covered in the next chapter.

In a patient with pancreatitis, the demonstration of cholelithiasis is generally viewed as sufficient indication for elective cholecystectomy. If the patient does well after an attack of acute pancreatitis, the operation is performed on an elective basis. Emergency surgery to remove an impacted ampullary calculus in severe acute pancreatitis is advocated by some, but is more controversial.

Carcinoma of the Gallbladder

A rare complication of cholelithiasis and chronic cholecystitis is carcinoma of the gallbladder. There are fewer than 7,000 cases per year but 80% of these have coexisting gallstones. The incidence of gallbladder cancer is four times greater in women than in men, as one would expect from the prevalence of gallstones in each sex. Because of the nonspecific nature of symptoms, the diagnosis is rarely made before operation. Usually acute cholecystitis or choledocholithiasis is suspected clinically.

Carcinoma of the gallbladder is found in about 1% of all patients who undergo cholecystectomies and in 5% to 10% of those over 65. Most patients (75%) are found to have widespread metastases. If the tumor is localized to the gallbladder and recognized, a more extensive lymph node dissection and wedge resection of the gallbladder bed should be performed. The one-year mortality of 90% reflects the usual situation of inoperable spread before recognition. The 5% five-year survival is accounted for almost entirely by patients whose tumor is discovered incidentally at a time when it is still confined to the gallbladder.

SELECTED READING

Gagic N, Frey CF, Gaines R: Acute cholecystitis. *Surg Gynecol Obstet* 140:868–874, 1975.

Lund J: Surgical indications in cholelithiasis: prophylactic cholecystectomy elucidated on the basis of long-term follow-up on 526 nonoperated cases. *Ann Surg* 151:153–162, 1960.

Schoenfield LJ: *Diseases of the Gallbladder and Biliary System.* New York, John Wiley & Sons, 1977.

Wenckert A, Robertson B: The natural course of gallstone disease: eleven-year review of 781 nonoperated cases. *Gastroenterology* 50:376–381, 1966.

Wilson ID, Delaney JP, Duane WC, et al: Choledocholithiasis: clinical conference. *Gastroenterology* 75:120–128, 1978.

CLINICAL PROBLEMS

I. A 38-year-old woman complains of recurrent epigastric pains that occur two to three times a month. The pain is steady and lasts one to two hours. It is usually associated with nausea. During the period of pain, the patient tends to move from one position to another, but she is unable to find one that helps the discomfort. She denies fever or chills. The physical examination is unremarkable. The initial impression is that she has gallstone disease.

1. How do the stones produce this symptom complex?
2. How does one establish the diagnosis?
3. What treatment would be offered?

II. The patient refuses operation and continues to be followed. Five months later she goes to an emergency room with a different pain syndrome. The abdominal discomfort, while still steady, is now in the right upper quadrant, and motion aggravates it. There is an associated fever of 101 F. Physical examination now reveals right upper quadrant tenderness and rebound. The bowel sounds are hypoactive. Murphy's sign is present.

1. What is causing the pain now?
2. How should the diagnosis be established?
3. What treatment could be offered?

III. The patient's 36-year-old sister, having noticed heartburn after eating greasy foods and knowing of her older sister's problems, asks to be evaluated for gallstones. She denies any abdominal pain, jaundice, or other intestinal symptoms. Her physical examination is normal.

1. Are stones producing the symptoms?
2. How should the diagnosis of gallstones be established?
3. What treatment should be offered?

Discussion

I. 1. The symptoms are probably due to intermittent impaction of stones in the cystic duct or passage through the duct system. The "restless" nature of the pain and the absence of fever suggest the lack of a clinically important acute inflammatory component.

2. A number of tests might be employed to establish the diagnosis, but the oral cholecystogram or the ultrasound should be ordered first. Occasionally (especially if the symptoms are due to transient stone impaction in the common bile duct) ERCP or intravenous cholangiography may be required. Finally stones may be sought by screening the stool.

3. Once the diagnosis is established, the patient should have elective cholecystectomy. Chenodeoxycholic acid stone dissolution should not be considered unless operation is strongly contraindicated.

II. 1. The patient now has acute cholecystitis. The stone remains impacted in the cystic duct; edema and inflammation develop in the wall, possibly worsened by subsequent ischemia. A tender inflamed gallbladder manifests itself with the finding of fever, peritonitis, and Murphy's sign.

2. The diagnosis can be established by intravenous cholangiography or cholescintigraphy. Visualization of the biliary tree without localization of contrast material in the gallbladder indicates cystic duct obstruction and presumed resultant cholecystitis.

3. The patient should be hospitalized and treated with nasogastric suction and intravenous hydration. If sepsis is suspected, antibiotics should be added to the regimen. If the patient responds favorably, operation can be performed electively; if deterioration continues, emergency cholecystectomy should be undertaken.

III. 1. This patient's symptom, as well as other variations of "fatty food intolerance," is not caused by gallstone disease. Rather some other gastrointestinal disorder (in this case, possibly reflux esophagitis) is responsible.

2. An oral cholecystogram or ultrasound would be obtained to answer the patient's question, "Do I have gallstones?" It should be explained to her that the symptoms are not caused by stones, however.

3. If stones are present, they should be considered to be asymptomatic. Because of the patient's young age, it would be appropriate to offer cholecystectomy, but care should be taken to make sure she understands that her current symptoms are not likely to be affected by the operation.

19 MARTIN A. POPS

Pancreatitis

Before beginning a discussion of inflammatory disease of the pancreas, it is imperative that clear definitions of certain terms be established. "Acute pancreatitis" will refer to the clinically apparent disease involving the acute onset of abdominal pain often accompanied by a host of other manifestations. This process is self limited, but may recur, especially if the underlying etiologic process is not corrected. "Chronic pancreatitis" is, technically, a histologic diagnosis with the pancreas demonstrating fibrosis and inflammatory round-cell infiltration. Histologic verification is rarely available, but the diagnosis can be inferred from either clinical evidence of pancreatic exocrine insufficiency or the radiologic demonstration of pancreatic calcifications. Patients with chronic pancreatitis who also suffer recurrent bouts of abdominal pain are classified as having "chronic relapsing pancreatitis." Acute and chronic pancreatitis will be considered separately.

Acute Pancreatitis

HOW DO I MAKE THE DIAGNOSIS?

Acute pancreatitis is an inflammatory reaction in and around the pancreas that results from escape of activated enzymes into the interstitial tissues. Depending on the degree of such enzymatic activation, the disease can be subdivided further into edematous, suppurative, necrotizing, or hemorrhagic forms in the order indicating the severity of the process. The diagnosis is made by recognition of the most important historical, physical, and laboratory findings, which vary according to the severity of the disease.

Abdominal pain is invariably the major presenting complaint. Pain is felt in the epigastrium or left upper quadrant, often radiating through to the back. The pain is characteristically constant and severe, and the patient tends to lie still with the legs brought up so as to open the retroperitoneal space. There is associated nausea and vomiting. Obstipation is due to the ileus, which occurs reflexively near the adjacent pancreatic inflammation.

Physical examination usually reveals tenderness in the upper abdomen, although rebound is variable and often absent. Bowel sounds are reduced or absent. Discoloration of the flanks (Grey-Turner sign) or of the umbilicus (Cullen's sign) are helpful when seen but are not usual. Both signs indicate retroperitoneal hemorrhage. Massive retroperitoneal edema and hemorrhage, along with the release of potent vasoactive substances such as kallikrein, may lead to hypotension and shock in the most severe forms of the disease. Occasionally, the release of activated pancreatic lipase into the circulation can cause lipid necrosis in distant sites, such as the subcutaneous tissue or the central nervous system.

Several laboratory diagnostic tools are available for the diagnosis of acute pancreatitis. The most important is the serum amylase concentration, which is abnormally high in most cases. Amylase, excreted by the kidney, can be measured in the urine (diastase); it remains elevated for a few days beyond the time when the serum amylase returns to normal (Fig. 1). Unfortunately, false-positive amylase elevations in serum or urine occur in many conditions other than pancreatitis (Table 1). Macroamylasemia is an infrequently en-

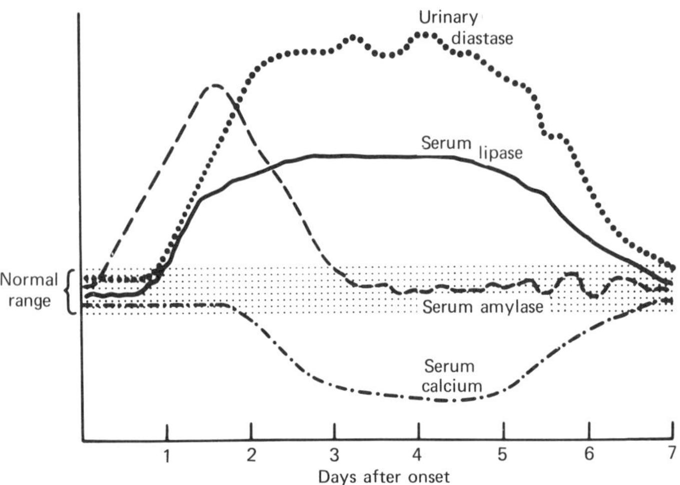

Figure 1 Acute pancreatitis: laboratory abnormalities. Time course of amylase elevation and lipase and calcium levels.

countered phenomenon that is not associated with any of the other diseases listed in Table 1. Individuals who have macroamylasemia produce two types of amylase, one that is filtered normally by the kidney and another, larger than normal, that is not filtered. (Conversely, it is not uncommon to see the serum or urine amylase fail to rise in patients with an acute exacerbation of chronic pancreatitis, presumably on the basis of previous widespread pancreatic acinar cell destruction.)

Because "normal amylase pancreatitis" occurs, a more sensitive test for acute pancreatitis has been sought. Urinary amylase increases in pancreatitis because the molecule is lost more rapidly, that is, the clearance of amylase is increased. If amylase clearance is expressed as a function of creatinine clearance (to compensate for potential artifacts caused by aberrations in renal function and to allow for a calculation based on a spot urine specimen instead of a timed one), the amylase/creatinine clearance ratio may provide a more sensitive index of acute pancreatitis than either the serum or urine amylase concentration alone. This ratio is easily calculated by the formula:

300   DISEASE ENTITIES

Table 1 Causes of Amylase Elevations

In serum:

Acute pancreatitis	Hepatitis
Cholecystitis	Acute parotitis
Diabetic ketoacidosis	Perforated peptic ulcer
Macroamylasemia[a]	Renal insufficiency
Opiate administration	Ruptured aortic aneurysm
Paralytic ileus	Ruptured ectopic pregnancy
Intestinal obstruction or perforation	

In urine:

All of the above except macroamylasemia and renal insufficiency (where urine amylase levels are low compared to serum amylase)

In amylase/creatinine clearance ratio:

Acute pancreatitis

Low molecular weight proteinuria
  Burns
  Diabetic ketoacidosis
  Light-chain proteinuria (multiple myeloma)
Proximal renal tubular dysfunction

[a] See text.

$$\frac{\text{Urine amylase concentration}}{\text{Serum amylase concentration}} \times \frac{\text{serum creatinine}}{\text{urine creatinine}}$$

The value of this test is being argued in the medical literature with discrepant results reported from various investigators. A growing list of diseases other than acute pancreatitis has been reported as causing an increase in the amylase/creatinine clearance ratio, and several reports of false negatives in acute pancreatitis have also been reported. At the present time, therefore, the value of this test is debatable.

Additional information contributed by other laboratory tests is limited and serves more to describe the severity of the pancreatitis than to diagnose it. An elevated serum lipase generally corroborates the involvement of the pancreas. A fall in the serum calcium level tends to correlate with the severity of the attack, with levels below 7 mg% indicating a very poor prognosis. Methemalbumin, a metabolite of heme attached to circulating albumin, has been mentioned as an indicator of hemorrhagic pancreatitis. However, the non-specificity of this test casts doubt as to its value. Rises in serum bilirubin, alkaline phosphatase, and transaminases may be seen secondary to constriction of the common duct by the edamatous pancreas but are also elevated in other forms of acute duct obstruction, such as gallstones, as well as nonspecifically in many intraabdominal conditions. A falling hemoglobin concentration may indicate hemorrhagic pancreatitis.

The chief value of radiologic examination in acute pancreatitis is to eliminate other diagnoses, particularly perforation of a viscus. The upper gastrointestinal contrast x-ray frequently suggests an enlarged head of the pancreas by the demonstration of distortion and widening of the duodenal sweep and the antrum of the stomach (Fig. 2). An intravenous cholangiogram (IVC) may help to differentiate acute pancreatitis alone from common duct or gallbladder stone with associated pancreatitis by visualizing the biliary tree and gallbladder in the former but not in the latter. In our experience the IVC seldom visualizes the duct system in either condition well enough to be of routine value. Ultrasonography has been a valuable adjunct in confirmation of the diagnosis when it demonstrates enlargement of the pancreas. Ileus with resultant overlying bowel gas often defeats the ultrasonographer's attempt to visualize the pancreas when the patient is acutely ill. Its main use would appear to be to detect pseudocysts presenting with acute symptoms and to serve as a baseline to monitor the possible development of a pseudocyst later in the course of disease. Endoscopic retrograde cholangiopancreatography (ERCP) is not performed during an acute attack of pancreatitis.

On occasion, especially if biliary tract disease is the cause of the pancreatitis, straining the stools subsequently passed will identify the responsible gallstone. In order to accomplish this, the entire stool specimen is washed through a fine mesh screen.

In summary, the diagnosis is established in most cases with history and physical examination. The serum amylase is usually elevated; it is the best initial confirmatory laboratory test to obtain.

WHAT ADDITIONAL WORKUP DOES THE PATIENT REQUIRE?

Because acute pancreatitis may result from a variety of causes, each patient should additionally be diligently evaluated in a search

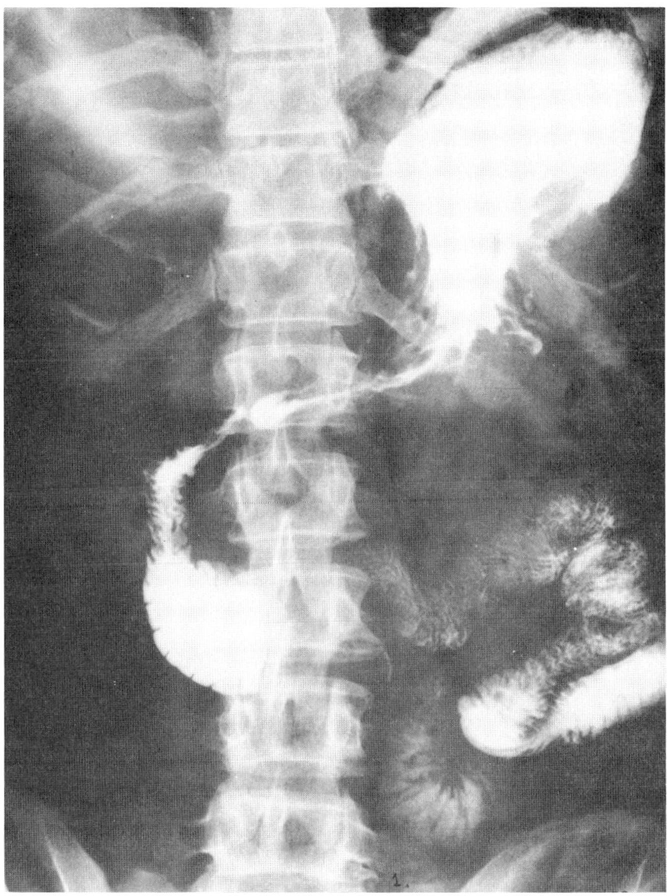

Figure 2 Acute pancreatitis; upper gastrointestinal series demonstrating changes in mucosa and contour of adjacent stomach and duodenum.

for an underlying etiology. The most important underlying causes are alcohol and gallstones. Other important, though less frequent, causes are listed in Table 2.

The appropriate tests for these underlying causes should be carried out. This is usually done after the acute pancreatitis subsides because the pancreatitis in and of itself often causes abnormalities that might be confusing. Examples of this are the secondary hyper-

Table 2   Etiologies of Pancreatitis

Gallstones

Alcohol

Drugs (thiazide diuretics, steroids, azathioprine)

Infection (mumps, hepatitis, Coxsackie, *Salmonella*, *Strongyloides*, *Ascaris*)

Hypercalcemia

Hyperlipidemia (especially hypertriglyceridemia)

Scorpion bites (Trinidad)

Vasculitis

Familial

Traumatic (including postoperative)

Penetrating ulcer (especially duodenal)

Carcinoma of the pancreas

Uremia

Duodenal diverticulum

Abnormalities of pancreatic duct

Idiopathic

lipidemia that is sometimes caused by pancreatitis or a hypercalcemic state that is masked by lowering of the serum calcium level because of the pancreatitis itself.

ERCP may be very useful in evaluating certain patients with recurrent pancreatitis in whom no underlying process is apparent. This examination should be conducted during a quiescent time, not during an acute attack. In spite of a thorough workup, however, a group remains without any known causes; this idiopathic group accounts for between 20% and 30% of all causes.

HOW SHOULD I TREAT THE PATIENT?

Treatment can be divided into medical or surgical therapy. The medical measures are based on general physiologic support and on the specific concept of slowing pancreatic secretion, thereby "putting the pancreas at rest." Fluid requirements may be enormous (up to 8 to 10 liters or more per 24 hours) in these patients. Fluid needs must be monitored carefully with the usual vital signs (including central venous pressure in the most severely ill patients), hourly urine outputs, and serial hematocrit values. Intravenous volume may be maintained with crystalloids or colloids, or both. Colloid loss is replaced with human albumin, plasma, or whole blood. Seriously ill patients will require between four and six units (25 gm per unit) of albumin, whole blood, or plasma in the first 24 hours in order to maintain good peripheral perfusion. Analgesics are used for control of pain. Meperidine seems to be effective in most patients. Morphine should be avoided because it is a potent constrictor of the sphincter of Oddi; it can worsen the pancreatitis by increasing pressures in the pancreatic ductal system.

In case of hypocalcemia with tetany, intravenously administered calcium will alleviate the tetany without necessarily restoring the serum calcium to normal. If there is significant hyperglycemia or hyperosmolar coma, insulin therapy is necessary.

Antibiotics have been advocated as prophylaxis against the development of pancreatic abscesses. In the milder form (edematous pancreatitis), however, recent studies have shown no benefit from their use. In severe disease, or in cases where an abscess is already suspected, broad-spectrum combination antibiotic therapy with agents directed mainly at gastrointestinal aerobic and anaerobic bacteria is conventionally employed and currently recommended. A combination of penicillin, gentamicin, and clindamycin (or chloromycetin) would be appropriate in this setting.

It has been accepted that pancreatic secretion should not be stimulated during an acute attack. Patients are usually fasted during the period of pain and are not permitted to eat until the pain and ileus have subsided and serum amylase levels have returned to nor-

Table 3   **Measures Not Shown to be Effective in the Management of Acute Pancreatitis**[a]

Measures to keep acid out of the duodenum:
    Nasogastric suction (trials in mild pancreatitis)
    Cimetidine

Measures to reduce pancreatic secretion:
    Glucagon
    Aprotinin (Trasylol, a pancreatic enzyme inhibitor)

Measures to accomplish both: anticholinergics

---

[a] In controlled prospective trials.

mal. An indwelling nasogastric tube is connected to low suction during the attack so as to decrease pancreatic secretion by removing gastric acid. It is therefore of note that, in several trials, measures that inhibit pancreatic secretions, either directly or by attempting to keep acid out of the duodenum, have not been shown to be beneficial. A summary of these techniques is found in Table 3. Nasogastric suction would still be appropriate in cases where ileus is present; its role in the milder disease is unproved.

WHAT SHOULD I EXPECT FROM SUCCESSFUL TREATMENT?

In spite of the limited means of controlling the disease, more than 95% of cases are self limited and subside spontaneously, usually within one to three days after treatment is initiated. Less than 5% of patients develop the fulminant form of the disease, which causes most of the deaths. (Mortality rates of as high as 80% have been reported in the fulminant or necrotizing hemorrhagic forms.) Several prognostic indicators have been found to correlate with the severity of the acute episode. These are listed in Table 4.

Table 4 **Initial Findings Indicating Severe Pancreatitis**[a]

On admission:
  Age over 55
  White cell count over 16,000/mm^3
  Blood glucose over 200 mg/100 ml
  Lactic dehydrogenase over 350 IU
  SGOT over 250 units per 100 ml

During initial 48 hours:
  Hematocrit decrease greater than 10% over admission
  BUN elevated more than 5 mg/100 ml over admission
  Serum calcium falls to below 8 mg/100 ml
  Arterial O$_2$ below 60 mm Hg
  Base deficit over 4 mEq/liter
  Estimated fluid sequestration over 6 liters

Reprinted with permission from Ranson JH, Rifkind KM, Turner JW: Prognostic signs and nonoperative peritoneal lavage in acute pancreatitis. *Surg Gynecol Obstet* 143:209–216, 1976.

[a] Patients with three or more of these findings had a significantly greater chance of dying.

The frequency of recurrent attacks varies according to the underlying precipitating factors and ranges from 30% without such factors to 90% to 100% in alcoholics who continue to drink. It is not clear whether abstention from alcohol reduces the incidence of recurrent attacks, although most clinicians believe that successful reformed drinkers tend to have fewer and less severe attacks.

WHAT MIGHT CAUSE A FAILURE OF TREATMENT? WHAT SHOULD THEN BE DONE?

As mentioned previously the majority of patients recover from an attack of acute pancreatitis unless the fulminant form is present. In these cases the two most common causes of death are vascular collapse during the first few days of the disease and superimposed infection as a late complication (weeks) after the onset.

Operation has a role in the management of acute pancreatitis at these possible points: at diagnosis, resuscitation from acute cardiovascular collapse in the most severe cases, and debridement of necrotic tissue or drainage of abscesses.

In a few patients peritonitis is prominent with marked direct and rebound tenderness and rigidity of abdominal wall musculature. Diagnostic paracentesis may not reveal much more than blood-tinged fluid with a high amylase content. Under such circumstances it is impossible to be sure that the patient does not have a perforated viscus or gangrenous bowel. The most useful course of action is to obtain a definite diagnosis via laparotomy. Recently it has been shown that laparotomy under such conditions does not worsen the already grim prognosis.

When fulminant pancreatitis pursues an unremitting course, a patient can sequester enormous amounts of plasma and blood. Hypotension and renal failure may not be reversed by vigorous, intravenous fluid therapy. More than 70% of patients with the combination of hypotension, hypocalcemia, and renal insufficiency die of the disease. For this reason we advocate surgical drainage to remove the exudate, which contains large quantities of the enzymes and vasoactive substances. Peritoneal lavage has its advocates, who cite the relative ease with which this accomplishes removal of the injurious products of pancreatic digestion from the abdominal cavity. The removal of this exudate will often reduce the fluid needs of the patient and correct the hypovolemia, hypotension, and hypocalcemia. It remains to be demonstrated whether such therapy improves overall survival.

Some physicians who have experience with these surgical forms of intervention (either laparotomy with drainage or closed peritoneal lavage) fear that they may actually favor the formation of pancreatic abscess. It is impossible to answer that question for certain since the procedure itself is usually performed only on the sickest patients. In patients with evidence of biliary tract obstruction and fulminant pancreatitis, laparotomy may be life saving when it is undertaken to accomplish biliary decompression, usually by cholecystostomy.

WHAT ARE THE SIDE EFFECTS OF THERAPY?

Since medical therapy (nasogastric drainage, intravenous fluids, colloids, etc.) is almost entirely supportive in nature, very few side effects are seen when the patient is monitored properly, usually in an intensive care area of the hospital. Placement of a central venous catheter for pressure recording will reduce the possibility of fluid overload and pulmonary edema in aged and cardiac patients. The complications of broad-spectrum antibiotic therapy are well known. A wide variety of side effects of surgical therapy have been described (e.g., pancreatic fistulas, wound abscess) but, as has already been pointed out, operation probably does not worsen the already serious prognosis in hemorrhagic pancreatitis and may improve it.

HOW SHOULD THE PATIENT BE FOLLOWED?

Feeding may be resumed when the attack has subsided, that is, when the pain has disappeared and the serum amylase level has returned to normal. It should be resumed cautiously with clear fluids followed by small feedings of solid foods and should be discontinued if the patient complains of abdominal pain, if fever reappears, or if the serum amylase concentration again begins to rise. The patient may be discharged from the hospital once gastrointestinal function returns to normal and remains normal after feeding has resumed.

The timing of follow-up examinations is variable depending on the suspected underlying case. An oral cholecystogram should be performed no sooner than three weeks after the attack of pancreatitis subsides, since it is unlikely that visualization of the gallbladder will occur before that time. A repeat abdominal ultrasound examination is indicated within six to eight weeks to monitor the possible development of a pseudocyst. A routine computerized axial tomography (CAT) scan is not necessary unless underlying carcinoma is suspected. Analgesics should not be continued beyond the period of hospitalization for treatment of a given attack of pancreatitis. It is a serious mistake to prescribe narcotic analgesics to be used as needed at the discretion of the patient because of the danger of narcotic abuse.

WHAT COMPLICATIONS OF THE DISEASE CAN OCCUR?

Complications of acute pancreatitis can appear early in the course of the disease, usually within the first few hours or days, or they may not become mainfest until weeks after the onset. These complications are all enumerated in Table 5.

Pseudocysts follow approximately 5% of attacks of acute pancreatitis. They are so designated because they do not contain an epithelial lining and therefore are not true cysts. Rather they represent localized collections of pancreatic fluid and debris, usually in direct contact with a major pancreatic duct. The clinical features of pancreatic pseudocysts are highly variable and often misinterpreted. Pseudocysts may bleed, erode into other organs, or rupture into the peritoneal cavity, the mediastinum, or the portal vein. A grave complication of pancreatic pseudocysts is bleeding into the cyst, with subsequent rupture into the stomach, bowel, or biliary tree producing massive gastrointestinal hemorrhage or hemobilia. Occasionally, they may cause obstructive jaundice, mimic a neoplasm, or dissect into the mediastinum.

Often pancreatic abscesses and lesser omentum fluid collections are difficult to separate from pseudocysts. In fact, even when masses are clinically appreciated, subsequent evaluation (usually surgical) reveals that it is difficult to distinguish any of these liquid masses from edematous pancreatic tissue, the so-called "phlegmon." Massive

Intraabdominal
   Pancreatic pseudocyst[a]
   Abscess/fluid collections[a]
   Colonic obstruction/fistulization
   Mesenteric vascular thrombosis ($\pm$ small-bowel infarction)
   Splenic rupture
   Portal vein thrombosis
   Intraperitoneal bleeding

Thoracic
   Acute respiratory distress syndrome
   Basilar atelectasis
   Pleural effusion
   Pneumonia
   Pulmonary embolus ($\pm$ infarction)
   Empyema
   Esophageal rupture

Neurologic
   Confusion/disorientation
   Central nervous system demyelinization

Others
   Shock
   Renal failure
   Subcutaneous fat necrosis
   Intramedullary fat necrosis

[a] Usually not seen until days or weeks after the onset of illness.

intraperitoneal bleeding is usually associated with frank arterial erosion, usually of the splenic or left gastric arteries.

An acute respiratory distress syndrome (ARDS) has been reported as a particularly grave complication of pancreatitis. This is probably due to the effect of proteolytic enzymes released into the pulmonary circulation with resultant damage to pulmonary alveoli. Patients with acute pancreatitis have been observed to become acutely confused during the course of the attack. Restlessness and disorientation may be difficult to control. This syndrome is probably due to the effects of circulatory toxins on the brain.

A variety of pathologic defects of the nervous system have been reported, including widespread demyelinization and small hemorrhages as well as pontine myelinolysis. Neurologic signs are variable under these circumstances. Obviously signs of midbrain dysfunction imply a very serious prognosis.

Shock complicating pancreatitis is also an ominous sign. Its mechanism is at least in part a reduction of plasma volume. It may also be a toxic phenomenon due to gram-negative bacterial sepsis or to circulating enzymes acting as vasoactive substances.

Renal failure is probably also multifactorial with the same mechanisms involved. It develops in a certain number of patients in spite of prompt restoration of plasma volume implying some type of humoral factor involvement.

HOW SHOULD THESE COMPLICATIONS BE MANAGED?

Pseudocysts may require surgical drainage but often do not. During their development, in the early phase, they lack a fibrous capsule. Until this develops (several weeks), the pseudocyst may resorb spontaneously. The capsule, once it forms, makes spontaneous resolution unlikely. Small, early, and uncomplicated pseudocysts are thus best left alone. When pseudocysts become very large, compress adjacent structures, or become infected, they must be drained surgically. This is preferably accomplished by permanent internal drainage into the stomach, duodenum, or a defunctionalizing (Roux-en-Y) loop of jejunum.

Infections and abscess formation in and around the pancreas always require vigorous therapy or the patient will die. Laparotomy and drainage with institution of appropriate antibiotic coverage is essential because the mortality in patients with undrained abscesses approaches 100%. Multiple abscesses occur in about 30% of these cases and the need to reoperate for further drainage is common. The acute abdominal complications such as thrombosis of major vessels with bowel infarction, organ rupture, or massive hemorrhage are all fatal unless surgical intervention is successful.

Pleural effusions should be aspirated in order to determine the nature of the effusion and examined by gram stain and cultured to exclude empyema; empyemas require surgical drainage. The acute respiratory distress syndrome is managed by positive-pressure oxygen therapy. Because of its seriousness, these patients always require tracheostomy.

Treatment of hypotension should be vigorous, with replacement of lost plasma volume as soon as possible. If the hypotension is unresponsive to aggressive fluid therapy, removal of necrotic pancreas via laparotomy and drainage or peritoneal dialysis should be instituted.

Renal failure is usually managed supportively. Peritoneal or hemodialysis can play a role in management of renal failure.

Acute pancreatitis and its many complications can produce a wasting illness of several weeks' duration. Some clinicians believe that nutritional support is an important component in the long-term management of such patients, although no prospective controlled trial is currently available to substantiate (or refute) this thesis. Provision of sufficient calories (which may amount to more than 4,000 a day) may be difficult unless intravenous hyperalimentation is instituted. Parenteral nutrition offers the further theoretical advantage of less pancreatic stimulation than enteral feeding. There have been some favorable reports on the use of elemental diet supplements as adjunctive therapy in the follow-up period, but it is usually not possible to supply large numbers of calories in this way.

Chronic Pancreatitis

HOW DO I MAKE THE DIAGNOSIS?

Chronic pancreatitis takes two forms: chronic relapsing pancreatitis and chronic pancreatitis per se. Chronic relapsing pancreatitis is chronic pancreatitis with acute symptomatic exacerbations characterized primarily by abdominal pain. Chronic pancreatitis is irreversible pancreatic destruction with its associated complications, and may or may not be associated with significant abdominal pain.

Some generalizations about chronic pancreatitis are possible: (1) The most common form, alcoholic chronic pancreatitis, requires heavy drinking for five to 15 years before problems develop. Temperate and occasional binge drinkers do not get the disorder. (2) When clinical symptoms first begin, the patient already has severe and chronic pathologic changes in the pancreas. (3) Although pain is the major symptom, it is variable and severe complications can occur without pain. (4) The diagnosis is usually made by recognition of the complications of the disease. The major complications are unremitting or remitting abdominal pain with a high incidence of opiate addiction, pancreatic exocrine insufficiency causing steatorrhea and weight loss, and diabetes mellitus. Less common complications include peptic ulcer disease (up to 20% in some series), vitamin B_{12} malabsorption, pseudocysts, biliary obstruction, and intraabdominal leakage of pancreatic juice (pancreatic ascites).

Invariably the patient loses weight unless the steatorrhea is treated. (In children a similar symptom complex may be seen but it is usually the result of cystic fibrosis involving the pancreas.) The stools are usually described as loose to formed, foul smelling, and containing recognizable globules of fat (due to unhydrolyzed triglycerides).

The physical examination may demonstrate only evidence of weight loss. Abdominal x-rays often reveal calcifications in the pancreas. This pathognomic sign confirms the diagnosis. Many patients will be overtly diabetic with the usual symptoms of hyperglycemia and glycosuria, while others have mild or "chemical" diabetes detectable only by performing a glucose tolerance test.

WHAT ADDITIONAL WORKUP DOES THE PATIENT REQUIRE?

In the classic situation, in which abdominal pain is not a significant factor, the previously discussed findings are sufficient cause to proceed directly to a therapeutic trial (pancreatic enzyme replacement with or without insulin). In other instances the cause of the weight loss or abdominal pain, or both, will require a more extensive evaluation.

The fecal fat collection has been discussed previously (see chapter on weight loss). Often in patients with coexistent abdominal pain, the weight loss may be due more to inadequate oral intake, which is caused by the pain itself or by the anorexia induced by narcotics.

In cases in which the major problem is abdominal pain, especially of recent onset, pancreatic carcinoma becomes a diagnostic possibility. In these cases abdominal ultrasound or a CAT scan of the upper abdomen may reveal an abnormal pancreas, a pseudocyst, or nothing at all to suggest a pancreatic process.

The scans are helpful in a confirmatory way but are often not definitive enough to be of more than adjunctive diagnostic value. Of more potential value is endoscopic retrograde cholangiopancreatography (ERCP). Visualization of the pancreatic duct may suggest a diagnosis of chronic pancreatitis by demonstrating the characteristic "chain-of-lakes" appearance (alternating areas of stricture and dilation of the major pancreatic duct). ERCP may also show acinar filling of the pancreas in chronic pancreatitis, which is not seen in the normal pancreas.

Not all patients with chronic pancreatitis will require ERCP, especially those with already obvious manifestations of the disease. Its most useful role may be in excluding the diagnosis of chronic pancreatitis in those patients with long-standing, severe abdominal pain.

Another set of tests that are invariably positive in chronic pancreatitis are those that measure stimulated pancreatic output. After duodenal intubation, the pancreas is caused to secrete either with a standard meal or with hormone (secretin) infusion. The output of pancreatic enzymes and bicarbonate, as well as fluid volume, can then be assessed. Since 90% of the pancreas must be destroyed before clinical sequelae of pancreatic insufficiency are seen, patients with pancreatic insufficiency always have reduced pancreatic fluid concentrations of enzymes and bicarbonate.

The secretin test has been advocated as useful in distinguishing between chronic pancreatitis and occlusion of the main pancreatic duct by a carcinoma. These theoretical differential responses to secretin are enumerated in Table 6. In chronic pancreatitis the fluid volume should be normal, but the digestive components are reduced. Since the pancreas proximal to a malignant obstruction is normal, the concentrations of both enzymes and bicarbonate are normal, but the total volume secreted is reduced. Unfortunately, this theoretical separation does not always occur in patients. The real value of the secretin test in this case may be to obtain pancreatic fluid for cytologic examination.

As in acute pancreatitis, a diligent search for an underlying cause of the chronic pancreatitis should be carried out. Successful treatment of such underlying disorders as alcoholism (difficult at best), hyperparathyroidism, gallbladder, and biliary tract disease or

Table 6 Secretin Test in Pancreatic Insufficiency and Carcinoma

Measurement	Chronic Pancreatitis	Carcinoma
Enzyme	Reduced	Normal
Bicarbonate	Reduced	Normal
Volume	Normal	Reduced
Malignant cells	Absent	Present

of possible mechanical problems such as stricture of the pancreatic ductal orifice can prevent relapsing attacks of pain and potentially fatal complications.

HOW SHOULD I TREAT THE PATIENT?

Treatment consists of reversal of the underlying cause (if possible), alleviation of pain, and correction of pancreatic exocrine and endocrine deficiency. Medical treatment should be directed toward prevention of recurrent attacks, most importantly eliminating alcohol, which is by far the most common cause of chronic pancreatitis in our society. Gallbladder or biliary tract disease, if present, must be corrected surgically.

Management of pain is difficult because of the chronic nature of the disease. Most experts agree that abstinence from alcohol will lessen the severity of pain or eliminate it. Because of the problem of narcotic addiction, these drugs are best not used in pain management, and if they are used should be withdrawn gradually from addicted patients.

A variety of surgical approaches for relief of pain have been tried but no one form of surgical therapy has been uniformly successful. These operations range from papillotomy or sphincteroplasty of the sphincter of Oddi to various pancreatic ductal drainage procedures all the way to subtotal or total pancreatectomy. In evaluating the effect of operation, one must keep in mind that spontaneous relief of pain occurs in about 40% of patients simply with passage of time, that cessation of alcohol will relieve pain in many patients, and that surgical treatment may relieve pain by virtue of a placebo effect in about 30% of operated patients. Although much disagreement exists about the efficacy of surgery, most experts at least agree that patients free of narcotic addiction are more likely to have a good result from operation than are patients currently addicted.

Steatorrhea is best treated by adequate replacement with pancreatic enzyme preparations such as Viokase or Cotazym. Since the enzymes must be in an alkaline medium to be effective, the problem of gastric acid inactivation is of real concern. A newer preparation (Pancrease), may be more resistant to gastric acid inactivation. Usual doses are: Viokase, four tablets, or Pancrease, three tablets, at the beginning of each meal; individualization of therapy is necessary. If the patient continues to lose weight and observes greasy stools, the enzymes may be given at intervals during the meal. If this is not effective, the dose may have to be increased. (Hyperuricemia has been reported with large doses of pancreatic enzymes.) Finally, antacids or cimetidine may be used in conjunction with the pancreatic enzymes.

Treatment of diabetes often requires the use of insulin and patients with chronic pancreatitis may be difficult to control.

WHAT SHOULD I EXPECT FROM SUCCESSFUL THERAPY?

Cessation of pain, weight gain by reducing malabsorption, and control of diabetes are considered the end points of successful therapy. Too often, however, patients will relapse because of insufficient attention to chronic administration of medicines, inadequate follow-up evaluation, or return to drinking.

WHAT MIGHT CAUSE A FAILURE OF THERAPY? WHAT SHOULD THEN BE DONE?

Chronic pancreatitis is a difficult disease to manage and we are often not successful because of the insidious progression of pancreatic insufficiency, further complications, or return to drinking. The following directions are suggested for management of the patient with chronic pancreatitis who is doing poorly:

1. Try hard and repeatedly to get the patient to stop drinking. Showing him or her life expectancy data may help.
2. Do not use narcotics. Use salicylates to tolerance.
3. If the pain continues even after the patient stops drinking, search for a pseudocyst and drain internally if one is found. Ultrasound is the single best test for diagnosis.
4. Do not rush into more extensive pancreatic operation even if pain continues. Try to tide the patient over, hoping for a spontaneous remission.

HOW SHOULD THE PATIENT BE FOLLOWED?

The patient should be referred to an alcohol detoxification program if appropriate, followed by a rehabilitation program such as Alcoholics Anonymous. Frequent office visits necessitated by refills of medication prescriptions provide the opportunity to monitor patients with respect to weight, fasting blood sugar, urinalysis for glucose, and abdominal examination (searching for masses suggesting pseudocysts).

WHAT COMPLICATIONS OF THE DISEASE CAN OCCUR?

Two potential problems of chronic pancreatitis need to be considered, pancreatic carcinoma and biliary duct obstruction. Although some believe that patients with chronic pancreatitis are at increased risk of developing cancer, very few data actually support this concept. As noted earlier, however, the diagnosis is often entertained when patients with chronic pancreatitis are first evaluated.

The fibrosing process in the head of the pancreas may entrap the common bile duct with subsequent ductal stricture. The chronic bile duct obstruction may result in secondary biliary cirrhosis in some patients. The problem of determining the cause of cirrhosis in a patient who is also an alcoholic is, however, obvious. Such patients need to be followed carefully, usually with gastroenterologic consultation. Any decision concerning operation must be individualized.

SELECTED READING

Carey LC: *The Pancreas.* St. Louis, CV Mosby Co, 1973.

Graham DY: Enzyme replacement therapy of exocrine pancreatic insufficiency in men. *N Engl J Med* 296:1314–1317, 1977.

Meyer JH: Acute pancreatitis, in Sleisenger MH, Fordtran JS: *Gastrointestinal Disease. Pathophysiology, Diagnosis, Management.* Philadelphia, WB Saunders Co, 1973, pp 1398–1439.

Paloyan D, Simonowitz D: Diagnostic considerations in acute alcoholic and gallstone pancreatitis. *Am J Surg* 132:329–337, 1976.

Warshaw AL, Imhembo AL, Civetta JM, et al: Surgical intervention in acute necrotizing pancreatitis. *Am J Surg* 127:484–491, 1974.

CLINICAL PROBLEMS

I. A 40-year-old woman with known gallstones is admitted to the hospital complaining of severe, steady epigastric pain that has been present for 18 hours. She has noticed that the pain is aggravated by movement, and that it is somewhat relieved if she sits up and draws her knees to her chest. Her physical examination reveals a temperature of 101 F, a blood pressure of 90/60, and a pulse rate of 130; abdominal findings include hypoactive bowel sounds, mild distention, and tenderness especially in the epigastrium.

   1. What pancreatic disorder is producing this clinical picture?
   2. How can it be diagnosed?
   3. How should it be treated?

II. A 45-year-old man presents with a gradual weight loss of 15 to 20 pounds over the past six to 12 months. He has maintained a good appetite and his usual food intake. He denies abdominal pain, but has noted some diarrhea over the same time period.

Upon close questioning he remembers seeing fat globules in the diarrheal stool. He has a long history of alcohol ingestion and he had two episodes of acute pancreatitis one and two years earlier. His physical examination is unremarkable except for evidence of weight loss.

1. What pancreatic disorder is producing this clinical picture?
2. How can it be diagnosed?
3. How should it be treated?

III. A 47-year-old alcoholic man is evaluated for chronic epigastric pain and weight loss. The pain is described as having been present virtually all the time for the past four years. Before that the patient had multiple episodes of intermittent abdominal pain usually diagnosed as "acute pancreatitis." Since the pain became constant, he has been unable to find any relief. He is currently consuming four to eight analgesic medications per day, each containing 30 mg of codeine. He has lost his appetite and has lost 25 pounds over the past two years. His physical examination reveals only evidence of weight loss and depression. Preliminary laboratory evaluation demonstrates pancreatic calcification and a normal serum amylase, urine amylase, and amylase/creatinine clearance ratio. The blood sugar is normal. Liver tests are all within normal limits.

1. What pancreatic disorder is producing this clinical picture?
2. How can it be diagnosed?
3. How should it be treated?

Discussion

I. 1. This patient has acute pancreatitis, presumably due to gallstone disease. The fever, tenderness, decreased bowel sounds, and pain with movement point to an intraabdominal inflammatory process. The assumption of a fetal position implies retroperitoneal involvement. Her tachycardia and low blood pressure indicate relative hypovolemia.

   2. The major diagnostic test is the history and physical examination. The serum amylase, urine amylase, and amylase/cre-

atinine clearance ratio are all likely to be elevated. Other tests that should be performed include an abdominal flat plate and upright (to rule out the presence of a perforated viscus), a blood sugar, a serum calcium, and a hematocrit. (These latter three tests really measure the severity of the pancreatitis.) Other tests, such as a barium upper gastrointestinal series or ultrasound, are not important to the patient's immediate management; they may be obtained later in the hospitalization to provide additional information concerning possible pancreatic masses. Straining the stool may identify the causative stone.

3. The patient should be treated supportively with observation, analgesics, intravenous fluids, and any of the following that are necessary: nasogastric tube (ileus), insulin (marked hyperglycemia), and intravenous calcium (hypocalcemia). If her condition improves, elective cholecystectomy should be undertaken in the future; if it deteriorates, antibiotics and emergency laparotomy may be necessary.

II. 1. This is a typical story for pancreatic insufficiency unassociated with abdominal pain. The presence of oil globules suggests undigested triglycerides in the stool (pancreatic lipase deficiency).

2. An abnormal fecal fat collection (see the chapter on weight loss), the presence of calcifications on an abdominal flat plate, and the absence of a pancreatic mass lesion on ultrasound or CAT scan (ruling out pancreatic carcinoma) would be an adequate workup, and an empiric trial of therapy could be undertaken. More specific diagnostic testing would include a pancreatic stimulation test and an ERCP. It would be appropriate also to obtain a blood sugar to evaluate the patient for concomitant diabetes.

3. Treatment revolves around the adequate supply of pancreatic enzymes. If the standard dose fails to correct the weight loss, the various maneuvers described in this chapter (increasing the dose, changing the timing of administration, or adding cimetidine or antacids) will need to be tried. If significant problems with the blood sugar are present, insulin may also need to be added.

III. 1. Although chronic pancreatitis occasionally produces constant abdominal pain, this clinical picture is more likely due to drug and alcohol addiction or functional bowel disease, or both. Pancreatic carcinoma would be unlikely to pursue a four-year course.

2. An abdominal ultrasound or CAT scan would probably be obtained to rule out the presence of a mass lesion or other hepatopancreatic pathology. In order to ascertain whether the pain is due to chronic pancreatitis, the patient would have to be off all narcotics and alcohol for a period of several months. Usually, if this can be accomplished, the pain becomes less severe and episodic, appetite returns, and a general improvement is seen.

3. Treatment consists of psychological support and drug and alcohol withdrawal. If weight gain cannot be accomplished as the appetite returns, pancreatic enzyme supplementation may be required. Operation should only be offered when it is clear that all other modalities have failed (after successful drug and alcohol withdrawal) for many months; it is rarely required.

WILFRED M. WEINSTEIN

Gastrointestinal Cancer

Carcinoma of the colon is the second most common malignancy in men and women. Pancreatic carcinoma appears to be increasing and gastric carcinoma is decreasing. Esophageal carcinoma is less common than the other three. Of these tumors, carcinoma of the colon holds the greatest hope for early diagnosis and curative surgery. Carcinomas of the esophagus, stomach, and pancreas often present at an advanced stage so that curative surgery is usually impossible. They respond poorly to other measures such as radiotherapy or chemotherapy. Only carcinomas of these organs will be considered. The more uncommon neoplasms, such as lymphomas and endocrine cell tumors, will not be covered.

The emphasis in this chapter will be on the local signs and symptoms and on the optimal approach to obtain a precise rapid diagnosis. Any of the tumors may present, de novo, with metastases. Favored sites are liver, regional lymph nodes and organs, peritoneum (malignant ascites), supraclavicular nodes, lungs, and bones. Rarely, patients may present with systemic or constitutional symptoms such as fever of unknown origin or certain endocrine manifestations, but these are rare. Rapid, nonoperative diagnosis is especially important when a cancer is untreatable or metastatic. It permits patients to spend their remaining limited time with more meaningful endeavors than undergoing batteries of tests or recovering from surgery.

The major advances have been in the area of diagnosis rather than therapy. For the hollow-organ tumors an important development has been fiberoptic endoscopy with direct-vision biopsy and cytology. In the case of carcinoma of the pancreas, there are more sophisticated imaging techniques such as ultrasound, computerized tomography (CAT) scans, and endoscopic retrograde cholangiopancreatography (ERCP). Chest x-ray, liver function tests, liver scan, ultrasound, CAT scans, and bone scans often detect metastases and prevent unnecessary surgery. Laparoscopy can be performed with the patient under local anesthesia and permits examination and biopsy of the liver to confirm metastatic disease. As a result, fewer laparotomies are now required simply to provide a "tissue diagnosis" when obvious metastatic disease is present.

When surgery for cure is planned, it is extremely important to search carefully in advance for evidence of metastatic disease. If metastatic disease is found, some patients will not require palliative operation for the primary tumor because it, per se, may not be causing symptoms such as obstruction or persistent hemorrhage.

Some of the newer diagnostic techniques theoretically provide an opportunity for earlier detection. Hopefully this will result in prolonged survival. Of the tumors to be considered here, this hope applies realistically only to carcinoma of the colon.

Why does the primary care physician need to be aware of the various diagnostic and therapeutic options available for carcinoma? The reason is clear: the patient with carcinoma may encounter a host of consulting physicians (surgeons, gastroenterologists, medical oncologists, and radiotherapists) and potentially conflicting recommendations may follow. The patient's own physician is usually in the best situation to distill the various judgments and translate the recommendations to the patient in a supportive fashion. This is especially important for the tumors considered in this section because most of them carry a poor prognosis. Often the decisions are of the value judgment type. One example is the patient with gastric adenocarcinoma and extensive metastatic liver disease. The gastric tumor may have been discovered because of anemia and occult gastrointestinal bleeding. One consultant may urge that the tumor be removed because it might bleed more dramatically. However, the patient's own physician should legitimately argue that the patient already has a limited life span and that some of that remaining time should not be spent recovering from palliative surgery simply to forestall an event that might not occur. The primary care physician should be more assertive in guiding the overall approach to the patient's management.

The general principles of supportive therapy apply to all the tumor states. These principles include correction of anemia, attempts to maintain optimal nutrition, management of pain, and mobilization of family and community resources for maximal psychological support when tumors are untreatable or advanced. The risk factors to be emphasized are those that the physician can do something about by recommending changes in habits or by having screening tests performed. Tables summarizing the important symptoms, diagnostic tests, and risk factors accompany the discussion of each tumor.

CARCINOMA OF THE ESOPHAGUS

Clinical Presentation

Progressive dysphagia is the most common presenting manifestation (Table 1). Typically, progressive dysphagia develops first with solids, then liquids. Pain is usually not prominent although discomfort is often associated with the dysphagia. Occasionally the presenting manifestation is a brisk or slow (anemia) hemorrhage. Even when bleeding appears to be the presenting manifestation, there

Table 1 Carcinoma of the Esophagus: Important Features

Cardinal symptoms
    Dysphagia
Diagnostic tests
    Barium esophagogram
    Esophagoscopy with biopsy and brush cytology
Risk factors
    Smoking
    Alcoholism
    Esophageal disease: achalasia, Barrett's esophagus, lye strictures

has often been a prior history of dysphagia, which has been mild or ignored by the patient. Weight loss is usually commensurate with the amount of dysphagia and reduced food intake that has occurred. Chest x-ray may reveal that aspiration pneumonitis has occurred.

Diagnosis

Everyone who presents with dysphagia must be evaluated carefully for evidence of an organic lesion. A barium esophagogram with an upper gastrointestinal x-ray should be ordered. The radiologist should be alerted that dysphagia is the problem, and if no obstructing lesion is seen, the examination should be extended by having the patient take a solid such as bread soaked in barium to look for an area of "holdup." Endoscopy is also indicated in all patients with clear-cut dysphagia. When lesions are encountered at endoscopy, biopsies and brush cytology are performed. Even with direct-vision techniques the diagnostic accuracy may only be 85% to 90%. This is because many of these esophageal cancers create an intense surrounding inflammatory infiltrate. Biopsy and cytology specimens may merely sample this shield of inflammation and miss the carcinoma. Sometimes it is necessary to reexamine these patients if the clinical suspicion of carcinoma is strong.

Differential Diagnosis

Because the tumors usually present as strictures or ulcerative lesions, the usual differential diagnosis is benign esophageal stricture associated with esophagitis. Other lesions to be considered are esophageal motility disorders, benign submucosal lesions (e.g., leiomyomata), and extrinsic compression from bronchogenic carcinoma. These can generally be differentiated with endoscopy and chest x-ray. The esophagus is lined by squamous epithelium and more than 90% of the carcinomas are of the squamous type. When an adenocarcinoma is found in the lower esophagus, it raises the possibility that the actual primary site is high in the stomach with secondary invasion of the lower esophagus. Primary adenocarcinomas rarely arise in the esophagus and are often associated with underlying Barrett's epithelium. Barrett's esophagus is a condition in which the normal, squamous epithelial lining of the esophagus is replaced by a columnar type in patients with prolonged gastroesophageal reflux. Barrett's esophagus carries with it an increased risk of primary adenocarcinoma of the esophagus.

Treatment and Prognosis

Only 20% of the patients with carcinoma of the esophagus have potentially resectable lesions and, in this group, five-year survival after operation is only 10%. Similarly dismal results are obtained with radiotherapy. There is no chemotherapy regimen that significantly alters outcome.

The most significant advance in those with obstructing untreatable tumors has been the development of tubes that can be positioned through the tumor-obstructed lumen under direct vision at endoscopy. This permits the patient to swallow and to eat. Formerly, many of these patients literally drowned in their own secretions.

Risk Factors

Smoking and alcoholism appear to be risk factors for the development of carcinoma of the esophagus. Preexisting conditions that are associated with an increased risk of carcinoma of the esophagus are lye strictures, achalasia of the esophagus, and Barrett's esophagus. Screening endoscopy and biopsy can be performed in these individuals but there are no reliable guidelines. This is because fiberoptic endoscopy has only been widely available for approximately 10 years. No studies have been done to demonstrate whether intensive screening will detect esophageal carcinomas at an earlier stage and, more importantly, whether earlier detection will result in prolonged survival. At present, the situation is quite ad hoc and depends entirely on the enthusiasm of individual physicians and patients.

CARCINOMA OF THE STOMACH

Clinical Presentation

Most patients have incurable lesions when they first present to physicians (Table 2). The most common symptoms are "indiges-

Table 2   **Carcinoma of the Stomach: Important Features**

Cardinal symptoms
   Upper abdominal pain
   Occult bleeding
   Weight loss
   Disordered emptying (vomiting, "indigestion," anorexia)
   Dysphagia
Diagnostic tests
   Barium upper gastrointestinal x-ray
   Gastroscopy with biopsy and cytology
Risk factors
   Adenomatous polyps
   Pernicious anemia
   Strong family history
   Partial gastrectomy ($>$ 10 years earlier, Billroth II)
   Immigrants from high-risk area (e.g., Japan)

tion," upper abdominal pain, and weight loss. The pain may mimic that of peptic ulcer. Anorexia and vomiting occur in at least half of the patients. Vomiting is especially prominent with tumors that are located in the distal stomach and interfere with gastric emptying. The weight loss is primarily due to anorexia but there may also be a component of early satiety. Dysphagia is a leading symptom in patients who have cardia tumors, that is, lesions of the fundus and gastric cardia zone, that encroach on the lower esophagus. Frank hematemesis is unusual but occult bleeding and anemia are common.

The physical examination may be negative or reveal abdominal tenderness. When other findings (epigastric mass, hepatomegaly, ascites, and supraclavicular adenopathy) are present, they usually indicate advanced cancer.

Diagnosis

Barium x-ray and endoscopy with biopsy and cytology usually provide a definitive diagnosis. The tumors usually appear as ulcers or masses (with or without associated ulceration). A linitis plastica pattern is less common. This is a tumor growth within the gastric walls, resulting in loss of pliability and impaired peristalsis. The rarest pattern is a superficial "spreading" carcinoma, which involves only the mucosa and appears as shallow ulcerations or nodular plaques. When a gastric carcinoma is suspected and barium x-rays are negative or equivocal, the patient should be referred for an endoscopic examination.

Differential Diagnosis

Benign gastric ulcer that is slow to heal, polyp, and gastric lymphoma are the usual entities that need to be excluded at endoscopy, with biopsy and cytology.

Therapy and Prognosis

The only hope for cure is surgical resection. Therapy for resectable lesions consists of partial or total gastrectomy. Unfortunately only approximately half of patients are resectable at surgery and many of them have regional lymph node involvement. The operative mortality may be as high as 10% and the overall five-year survival is approximately 10%. Therefore, surgery for cure is attempted, but the biology of gastric cancer is such that long-term survival is infrequent. The tumors that carry the most favorable prognosis are those confined to mucosa or submucosa and smaller (less than 2 cm) lesions with no lymph node involvement. Surgery for palliation is sometimes necessary when there is total obstruction or hemorrhage, even in the presence of obvious metastases.

Chemotherapy, as adjunctive therapy after surgery or alone for metastatic disease, offers little. Occasional "responses" are observed, but some patients have increased discomfort and no prolongation of life.

Risk Factors

There is an increased risk of gastric cancer in those with adenomatous gastric polyps, pernicious anemia, a strong family history of gastric cancer, a Billroth gastrectomy 10 years previously, and in immigrants from countries where gastric cancer is more frequent (e.g., Chile, Japan). In those with adenomatous polyps or a previous history of same, periodic screening with endoscopy is justified. In the others, stool guaiac examinations after the age of 40 and advice to seek medical attention promptly for the symptoms referred to previously seem the most reasonable approaches at present.

Some would favor more vigorous screening with endoscopy and biopsy in all of the risk factor settings referred to previously. Nevertheless, as for esophageal cancer, the question concerning yield and prolongation of life with earlier detection is unanswered.

CARCINOMA OF THE PANCREAS

Clinical Presentation

Abdominal pain, weight loss, and jaundice in a middle-aged person are the classic symptoms of carcinoma of the pancreas (Table 3). The pain is usually in the epigastrium and often radiates to the right and left and to the back. It is constant and boring in quality, sometimes worsened or provoked by meals. Jaundice is common with tumors of the head of the pancreas. The tumors occur in the head in 70% of those with carcinoma of the pancreas, in the body in 20%, and in the tail in 10%. Weight loss is due to anorexia, pain, and

Table 3 **Carcinoma of the Pancreas: Important Features**

Cardinal symptoms
    Upper abdominal pain
    Weight loss
    Jaundice
Diagnostic tests
    Barium upper gastrointestinal x-ray
    Ultrasound
    Computerized axial tomography scan
    Endoscopic retrograde cholangiopancreatography with cytology
    Angiography
    Percutaneous biopsy (if inoperable)
Risk factors
    Smoking
    Alcoholism (?)
    Chronic pancreatitis (?)
    Diabetes (?)

sometimes malabsorption. The latter occurs when the major pancreatic duct is obstructed. In these instances diarrhea and steatorrhea may be accompanying symptoms. Recent-onset or accompanying diabetes may indicate involvement of the endocrine pancreas. Disorders of affect have been described, both at the time of presentation and sometimes preceding the onset of local symptoms. Traditionally, recurrent or migratory thrombophlebitis has been considered a premonitory presentation of pancreatic carcinoma. However, other visceral malignancies may also be associated with this.

The physical examination may reveal an upper abdominal mass. When jaundice is present the gallbladder may be visibly or palpably distended. Splenomegaly is sometimes found and results from compression of the splenic vein.

Diagnosis

The usual approach in suspect cases is to first perform an upper gastrointestinal barium x-ray. It may reveal widening of the duodenal loop, encroachment on the medial aspect of the descending (second) portion of the duodenum, or displacement of the stomach. Ultrasound is the next test to perform and if results are equivocal the order of investigations should be CAT scan, ERCP with cytology, and angiography. Sometimes the diagnosis remains elusive for months.

Many inoperable patients can be spared surgery simply for tissue diagnosis by having a percutaneous aspiration biopsy under ultrasonic guidance. If this is unsuccessful, laparotomy and biopsy may be required. Even then, it may be difficult to differentiate chronic pancreatitis from carcinoma because the tumors (like those in the esophagus) may be surrounded by a zone of inflammation.

Differential Diagnosis

When pain and marked weight loss are the presenting manifestations, other intraabdominal malignancies, especially gastric, need to be excluded. In the alcoholic, chronic pancreatitis is a frequent consideration. When jaundice is present, other causes of extrahepatic obstruction enter into the differential diagnosis; these include stones in the common bile duct or hepatic duct, duct tumors, and tumors of the ampulla of Vater. To exclude these, percutaneous transhepatic cholangiography or ERCP, or both, are invaluable.

Treatment and Prognosis

The tumors are usually inoperable at the time of presentation because of regional extension. In rare instances when they are resectable a pancreaticoduodenectomy can be performed. This operation carries a 15% to 20% mortality rate and survival is often unaffected. Bypass procedures may be performed to alleviate jaundice with pruritus or cholangitis, or both. Overall survival is 10% at one year and one to two percent at five years. No effective chemotherapy is available.

A nonoperative approach is being evaluated in patients with carcinoma of the head of the pancreas who have jaundice because of common bile duct obstruction. This consists of the placement of a drainage catheter into the common bile duct with an endoscope. The intent is to avoid bypass surgery for intractable jaundice. The efficacy of this approach remains to be established.

Risk Factors

Risk factors are said to be smoking, alcoholism, chronic pancreatitis, and diabetes. Smoking appears to be the risk factor with the most convincing data.

CARCINOMA OF THE COLON

Clinical Presentation

The most common symptoms of carcinoma of the colon are altered bowel habits and occult or overt lower gastrointestinal bleeding (Table 4). In tumors of the cecum, the lesions have more room to grow before local symptoms develop. Therefore, blood-loss anemia is often the first mode of presentation. In tumors of the descending and sigmoid colon and rectum, altered bowel habits (constipation or alternating constipation and diarrhea) and abdominal pain are frequent. In these "left-sided" sites there may be

Table 4 **Carcinoma of the Colon: Important Features**

Cardinal symptoms
    Altered bowel habits
    Lower gastrointestinal bleeding (occult or overt)
    Lower abdominal pain
Diagnostic tests
    Stool for occult blood
    Sigmoidoscopy
    Air-contrast barium enema
    Colonoscopy
Risk factors
    Stool positive for occult blood (patient older than 40)
    Recurrent adenomatous polyps
    Ulcerative colitis
    Familial polyposis
    Gardner's syndrome
    Villous adenomas

accompanying bright-red rectal bleeding. The latter is sometimes wrongly attributed to hemorrhoids. A more dramatic but less common form of presentation is bowel obstruction or localized perforation. Some presymptomatic carcinomas are detected in the course of screening high-risk groups and through general screening programs.

The most common local physical findings are abdominal mass or a palpable lesion on rectal examination. Stool guaiac examinations are necessary whenever carcinoma of the colon is suspected.

Diagnosis

Sigmoidoscopy is essential in suspect cases. Approximately one-half of all large-bowel cancers are within reach of the rigid sigmoidoscope. Flexible fiberoptic sigmoidoscopes will probably replace the rigid sigmoidoscopes because they reach further, as far as 60 cm.

An air-contrast barium enema is mandatory. Many radiologists are still reluctant to perform this more time-consuming but clearly superior examination. However, the tide is swinging. The preparation of the patient for x-ray is important in order to obtain optimal x-ray visualization. Patients without major obstructive symptoms can take clear liquids for two days before the procedure and laxatives to the point of watery diarrhea on each of these two days. The radiologist must be alerted when patients have symptoms of partial obstruction so that they do not fill the colon with barium proximal to the lesion. When a cancer of the rectum has been diagnosed on sigmoidoscopic biopsy, an air-contrast enema should still be done because second colonic neoplasms sometimes coexist.

The patterns of neoplasia on x-ray are generally either polypoid masses or constricting lesions. The latter are more common in the left colon.

Colonoscopy has simplified the definitive diagnosis immensely. It provides visual and biopsy access to lesions beyond the reach of the sigmoidoscope. It is also used when x-rays are negative or equivocal in suspect colonic cancer and for screening high-risk groups.

Differential Diagnosis

The usual problem with differential diagnosis is in the person with one or more colonic polyps. Here, excisional biopsy at colonoscopy is often the final arbiter. In ulcerative colitis, benign strictures need to be differentiated from cancer. Patients with diverticular disease may have gross deformity of the bowel necessitating visual access with endoscopy to rule out carcinoma.

Other inflammatory lesions may enter into the differential diagnosis. They are Crohn's disease and less common disorders such as tuberculosis and amebiasis.

Treatment and Prognosis

Surgery for cure entails resection and reanastomosis. Tumors of the rectum usually require an abdominoperineal resection and a permanent colostomy. When surgery is performed for palliation in the presence of known metastases, proximal colostomy may be required. In some patients with inoperable carcinomas, staged fulguration via endoscopes may maintain an open lumen and reduce the rate of hemorrhage.

When it is anticipated that a patient will require a permanent colostomy he or she should meet others who have had a successful result. In many centers there are ostomy societies that provide a forum for practical information about day-to-day life with an ostomy.

Five-year survival depends on the site of the cancer, whether regional lymph nodes are positive, and how far into the bowel wall the tumor has penetrated. The five-year survival figures for resectable lesions with no adjacent or distant organ involvement are: 80% for lesions confined to the mucosa alone and 25% when there is lymph node involvement. When there are distant metastases, the five-year survival outlook is five percent or less.

Treatment for metastatic disease only benefits a few. There is no increase in overall median survival. 5-Fluorouracil alone or in combination with other drugs is the approach taken when chemotherapy is instituted.

Risk Factors

Because carcinoma of the colon is so common and because early detection and treatment appear to prolong life, we can all be considered at risk. Recommendations vary. One approach is that all persons over age 40 have annual stool guaiac tests and an annual digital rectal examination. After age 50 sigmoidoscopic examinations could be added, at a rate of every two years. All agree that screening is important. Opinions concerning intensity and frequency vary from the more relaxed approach of the Canadian Task Force on the Periodic Health Examination to the more rigorous guidelines of the American Cancer Society.

Stool guaiac tests have been simplified with the Hemoccult cards. Patients take two specimens from different parts of the same stool for three consecutive bowel movements. The cards should be returned promptly for testing. Some recommend a meat-free diet for three days before testing. I test first with the patient on a regular diet, then repeat the tests with the patient on a meat-free diet in those with positive tests. False-negative results may occur when samples age for four or five days before testing and when patients take high doses of vitamin C. Positive tests dictate the need for investigation. Approximately one percent of those over age 40 will have a positive test and of these approximately 10% are found to have cancer.

More intensive screening with regular (every one to two years) air-contrast barium enemas and colonoscopy is necessary in those with a history of villous adenomas or previous resections of adenomatous polyps, ulcerative colitis after 10 years, or familial polyposis syndromes.

FOLLOW-UP STUDY AFTER SURGERY

When surgery for cure has been performed, the physician should, in conjunction with the surgeon, formulate a plan for the type and frequency of follow-up study. This will often entail chest x-rays, hemoglobin determinations, barium x-rays after resection of hollow-organ tumors, endoscopy, and stool guaiac tests.

What is the role of carcinoembryonic antigen (CEA)? The main value of this test is in follow-up study after colorectal surgery. A rise in circulating CEA levels may indicate the presence of recurrent disease. We do not know whether recurrent disease that is detected in this way, and is treated, results in prolonged survival.

SELECTED READING

Rubin CE, Silverstein FE, McDonald GB: Indications for fiberoptic endoscopy. *Viewpoints on Digestive Diseases* 10: #5, 1978.

Sarna G: *Practical Oncology*. Boston, Houghton Mifflin Professional Publishers, 1980.

Taylor WC, Delbanco TL: Looking for early cancer. *Ann Intern Med* 93:773–775, 1980.

Winawer SJ: Gastric immunoreactive CEA as a potential marker of malignancy. *Gastroenterology* 76:870–879, 1979.

CLINICAL PROBLEMS

I. A 61-year-old man complains of upper abdominal pain and a 10- to 15-pound weight loss over the past two to three months, which he attributes to a sharp decline in his appetite. His physical examination is unremarkable except for the presence of occult blood in his stool. Preliminary laboratory data reveal a mild anemia and normal liver tests. A barium upper gastrointestinal x-ray demonstrates a large ulcerated lesion on the greater curvature of the stomach.

1. What further diagnostic tests should the patient undergo?
2. If the lesion is malignant, what is his prognosis?
3. If the lesion is malignant, how should he be followed?

II. A 53-year-old former alcoholic has noted anorexia, progressively increasing abdominal pain, and weight loss for eight weeks. He has noted mild pruritus for a week. He presents with icterus and has a palpable, hard, mid-to-right upper quadrant abdominal mass. A barium upper gastrointestinal series demonstrates a widening of the duodenal sweep with an irregular mucosal pattern on the medial side of the descending duodenum. An ultrasound examination reveals a large solid mass in the head of the pancreas, several solid intrahepatic masses, and a dilated biliary tree.

1. What further diagnostic tests should the patient undergo?
2. If the lesion is malignant, what is his prognosis?
3. If the lesion is malignant, how should he be followed?

III. A 67-year-old woman is found to have occult blood in her stool on routine evaluation. She denies any abdominal or systemic symptoms and her physical examination is entirely normal otherwise. Fiberoptic sigmoidoscopy reveals a 2-cm, sessile friable lesion in the sigmoid colon.

1. What further diagnostic tests should the patient undergo?
2. If the lesion is malignant, what is her prognosis?
3. If the lesion is malignant, how should she be followed?

Discussion

I. 1. The next step in the diagnostic evaluation is to assess the nature of the intragastric process. Endoscopy with multiple biopsies and cytology is usually effective in this regard. If a carcinoma is confirmed, the patient should be evaluated as a surgical candidate. If he is an acceptable general surgical risk, a metastatic workup (chest x-ray, liver scan, bone scan) can be undertaken. If this workup is negative, he is a candidate for an attempt at surgical cure.

2. Even if he has no overt evidence of metastatic disease preoperatively, the chances of a five-year survival are probably less than five percent. (One-half of operable patients are resectable; the five-year survival rate in resectable patients is only 10%.)

3. Whether or not he is an operable, or resectable, candidate, he should have continued follow-up study. This accomplishes several purposes: emotional support for a patient with a life-threatening process, objective professional advice concerning the various low-yield therapeutic options if the disease spreads, observation for potentially reversible complications or other illnesses (e.g., anemia, infections), and sympathetic and understanding care during the terminal phase of the illness, should that need arise.

II. 1. The clinical suspicion at this point is that the patient has metastatic pancreatic carcinoma. One approach is to undertake palliative surgical therapy; the histologic diagnosis can be established at laparotomy and the biliary tree (and potential duodenal obstruction) can be bypassed. If a nonoperative biliary decompression procedure is available, this can be employed instead. (In this latter case, many physicians would want histologic evidence of carcinoma; this can be obtained via laparoscopic, or even closed, liver biopsy or percutaneous thin-needle pancreatic biopsy.) The presence of the liver metastases disqualifies the patient from consideration for an attempt at curative pancreaticoduodenectomy.

2. His prognosis is extremely poor. The five-year survival rate of such patients is less than one percent.

3. The role of the primary physician in this patient's care is critical. He or she can help the patient to decide whether and when any oncologic therapy would be appropriate. The primary physician should coordinate the management of the various medical problems that arise, including the emotional ones, and should also be the one to provide terminal care.

III. 1. The patient should obviously have a biopsy of this suspicious
lesion and an air-contrast barium enema to look for synchronous disease elsewhere. In the absence of metastatic
disease (if this lesion is malignant) or other illness con-
traindicating surgery, she should undergo resection of this
area of the colon.

2. In the absence of lymph node involvement, her prognosis is
quite good.

3. Her follow-up study should consist of repeated examinations
of the stool for occult blood, six-monthly (then annual)
evaluations of the colon (air-contrast barium enema or
colonoscopy), and even periodic CEA determinations. Any
of these tests that become positive will require investigation.

21

RONALD L. KORETZ

Cirrhosis

HOW DO I MAKE THE DIAGNOSIS?

How often in our medical careers have we encountered middle-aged alcoholic patients who have been admitted to the hospital for bleeding esophageal varices and who, on examination, demonstrate jaundice, splenomegaly, ascites, spider angiomata, palmar erythema, and hepatic encephalopathy? Are there any among us who would even hesitate to make the clinical diagnosis of cirrhosis?

Strictly speaking, the term "cirrhosis" is one that should be used only by a pathologist viewing a section of liver. Nonetheless the diagnosis can often legitimately be made on the basis of clinical findings. The word is even familiar to the lay public, to many of whom it is synonymous with excessive alcohol consumption.

The histologic development of cirrhosis usually precedes its

Acknowledgments: The author is grateful to Sally Clement and Dorothy Emley for their endurance in preparing this manuscript.

339

clinical manifestations, as all of the clinical problems represent one or another of the complications of two processes, portal hypertension or hepatocellular failure. These two aspects of cirrhosis are important to differentiate from each other as other disease entities may present with either increased portal pressure (e.g., portal vein thrombosis) or liver cell dysfunction (e.g., hepatitis) alone. The various clinical findings of cirrhosis are so separated in Table 1. Patients with symptomatic cirrhosis will usually have evidence of both processes.

Subclinical cirrhosis (no overt evidence of portal hypertension or hepatocellular failure, but biopsy-established cirrhosis) does exist. Such individuals are rarely seen in day-to-day practice, however, and will not be considered further in this chapter.

WHAT ADDITIONAL WORKUP DOES THE PATIENT REQUIRE?

Cirrhosis, per se, is not a specific disease but rather a consequence of hepatic insult. As such, it is secondary to some other disease process. The causes of cirrhosis are enumerated in Table 2, and some of them are either potentially treatable or of import to patients or their families (e.g., for genetic reasons). Thus, the cause of the cirrhotic process should be found. This may often be established on the basis of history, as in the case of alcoholic liver disease.

Table 1   **Clinical Manifestations of Cirrhosis**

Portal Hypertension	Hepatocellular Failure
Esophageal (and other) varices	Spider angiomata
Caput medusae	Palmar erythema
Hemorrhoids	Gynecomastia
Splenomegaly ± hypersplenism	Absent nail lunulae
Ascites	Testicular atrophy
	Jaundice
	Encephalopathy
	Coagulopathy
	Ascites

Alcohol
Chronic active hepatitis
   Viral induced (hepatitis B; non-A, non-B hepatitis)
   Autoimmune (lupoid)
   "Idiopathic"
Metabolic diseases
   Wilson's disease
   Hemochromatosis
   Cystic fibrosis
   α_1-antitrypsin deficiency
   Galactosemia
   Glycogen storage disease
Drug induced
   Oxyphenisatin
   Methyldopa (Aldomet)
   Isoniazid (INH)
   Nitrofurantoin
   Methotrexate
   Chlorpromazine (Thorazine)
   Vitamin A excess
Secondary biliary cirrhosis
Primary biliary cirrhosis
Schistosomiasis
Obesity and/or jejunoileal bypass
Sarcoidosis
Cardiac (?)
Hydatid disease
"Cryptogenic"

Occasionally patients are seen for whom no readily apparent cause is obvious, and extensive workups may ensue to exclude some of the entities listed in the table. (It is beyond the scope of this chapter to discuss the diagnosis of each of the diseases listed.)

It is important to determine whether or not blood is present in the stool. If it is, then a source should be identified. Patients with cirrhosis have an increased incidence of peptic ulcer disease, and upper gastrointestinal x-rays are often helpful in this regard. It should be kept in mind, however, that, at least in the alcoholic cirrhotic patient, gastritis is a common cause of occult bleeding.

It is reasonable to obtain an initial set of liver tests, including serum transaminase, bilirubin, and alkaline phosphatase. The presence or absence of an inapparent coagulopathy can be determined with a prothrombin time, partial thromboplastin time, and platelet count.

Alcohol-induced disease is associated with multiple nutritional deficiencies. Thus, it is appropriate to investigate for evidence of anemia (possibly from reduced iron or folate stores) as part of the baseline evaluation.

Hyperglycemia is associated with cirrhosis and a blood sugar should be obtained. Electrolyte abnormalities are not uncommon in the cirrhotic patient with ascites, especially if he or she has recently received diuretics. In such patients serum electrolytes should be examined.

It is not necessary specifically to seek evidence for the presence or absence of the other various complications of cirrhosis beyond what is apparent from the history and physical examination. For example, if a patient presents with ascites, one need not prove or disprove that esophageal varices are present via x-ray or endoscopy. Similarly, clinically undetectable ascites is unlikely to be a problem, and need not be sought with other procedures such as ultrasound or paracentesis.

The liver-spleen scan is probably the most overused and unnecessary test employed in the evaluation of the patient with cirrhosis. Its major values are in establishing the presence of a small liver in a patient with ascites (in whom the liver cannot be palpated) and in seeking supportive evidence for the presence of hepatoma when it is strongly suspected. Even in these instances, the test is not highly sensitive or specific. For example, the regenerative nodules of cirrhosis may be interpreted as filling defects if they do not take up as much tracer as the neighboring tissue. Since the history and physical examination usually provide the same information, the scan should not be ordered routinely.

Finally, what is the place of a liver biopsy? By the time the patient becomes symptomatic, the diagnosis is usually not in doubt, and a liver biopsy becomes superfluous. (In fact, there may even be an increased risk due to the coagulopathy that is often associated with this liver disease.) Occasionally patients are seen in whom the presence of cirrhosis is in doubt (e.g., those with suspected portal or splenic vein thrombosis with associated variceal bleeding), and a liver biopsy is an appropriate component of the evaluation. Liver biopsy may also be used in cases in which hepatoma is strongly suspected or when the patient wishes to know if cirrhosis is definitely present. A liver biopsy may be of use in determining the etiology of the cirrhotic process when such information cannot be obtained by less invasive techniques.

HOW SHOULD I TREAT THE PATIENT?

Unfortunately no treatment is currently available to undo the fibrotic process. Hence therapy is directed at managing the complications and, where possible, at treating the cause.

Alcohol is the most common cause of cirrhosis in the United States. Some debate has recently been raised over the value of stopping alcohol ingestion once clinical cirrhosis has appeared. It has been argued that, by the time symptoms appear, liver disease has progressed to such an extent that it becomes the limiting factor for the patient. Any further damage is then inconsequential. No prospective trial has been done randomizing cirrhotic patients into abstaining or further drinking groups, and none is likely to ever be done. Retrospective reviews of the fates of such people who stopped drinking compared to those who did not would seem to indicate that, contrary to the previously mentioned thesis, the abstainers had better survival statistics (Table 3). It would be appropriate, therefore, to continue to employ whatever means are at hand to discourage the alcoholic cirrhotic from consuming any more ethanol.

As noted previously, uncomplicated cirrhosis is not usually a problem for the practitioner. Rather the patient is seen when some dramatic event of liver failure or portal hypertension supervenes (ascites, encephalopathy, or a variceal bleed). These complications will be discussed in the sections to follow.

WHAT SHOULD I EXPECT FROM SUCCESSFUL TREATMENT?

The fibrosis that occurs is irreversible. Successful management of the underlying cause would prevent further progression of the scarring, but the long-term prognosis is directly related to the amount of damage that has occurred.

Table 3 Consequences of Abstinence on Survival in Alcoholic Cirrhotics

Series (Reference)	No. of Patients	Survival	
		Numerical	Life Table (5 year)[a]
Yale (*Am J Med* 44:406–420, 1968)			
Alcohol	185	34 (18%)	41%
No alcohol	93	35 (38%)	63%
VA Proph[b] (*Am J Surg* 165:22–42, 1968)			
Alcohol	49	29 (59%)	NS
No alcohol	23	21 (91%)	NS
BILG Proph[c] (*Ann Intern Med* 70:675–688, 1969)			
Alcohol	38	23 (61%)	NS
No alcohol	43	25 (58%)	NS
Tufts[d] (*Gastroenterology* 74:64–69, 1978)			
Alcohol	76	46 (61%)	NS
No alcohol	68	41 (60%)	NS
Sepulveda Veterans Administration Hospital (S. Borowsky, personal communication)			
Alcohol	25	14 (56%)	NS
No alcohol	24	24 (100%)	NS

[a] NS, not stated in reference.
[b] Veterans Administration cooperative study of prophylactic portocaval shunts.
[c] Boston Interhospital Liver Group study of prophylactic portocaval shunts.
[d] Some of these patients may be from the BILG Proph group.

HOW SHOULD THE PATIENT BE FOLLOWED?

Again there is a wide variability depending on the severity of the illness. This material will be discussed separately for each of the complications.

WHAT COMPLICATIONS OF THE DISEASE CAN OCCUR? HOW SHOULD THEY BE MANAGED?

The three major complications of cirrhosis are ascites, variceal bleeding, and hepatic encephalopathy. The management of each of these will be discussed separately.

ASCITES

Diagnosis

The major consideration in evaluating a patient with ascites is the determination of the etiology. A diagnostic paracentesis should be performed whenever there is either the new appearance of ascites or some change in the clinical picture related to the ascites of a previously stable cirrhotic patient. Examples of this latter situation would include unexplained fever or increased fluid accumulation in the absence of dietary or drug regimen indiscretion. In cirrhosis, the fluid is the result of various hemodynamic forces, and it is usually a transudate, that is, the protein concentration is less than 3 gm/100 cc. It is of note that, in some patients, the protein content is higher than this in uncomplicated cirrhotic ascites, but, under these circumstances, other exudative processes must be considered.

The causes of exudative ascites are listed in Table 4. Although an exudate occurs only occasionally in patients with uncomplicated

Table 4   **Causes of Exudative Ascites**

Common
   Uncomplicated cirrhosis
   Infection (acute bacterial, chronic granulomatous)
   Malignancy
Unusual
   Pancreatic
   Lymphatic
Rare
   Hypothyroidism
   Congestive hepatopathy (especially constrictive pericarditis)

cirrhotic ascites, the relative rarity of the other processes makes cirrhosis a common cause of a high-protein ascitic fluid. On the other hand, acute bacterial infection of preexistent ascites (spontaneous bacterial peritonitis) may be seen in the presence of a low protein level in the fluid. Although a congested liver would be expected to produce a transudate, since only hemodynamic factors are at play, a high-protein fluid is seen at times. This may be due to increased lymphatic pressure (and subsequent protein extrusion) in addition to the venous hypertension, although the exact pathophysiologic processes have not been elucidated.

Therapy

One of the early experiences in medical school that most of us recall easily is the first time we evaluated a patient with cirrhosis and massive ascites. The unsightly appearance of these patients strikes a chord in all of us to do something about the water. However, ascites is not usually a medical emergency and the goal is to establish long-term control rather than rapid, short-term weight loss. In general, weight losses in excess of one to one and a half pounds a day should be avoided. Medical management is the mainstay in treating ascites. As in other water-retaining states, the important principles include sodium restriction and the judicious use of diuretics. One proceeds from the simplest to the most complicated regimens, stopping when a successful program is found.

Before initiating treatment, some prognostic information can be gleaned from an evaluation of the urinary electrolytes. This is summarized in Table 5. Three general patterns can be discerned. In the first, the one that is seen most commonly in the untreated patient, the urinary sodium and potassium are both in the normal range. In this situation the intravascular volume is adequate, but often only at the cost of the patient's consuming excessive amounts of sodium. The sodium load that is not excreted is reflected in the edema and ascites. Sodium restriction in this patient will result in either gradual loss of fluid (if the intravascular state can maintain itself with less sodium priming) or the development of hyperaldosteronism if the kidney "sees" a functional hypovolemia.

The second situation, which is common in the hospitalized patient, demonstrates a relatively pure form of secondary hyperaldosteronism. For reasons that are not entirely clear, the mechanisms that maintain intravascular volume view the ascitic state as "hypo-

Urine Concentration		
Sodium	Potassium	Interpretation
Normal	Normal	Normal electrolyte excretion, which may represent dietary sodium excess (good prognosis with sodium restriction $\pm$ aldosterone blockade)
Low	Normal/high	Hyperaldosteronism (good prognosis with aldosterone blockade)
Low	Low	Proximal tubular extraction of water and electrolytes (poor prognosis)

volemic," and this ultimately results in excessive aldosterone secretion. In this case, the urine sodium is low (less than 10 mEq/liter) and the urine potassium is normal or even high. This reflects an active aldosterone-induced sodium-potassium exchange in the more distal portions of the nephron. Since the urine already contains only small quantities of sodium, further sodium restriction is unlikely to be of benefit when used alone; rather sodium restriction should be employed in conjunction with aldosterone blockade.

The third situation is the most unusual, but is seen in association with the most intractable forms of ascites. In this situation the body is responding as though it were severely volume depleted, and most of the water and electrolytes are extracted in the proximal portion of the nephron, leaving no sodium to exchange for potassium. In such cases, some agent that is active on proximal tubular processes may have to be employed in addition to the measures already cited.

A point should be made concerning sodium flux. The ultimate aim is to have the patient go into a state of negative sodium balance, that is, the amount of sodium excreted is greater than the amount taken in. Water will follow the sodium out. In the situation in which the patient is excreting one liter of urine containing 5 mEq of sodium a day, his or her urinary sodium loss is only 115 mg. Thus, in order to stay even (excluding, for the moment, fecal and insensible loss), the patient's daily dietary intake of salt (sodium chloride) can only be 290 mg. On the other hand, patients who excrete 750 cc of urine that contains 35 mEq of sodium per liter (approximately 27 mEq of sodium per day) will be in negative sodium balance on a diet containing 1 gm of salt per day. (Note again the difference between sodium and salt.) Thus, in addition to baseline urinary sodium and potassium concentrations, it is often useful to periodically check the urinary sodium during therapy (low-sodium diet). A situation in which the urinary sodium is relatively high and the patient is not losing the excess water would suggest that dietary indiscretion is occurring. (In this regard, in an outpatient setting compliance with a salt restriction of less than 2 gm is almost impossible.)

What about water restriction? Although the ascitic fluid does represent water, the fluid is there only as a consequence of the salt. Hence, initial water (volume) restriction is unnecessary. Some patients with ascites will have problems with free water clearance and, on sodium restriction, the serum sodium will fall. Most patients can tolerate mild hyponatremia, but if the value falls below 125 mEq/liter this would indicate a problem. Fluid as well as salt may have to be limited in such patients.

For patients whose disease is alcohol related, abstinence (in or out of the hospital) will eventually allow resolution of the reversible components of their liver disease (e.g., fat accumulation) and spontaneous diuresis may occur, but only after weeks or months.

Diuretics are often required in the management of ascites. Again it is reasonable to begin with the least potent agent and change or add drugs as needed. One reasonable regimen is to begin with spironolactone at 100 mg per day and gradually increase the dose, in 100-mg increments, every four to five days, monitoring urinary sodium. (This presumes the urinary sodium concentration is low after the institution of sodium restriction; if it were high, then the salt restriction alone should have sufficed according to the reasoning discussed in the previous paragraphs.) The dose of spironolactone can be raised until side effects of the drug are encountered. Until the aldosterone effect is overcome, hyperkalemia is not usually a problem (when spironolactone is used alone). However, gynecomastia in men or breast tenderness in women may be limiting factors.

In the event of the failure of spironolactone (e.g., no response to 600 to 800 mg per day) and salt restriction, thiazide diuretics are then added. Again, a low dose is used initially and it is gradually raised. Strict attention to serum electrolytes is important. If thiazides fail, the more potent furosemide can be used. Very few patients fail to respond to this regimen. Those who do not are considered to have "intractable" ascites. (Such patients usually have also required hospitalization at some time to enforce stricter sodium restriction or to ensure compliance with the drug regimen, or both.) If the described sequential regimen is pursued, a significant period of time will have elapsed (consisting of one or two weeks of salt restriction, three or four weeks of spironolactone, and three or four weeks of the more potent diuretics) and reversible components of the liver disease should have resolved. Thus, these few patients who have failed to undergo a diuresis may be considered for more invasive treatment of the ascites.

Uncontrolled trials have claimed success for a variety of techniques. Some authors have observed a spontaneous diuresis after performing paracentesis and removing a liter of fluid. Usually this is not efficacious. In the past the ascitic fluid was reinfused into the patient with the hope that the increase in intravascular volume would promote a diuresis. In those older days, the problem of infection was significant. However, the principle is the one on which the peritoneovenous shunt is based. But more of this later.

Repeated paracentesis could be used to remove fluid. Unfortunately problems of infection and protein loss have resulted in the abandonment of this form of therapy. Albumin infusions may transiently increase urine output, but probably do not provide any long-term benefit. A decade ago side-to-side portocaval shunts were touted for the treatment of intractable ascites. This technique has also fallen from favor in recent years, as such patients usually have a high surgical mortality.

The currently popular treatment for medically refractory ascites is the placement of a subcutaneous catheter with a one-way valve that connects the peritoneal cavity to the internal jugular vein. Transient increases in intraabdominal pressure cause an opening of the valve and the passage of fluid into the venous system. Closure of the valve prevents reversal of flow. These peritoneovenous shunts, often referred to by the name of one of the developers (Leveen), are currently being evaluated in controlled trials, but they are also available commercially. Unfortunately, as is true about everything else in medicine, nothing comes free. Complications have been described, including systemic coagulation defects, sepsis, and variceal bleeding from the increased intravascular volume. It will remain for the controlled trials to determine the exact value of such shunts in the treatment of intractable ascites.

The complications of ascites are listed in Table 6. These occur infrequently and the major problem with ascites is usually cosmetic. (Again, this emphasizes the point that there is usually no urgency to remove the fluid rapidly.)

Occasionally patients are encountered in whom the tense ascites is actually interfering with respiration. The treatment is to remove enough fluid by paracentesis to allow for adequate air exchange.

Bacterial peritonitis is being recognized as an occasional problem in the ascitic patient. The clinical findings may be subtle, consisting of low-grade fever, mild abdominal pain, or encephalopathy. Physical findings may be scant. This diagnosis must always be considered when the patient with ascites complains of, or is observed to have, one of the previously discussed problems. Examination and culture of the ascitic fluid will establish or refute the diagnosis. There is a statistical association between the presence of infection and a peritoneal fluid leukocytosis (> 300 white blood cells/mm^3), especially if the white cells are predominantly polymorphonuclear. If there is a reasonable clinical index of suspicion, such patients should be empirically begun on antibiotics until the culture results are ascertained. The usual infecting organisms are enteric, and broad-spectrum coverage should be employed until the specific agent is identified and antibiotic sensitivities are completed. On the other hand, asymptomatic individuals with only a peritoneal leukocytosis can be observed without treatment.

The hepatorenal syndrome is defined as oliguria and renal failure (rising serum creatinine) in a patient with decompensated cirrhosis (usually at least ascites and jaundice). The etiology of the disorder is unclear, but the kidneys themselves are normal, as they have been transplanted and have functioned satisfactorily in chron-

Table 6 **Complications of Ascites**

Respiratory embarrassment
Spontaneous bacterial peritonitis
Hepatorenal syndrome
Abdominal wall rupture

ically uremic patients. It has been speculated that the liver is failing to metabolize some toxin (or the liver is producing some toxin) that alters the functional hemodynamic state in the kidney. Such a factor (or factors) has not been identified. The kidney behaves as though there is severe intravascular hypovolemia, and therapeutic attempts have been directed at increasing the plasma volume. The mortality from the hepatorenal syndrome is very high, but it should be noted that the actual cause of death is usually not uremia but rather some condition related to the liver disease. Many of the treatment modalities are the same as those noted for intractable ascites, but none has ever been tested in a prospective, randomized controlled trial. (Such a trial for peritoneovenous shunts is under way, however.)

The final complication, abdominal wall rupture, is also dramatic and carries a high mortality. Peritoneal infection may be a consequence, and surgical treatment may be required to seal the leak.

VARICEAL BLEEDING

Diagnosis

Gastrointestinal bleeding is also a common problem in patients with cirrhosis. However, in a large percentage (perhaps the majority), the site of bleeding is not a varix but rather some inflammatory mucosal lesion (e.g., gastritis or peptic ulcer disease). It is a generally held opinion that the site of bleeding should be identified specifically so that treatment can be applied more specifically; thus, such patients are subjected to early endoscopy when they present with upper gastrointestinal bleeding. It should be pointed out that there is no evidence favoring the concept that early diagnosis results in any long-term favorable outcome for the bleeding patient; some trials would, in fact, indicate that the concept is not true.

At times the bleeding varix may be located in the intestinal tract distal to the duodenum, and the clinical presentation is lower gastrointestinal bleeding only. Upper gastrointestinal endoscopy will therefore fail to establish a diagnosis. Occasionally the bleeding may be from hemorrhoidal veins and the diagnosis can be established by sigmoidoscopy. Otherwise angiography may be required to determine the bleeding site. Since the blood loss is usually relatively rapid, colonoscopy, because of its limited ability to clear the intestinal lumen, is not helpful in the acute phase.

The other important diagnostic issue to consider when confronting a patient with variceal bleeding is whether or not the portal hypertension is a consequence of cirrhosis. This issue should be raised in the patient with bleeding varices but no overt evidence of hepatocellular failure, as discussed earlier in the chapter.

Therapy

The initial treatment for bleeding varices is no different from that for any other gastrointestinal bleeding disorder, namely the prompt establishment of a normovolemic state. In this regard it must be remembered that almost any fluid will work, at least temporarily. The hematocrit does not reflect blood volume, but rather what percentage of the volume is occupied by red cells. It is common practice to transfuse a patient up to a certain hematocrit value, but this may be inappropriate and even dangerous both because of the risk of hepatitis and because overexpansion of the intravascular volume may cause the varices to rebleed; rather the patient should have his or her volume restored first. Blood should be employed judiciously. My experience has revealed that most patients can comfortably tolerate hematocrit levels below 25% if they are normovolemic.

After measures are undertaken to correct volume, consideration turns to stopping the bleeding. A variety of modalities has been used in this regard.

Patients with variceal bleeding often have associated coagulopathies related to the underlying liver disease. It has been traditional to provide vitamin K and various clotting factors if the coagulation tests are significantly abnormal. Although this practice is appropriate, coagulation abnormalities are usually only minimally altered by such therapy.

Nasogastric suction is usually a reasonable technique to employ in the management of the cirrhotic patient with upper gastrointestinal bleeding. The removal of the blood from the stomach prevents the presentation of this protein load to the colon, from whence hepatic encephalopathy may ensue. There is no good evidence that such tubes, used for short periods of time (up to a few days), have any direct adverse mechanical effect on the varices.

More complex tubes are available; they have inflatable balloons that can be used to tamponade the gastroesophageal junction. This in turn either directly compresses the bleeding vessel or at least blocks the retrograde portal flow from entering the esophageal venous system. Temporary control of the bleeding can usually be obtained, but only at a significant hazard of a tube complication, such as aspiration, esophageal erosion, or airway obstruction.

Vasopressin infusions have again found their way into regimens for managing bleeding varices. The vasopressin works by reducing mesenteric flow, which in turn reduces portal flow and, consequently, portal venous hypertension. Controlled trials have demonstrated that bleeding can be stopped by this technique. Unfortunately the studies indicate that no improvement in survival occurs even though the bleeding ceases. Intravenous vasopressin is as effective as intra-arterial. The medication is provided as a continuous infusion, and the lowest dose that is associated with the cessation of bleeding is employed. The recommended dosage varies from 0.1 to 1.5 units per minute, but the usual effective dose is 0.3 to 0.6 units per minute.

Techniques have recently been introduced to sclerose esophageal varices in much the same manner that hemorrhoids are injected. This can be accomplished via the endoscope or even by percutaneous transhepatic cannulation of the portal vein with retrograde passage of the catheter into the esophageal veins. The sclerotherapy appears to be effective for at least temporarily clotting the vein, but whether it is efficacious with regard to either the short- or long-term outcome in variceal bleeding remains to be shown.

Most of the time a variceal bleeding episode ceases on its own. If not, emergency portocaval surgical shunts may need to be performed. Under these circumstances, especially in patients with other evidence of hepatic decompensation, a sizable surgical mortality results. In fact, such emergency shunts carry a mortality rate that approaches 100% in patients with jaundice, ascites, and encephalopathy in combination; these individuals are not surgical candidates.

More often the issue of surgery is raised in patients with varices who are not bleeding and whose liver function is reasonably well compensated. There would not appear to be any question that the various surgical procedures decompress the portal circulation and reduce the incidence of bleeding. The question that it is not clear is whether such reductions can be translated to an improved survival in the patient.

The initial trials of portocaval anastomoses were conducted in patients who were known to have esophageal varices, but who had

Table 7 **Prophylactic Shunt Trials**

Study (reference)	Subject	No. of Patients	Mortality[a]	5-Year Survival[b]	Hepatic Failure	Rebleed
Yale 1[c] (*Medicine* 51:27–40, 1972)	Shunt	25	20 (80%)	31%	9 (36%)	1 (4%)
	Control	30	17 (57%)	64%	2 (7%)	6 (20%)
Yale 2[c] (*Medicine* 51:27–40, 1972)	Shunt	19	8 (42%)	50%	5 (26%)	1 (5%)
	Control	22	10 (45%)	50%	1 (5%)	5 (23%)
BILG[d] (*Ann Intern Med* 70:675–688,	Shunt	48	22 (46%)	52%	24 (50%)	1 (2%)
1969)	Control	45	19 (42%)	51%	16 (36%)	12 (27%)
	Shunt	37	19 (51%)	45%	17 (46%)	6 (16%)
VA[e] (*Am J Surg* 115:22, 1968)	Control	58	16 (28%)	64%	14 (24%)	11 (19%)

[a] Total number of deaths occurring after randomization.
[b] Life table analysis of survival statistics.
[c] The numbers after Yale refer to two different studies from the same institution.
[d] Boston Interhospital Liver Group study of prophylactic portocaval shunts.
[e] Veterans Administration cooperative study of prophylactic portocaval shunts.

Table 8 Therapeutic Shunt Trials

Study (reference)	Shunt[a]	No. of Patients	Mortality[b]	5-Year Survival[c]	Hepatic Failure	Rebleed
BILG[d] (Gastroenterology 67:843–851, 1974)	E-S	25	9 (36%)	64%	6 (24%)	1 (4%)
	S-S	21	11 (52%)	48%	7 (33%)	1 (5%)
	Control	25	12 (48%)	48%	2 (8%)	10 (40%)
France[e] (Lancet 1:655–659, 1976)	E-S	40	21 (53%)	47%[f]	8 (20%)	6 (15%)
	Control	49	23 (47%)	56%[f]	0 (0%)	35 (71%)
USC[g] (Arch Surg 108:302–305, 1974)	E-S	37	9 (24%)	60%	7 (19%)	3 (8%)
	Control	38	18 (47%)	10%	2 (5%)	15 (39%)
VA[h] (Ann Surg 174:672–701, 1971)	Shunt	67	30 (45%)	54%	23 (34%)	4 (6%)
	Control	51	32 (63%)	32%	21 (41%)	24 (47%)

[a] E-S, end-to-side portocaval anastomosis; S-S, side-to-side portocaval anastomosis.
[b] Total number of deaths occurring after randomization.
[c] Life table analysis of survival statistics.
[d] Boston Interhospital Liver Group study.
[e] Beaujon Hospital.
[f] Three-year survival.
[g] University of Southern California study.
[h] Veterans Administration cooperative study.

not bled from them. It was believed that "prophylactic" shunts might prolong survival by eliminating bleeding episodes. The data from four prospective randomized studies are displayed in Table 7. In all four studies no difference was seen in overall survival. However, the shunted patients usually died of complications of liver failure, whereas the nonshunted control subjects expired as a consequence of gastrointestinal hemorrhage. Prophylactic shunts have been abandoned.

The second generation of controlled trials evaluated cirrhotic patients who were thought to have bled from varices. It was believed that a "therapeutic" shunt might be of benefit if performed in the subpopulation of patients who had varices that had already bled. The data from the four studies are compiled in Table 8. Again the performance of the shunt reduced the subsequent incidence of bleeding. In three of the four studies, the patients who had the operation had a higher incidence of liver failure. Although the survival statistics appear to favor the operation in three of the four studies, in none of them (including the University of Southern California study) was a statistically significant difference observed. Therapeutic shunts are still being performed on patients at reasonable risk who have suffered from repeated variceal hemorrhages, even though there is a question as to whether survival is prolonged.

Both sets of studies have demonstrated that a shunt procedure reduces the subsequent incidence of hemorrhage. Unfortunately it would appear to be at the cost of hepatic decompensation. It has been believed that this problem is directly related to the shunting of portal blood from the liver and into the systemic circulation. Is there some way to selectively decompress the esophageal and upper gastric varices, which are the most likely to bleed?

The venous outflow from the esophagus and upper stomach is schematically diagrammed in Figure 1. Most of the veins drain directly into the superior mesenteric vein and the portal circulation. However, some of the blood drains through the spleen via the short gastric veins, and thence to the portal vein via the splenic vein. By ligating all of the venous drainage except the short gastric veins, and then by interrupting the splenic vein and allowing the splenic effluent to drain into the renal vein in an antegrade fashion, the gastroesophageal area is selectively decompressed (Fig. 2). This operation has been referred to as the distal splenorenal shunt or the Warren shunt. Note that this is conceptually an entirely different procedure from the standard splenorenal shunt, in which the splenic vein is

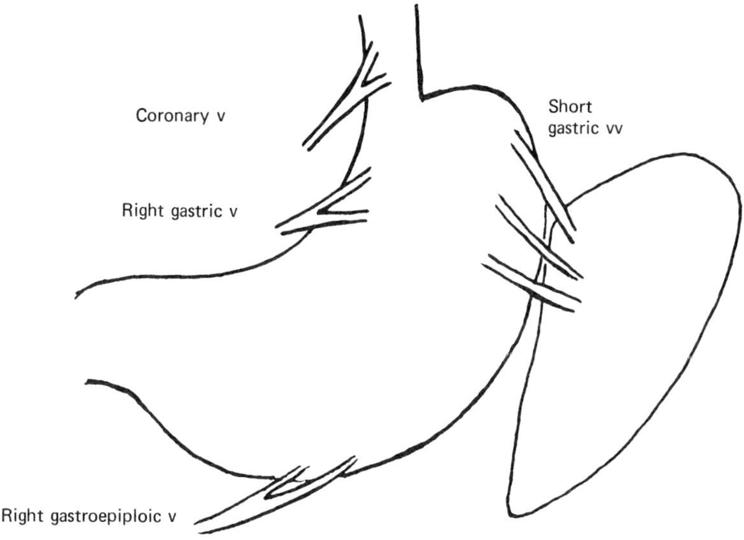

Figure 1 Veins of the lower esophagus and upper stomach drain directly into the portal system (via the coronary, right gastric, and right gastroepiploic veins) and indirectly via the short gastric veins to the spleen, and thence via the splenic vein to the portal vein.

divided and the proximal portion of it (before the anastomosis with the superior mesenteric vein) is connected end to side with the renal vein; the spleen is removed and the entire portal system is decompressed via retrograde flow through the proximal splenic vein.

The effectiveness of the distal splenorenal shunt has never been compared to that of medical therapy. Prospective controlled trials have been conducted comparing outcomes with this shunt and "total" shunts, those in which an attempt is made to decompress the entire portal circulation. These studies are summarized in Table 9. No significant difference in mortality or rebleeding has been observed. In three of the four studies, however, significant differences in the occurrence of hepatic failure, defined as hepatic encephalopathy, were seen. The operation is technically more difficult to perform, and the long-term outcome is not known. Again, although improvement in encephalopathy and bleeding may be expected, no evidence yet indicates any improvement in survival.

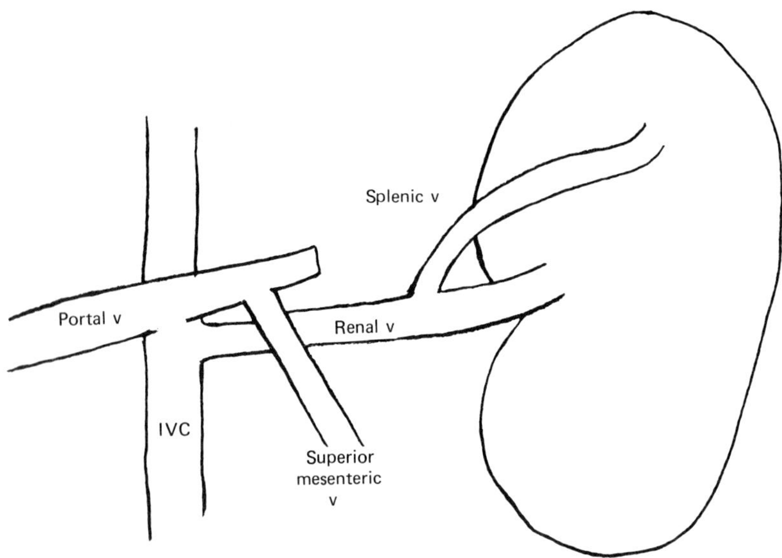

Figure 2 In the distal splenorenal shunt, the direct venous drainage of the lower esophagus and upper stomach is interrupted, and all of the blood traverses the short gastric veins into the spleen. The splenic vein is divided and the splenic effluent is drained into the renal vein. IVC, inferior vena cava.

A further note of caution should be mentioned. All of these studies looked only at one type of cirrhosis, alcoholic. It has been presumed that the data will apply to other types of cirrhosis, but this is not established.

Finally, what about hemorrhoidal bleeding in patients with cirrhosis? Although this is a common problem, very few data exist as to its management. Certainly such bleeding can be massive. However, accumulated individual experiences have indicated that local therapy (hemorrhoidal obliteration or excision) has been associated with subsequent variceal bleeding from higher in the gastrointestinal tract. Some have even proposed performing initial portocaval anastomoses for such hemorrhoidal problems. It should be noted that hemorrhoidal bleeding does not usually produce encephalopathy (as the proteinaceous material is passed directly out of the body) and the area of the gastrointestinal tract is easily available to direct compres-

Table 9 Comparisons of Distal Splenorenal and Total Portosystemic Shunts

Study (reference)	Shunt[a]	No. of Patients	Mortality	Hepatic Failure	Rebleed
Emory[b] (*Ann Surg* 188:271–282, 1978)	DSR	26	10 (38%)	3 (12%)	1 (4%)
	Other	29	8 (28%)	15 (52%)	2 (7%)
Temple[c] (*Am J Surg* 137:13–21, 1979)	DSR	13	4 (31%)	"Less"	NS[d]
	Mesocaval	14	4 (29%)		NS
BYLG[e] (*Gastroenterology* 77:A33, 1979)	DSR	16	4 (25%)	4 (25%)	NS
	Other	21	7 (33%)	3 (14%)	NS
Toronto[f] (*CMA Journal* 118:369–372, 1978)	DSR	22	6 (27%)	1 (5%)	NS
	Other	21	3 (14%)	6 (29%)	NS

[a] DSR, distal splenorenal; other, shunt not specified or several different systemic shunts performed.
[b] Emory University study.
[c] Temple University study.
[d] NS, not stated.
[e] Boston Yale Liver Group.
[f] University of Toronto.

sion. Perhaps this pop-off valve for portal hypertension is the safest one for the cirrhotic patient to use.

ENCEPHALOPATHY

Diagnosis

Hepatic encephalopathy is a syndrome consisting of a constellation of signs observed in a patient with known liver disease (Table 10). Unfortunately most of these signs are nonspecific. Usually the alteration in consciousness consists of somnolence, but other forms of more active bizarre behavior may be seen early in the course. Confusion is commonly observed. Asterixis is seen in other metabolic encephalopathies (uremia, respiratory failure, hypomagnesemia, congestive heart failure). The only specific finding, fetor, is often not detectable or masked and/or confused by a variety of other odors emanating from the patient's oral cavity.

Similarly, no laboratory test specifically identifies hepatic encephalopathy. Classically the blood ammonia level is used, but there is great variation from patient to patient, and some individuals with relatively low levels may be encephalopathic whereas others with even higher values are not. (Blood ammonia levels may be of more help when obtained serially in the same patient to follow the progression of therapy.) Similar problems exist for another touted test, the cerebrospinal fluid glutamine level. EEG evaluation has also not been found to be of much assistance in establishing the diagnosis. Thus, as is true for many other problems in clinical medicine, the diagnosis of hepatic encephalopathy is established at the bedside.

Table 10 **Signs Associated with Hepatic Encephalopathy**

Alteration of consciousness
Asterixis
Hyperreflexia
Fetor hepaticus

Therapy

Hepatic encephalopathy is usually seen as a consequence of some stress to the compromised liver. Thus, the first step in treatment is to identify and correct the precipitating cause(s). A list of the precipitants of hepatic encephalopathy in mnemonic form comprises Table 11. Some of these are situations rarely encountered in clinical practice. The common causes are gastrointestinal bleeding, sepsis, electrolyte and acid/base imbalances (especially as a result of diuretic therapy), dietary protein excess, and surgically created portosystemic shunts.

Before going on to specific steps designed to counter the syndrome, some attention should be paid to its pathogenesis. Encepha-

Table 11 Precipitants of Hepatic Encephalopathy

A: acid/base imbalance

H: hyperglycemia or hypoglycemia
E: electrolyte imbalance
P: protein excess (dietary)
A: anesthesia
R: renal failure

S: sedation
H: hyperalimentation
O: obstipation
U: ureterosigmoidostomy
L: liver disease (acute fulminant hepatitis in particular)
D: diuretics

S: sepsis
O: other coexisting metabolic or organ dysfunctions
P: portosystemic anastomoses

T: transfusion
H: hypovolemia
E: enzyme deficiency (ornithine transcarbamylase)

N: neurologic disease (subdural hematoma)
H_3: hemorrhage (gastrointestinal)

lopathy appears to arise from the failure of the liver to metabolize some toxins produced in the gastrointestinal tract. The detoxification failure may be due to portal blood bypassing the liver entirely (anatomic shunt) or to its flowing past nonfunctioning hepatocytes (functional shunt). The toxin is probably a product of intestinal bacterial action and it may be nitrogenous. Classically this noxious agent was thought to be ammonia. For a variety of reasons, not the least of which is the lack of correlation between blood ammonia levels and encephalopathy from patient to patient, other agents have been considered. These include short-chain fatty acids and various amino acids or their metabolic products.

In recent years a great deal of emphasis has been placed on the role of aromatic amino acids. According to this hypothesis, these amino acids are taken up by the brain and converted to aromatic compounds that function as false neurotransmitters. Although there is some experimental evidence favoring this hypothesis, other models argue against the role of such false transmitters.

Current standard therapy includes removal of nitrogenous material from the intestinal lumen. In the acute stage, this may be accomplished by catharsis. Chronically this manipulation is carried out by placing the patient on a low-protein diet. It appears, in this regard, that not all proteins are created equal. Some early work has indicated that more nonmeat protein can be tolerated than meat protein. As part of the dietary manipulations, emphasis should be placed on milk and vegetable protein sources.

Antibiotics have been available for years and have been used to "sterilize" the bowel. This, in fact, does not occur, but agents such as neomycin may rid the colon of the particular bacteria that produce the noxious agent. Neomycin has the further advantage of being relatively nonabsorbable, so systemic effects and toxicities are held to a minimum. Nonetheless when it is used on a chronic basis (4–8 gm per day), nephrotoxicity and ototoxicity are seen.

A more recent development has been the availability of lactulose. This is a synthetic disaccharide that cannot be absorbed by the human. In the colon, however, it is metabolized by the bacterial flora to organic acids. The reduction in pH appears to have some beneficial effect on the encephalopathy although the exact reason for this is not clear. Lactulose is used in doses of 60 to 160 gm per day. Its chief side effect is an osmotic diarrhea that is dose dependent. Lactulose is about as effective as neomycin.

Several drugs that presumably act at the level of the brain have been proposed as therapeutic agents. L-dopa has been used in uncontrolled trials in an attempt to overcome the proposed false neurotransmitter, but no controlled trial has yet been done. Special solutions containing high concentrations of branched-chain amino acids and low concentrations of aromatic ones are currently being tested. It is hoped that these will alter the peripheral blood amino acid levels such that fewer aromatic compounds will be available for uptake in the central nervous system. Bromocriptine, a dopamine receptor agonist, has also been proposed, but there is scant clinical information available regarding its efficacy.

Arginine infusions have been used in an attempt to stimulate the production of urea from ammonia. One controlled trial at USC using a two-hour infusion of arginine failed to demonstrate efficacy (*Am J Med* 25:359–367, 1958) and this therapy has been abandoned. Recently encephalopathy has been reported in hyperalimentation using amino acid formulations. These formulae had low concentrations of arginine and a state of arginine deficiency was presumably created. Under this circumstance arginine infusion appeared to be beneficial in reversing the clinical abnormalities.

Analogues of amino acid missing the amine portion (α-keto-analogues) have been proposed for use. These compounds would be available as substrates to which ammonia could be bound. In fact, the most recent attempt at designing an antiencephalopathy drug has been to produce the α-keto-analogue linked to arginine. It remains to be seen whether this compound is efficacious.

Hemodialysis has been employed but, even though the blood ammonia level may be lowered, no long-term benefit has seemed to occur. Currently much work is being expended on different dialysis membranes (which will allow the filtration of larger molecules) and absorbent compounds, but we remain a long way from an artificial liver.

SELECTED READING

Bar-Meir S, Lerner E, Conn HO: Analysis of ascitic fluid in cirrhosis. *Dig Dis Sci* 24:136–144, 1979.

Conn HO: Portal hypertension and its consequences, in Gitnick GL (ed): *Current Gastroenterology and Hepatology*. Boston, Houghton Mifflin Professional Publishers, 1979, pp 338–402.

Conn HO, Ramsby GR, Storer EH, et al: Intraarterial vasopressin in the treatment of upper gastrointestinal hemorrhage: a prospective, controlled clinical trial. *Gastroenterology* 68:211–221, 1975.

Gregory PB, Broekelschen PH, Hill MD, et al: Complications of diuresis in the alcoholic patient with ascites: a controlled trial. *Gastroenterology* 73:534–538, 1977.

Greig PD, Langer B, Blendis LM, et al: Complications after peritoneovenous shunting for ascites. *Am J Surg* 139:125–131, 1980.

Hoyumpa AM, Desmond PV, Avant GR, et al: Hepatic encephalopathy. *Gastroenterology* 76:184–195, 1979.

Kline MM, McCallum RW, Guth PH: The clinical value of ascitic fluid culture and leucocyte count studies in alcoholic cirrhosis. *Gastroenterology* 70:408–412, 1976.

CLINICAL PROBLEMS

I. A 52-year-old alcoholic is evaluated for abdominal swelling of three-weeks' duration. During this period the patient has also noted that his skin and urine have become darker and fluid has accumulated in his legs. He has gained 20 pounds despite no increase in his appetite. The physical examination reveals icterus, spider telangiectasias on his chest and back, palmar erythema, testicular atrophy, gynecomastia, and peripheral edema. A distended, tense abdomen is observed; spleen and liver are both ballottable. Shifting dullness is easily demonstrated.

Preliminary laboratory data reveal a total bilirubin of 14 mg%, a serum albumin of 2.3 gm%, and a prothrombin time of 17 seconds. Serum electrolytes show a sodium of 130 mEq/liter and a potassium of 3.8 mEq/liter. Urine sodium is 47 mEq/liter and urine potassium is 42 mEq/liter.

1. How can the ascites be diagnosed?
2. How can it be managed?
3. What complications may ensue?

II. A 58-year-old man is brought to the physician's office by his wife for changes in his behavior over the past four months. The problem reached a crisis point the previous day when he was arrested after driving up a freeway off-ramp. He was initially thought to be drunk but a subsequent blood alcohol was 0. The wife insists that her husband never drinks. Further medical history is unremarkable except for a history of posttransfusion hepatitis 20 years earlier. (This transfusion was administered for injuries sustained in an automobile accident.)

Physical examination reveals an elderly man who responds to questions slowly and whose memory is clearly impaired. A few spider telangiectasias and palmar erythema are present. There is no evidence of ascites, but a caput medusae is apparent on the abdominal wall. The liver cannot be palpated and can only be percussed as 4 cm in span. Splenomegaly is detected. Neurologic examination reveals hyperreflexia and asterixis. Examination of the patient's breath is hampered by garlic, which the patient habitually consumes.

Laboratory data demonstrate a prolonged prothrombin time, a low serum albumin, a positive hepatitis B surface antigen, and slightly elevated aminotransferases.

1. What liver disease is present?
2. How should the neurologic problem be evaluated?
3. How should this neurologic problem be managed?

III. A 38-year-old alcoholic is admitted for upper gastrointestinal bleeding. The patient drank heavily for 15 years until acute pancreatitis developed six months earlier. He subsequently "reduced" his alcohol intake to three to four beers per day. On the day of admission he began vomiting large quantities of blood and came to the emergency room.

Physical examination reveals a well-developed man who is anicteric. He has postural hypotension. There is no evidence of palmar erythema, gynecomastia, spider telangiectasias, or testicular atrophy. A caput medusae is present. There is no apparent ascites or encephalopathy. The liver and spleen are both slightly enlarged.

The initial laboratory evaluation demonstrates a hematocrit of 26%. The serum bilirubin, aminotransferases, albumin, and prothrombin time are all normal. Emergency endoscopy reveals actively bleeding esophageal varices.

1. What underlying liver disease is present?
2. How can it be diagnosed?
3. How should the bleeding varices be managed?

Discussion

I. 1. The diagnosis is established on the basis of the physical
examination. Although its presence can be inferred from
various radiologic procedures, this is not necessary. A diagnostic paracentesis would be appropriate to exclude other
causes of ascites besides the apparent cirrhosis.

2. Once other causes for ascites have been excluded, management should progress along the lines described in this chapter. Sodium restriction and bed rest alone can be introduced.
If the urine sodium stays at the pretreatment level, fluid may
mobilize and diuresis may occur without other therapeutic
manipulation. If the urine sodium falls, spironolactone in
increasing doses is added. If this is also unsuccessful,
stronger diuretics will be necessary. Unless the serum sodium
falls, no water restriction is needed. Almost all patients will
respond to this regimen.

3. The major complications are fluid and electrolyte imbalance
from the diuretics. Less commonly one of the primary complications of ascites (respiratory embarrassment, spontaneous
bacterial peritonitis, hepatorenal syndrome, or abdominal
wall rupture) may occur.

II. 1. The physical findings indicate both hepatocellular failure
and portal hypertension. These findings plus a small liver indicate severe cirrhosis. The etiology of the process is not
established, but the other laboratory data and the history of
hepatitis point to a slowly progressive, viral chronic active
hepatitis.

2. Although it would be appropriate to undertake a screening
neurologic evaluation (e.g., CAT scan) to rule out primary
intracranial lesions, the patient is presenting with a complication of his (previously asymptomatic) cirrhosis, hepatic
encephalopathy. The presence of the described findings (confusion, asterixis, and hyperreflexia) in the setting of cirrhosis
should establish the diagnosis.

3. The initial step in management is to exclude the various exogenous causes of encephalopathy enumerated in Table 11. If they are found, they should be treated. If the only apparent cause is progression of the cirrhosis per se, a protein-restricted diet (emphasizing nonmeat sources of protein) as well as neomycin or lactulose should be instituted.

III. 1. There is clinical evidence of portal hypertension but not of hepatocellular failure. The slightly enlarged liver may be due to fat accumulation. Although the cause of the portal hypertension may be cirrhosis, one must also consider the possibility of a portal vein occlusion (possibly the result of the previous pancreatitis).

2. Although cirrhosis could be diagnosed by a liver biopsy, the presence of a portal vein thrombosis could not be excluded. If there is a strong suspicion that this venous occlusion is present, its presence or absence can only be determined by angiography.

3. Before undertaking this evaluation, efforts should be directed toward restoring blood volume and stopping the bleeding. Intravenous fluids are begun. Since there is no coagulopathy, clotting factors are not necessary. If the bleeding does not cease spontaneously, vasopressin infusions can be attempted. If this fails, balloon tamponade can be tried. If surgery is needed, emergency angiography should be obtained. This is necessary to define the portal anatomy, since a standard portocaval shunt may not be possible if portal vein thrombosis is present.

NEIL KAPLOWITZ

Alcohol and Drug-Related Liver Disease

DRUG-INDUCED LIVER DISEASE

Whenever physicians are confronted with a patient who has suspected hepatobiliary disease, whether jaundice is present or not, they should consider the possibility of a drug etiology. Drugs and alcohol seem to cause liver disease selectively because the liver is the principal site of metabolism and biodegradation of these foreign compounds. Noxious intermediate metabolites often play a key role in mediating toxicity either by killing the hepatocyte, attacking a specific subcellular organelle or function (e.g., bile secretion) while sparing the rest of the cell, or by eliciting an immune response directed at the drug-liver complex. Drug effects can mimic any form of acute or chronic liver disease. Therefore, one should always take a careful history of such exposures and withdraw potential etiologic agents immediately.

Acknowledgment: I wish to thank Nick Onstott for his superb administrative assistance.

Table 1   Clinical Approach to Drug-Induced Liver Disease

Features Demonstrated	Trans-aminase	Alkaline Phosphatase	Clinically Resembles	Example
Hepatitis	↑↑	±	Viral hepatitis (including fulminant	Halothane Isoniazid Alpha-methyldopa Acetaminophen
Cholestatic	±	↑↑	Obstructive jaundice	Phenothiazines Erythromycin estolate Estrogens Androgens
Mixed	↑	↑	Atypical viral hepatitis or granulomatous disease	Para-aminosalicylic acid (PAS) Sulfonamides Diphenylhydantoin (Dilantin) Allopurinol Phenylbutazone Quinidine

↑↑ = markedly increased
↑ = mild to moderately increased
± = borderline increased

Classification

The approach that is most useful on a practical clinical level is the consideration of the clinical-biochemical pattern of injury (Table 1). This approach is of universal value in approaching hepatobiliary disease; that is, does the patient exhibit features of acute hepatitis resembling viral hepatitis, features of cholestasis resembling obstructive jaundice, or mixed or indeterminate features? The great value of this clinical classification rests on the consistency with which specific drugs are associated with specific patterns of injury.

The acute hepatitis presentation is usually indistinguishable clinically, biochemically, and even histopathologically from viral disease. There may be a typical prodromal period preceding jaundice and the serum transaminases usually are markedly elevated (> five to 10 times) with minimal increase in serum alkaline phosphatase and variable jaundice. This form of drug-related injury may produce life-threatening fulminant disease. The onset of symptoms follows within several days to several weeks after the patient starts the medication but may even be delayed for several months. This pattern is typical of the syndrome associated with halothane, alpha-methyldopa, isoniazid, or acetaminophen overdose, and, in milder form, salicylates (the latter is anicteric).

The cholestatic pattern may be associated with jaundice, pruritus, fever, and abdominal pain, and it closely resembles biliary tract disease. Biochemically, the alkaline phosphatase is disproportionately increased (> four times) with minimal transaminase increases. This pattern is produced by phenothiazines, erythromycin estolate, oral contraceptives, and certain androgens. The key issue in this case is to avoid unnecessary biliary surgical exploration and to recognize the drug association.

Mixed patterns of injury are often associated with moderate elevation of serum transaminases and alkaline phosphatase, producing the type of pattern frequently seen with infectious mononucleosis and granulomatous infiltration. Numerous drugs produce this picture; para-aminosalicylic acid, sulfonamides, diphenylhydantoin, allopurinol, phenylbutazone, and quinidine are a few of them.

Another way to view hepatotoxins is either as predictable or unpredictable. Predictable toxins are intrinsically toxic drugs or drug metabolites that produce injury in a dose-related fashion in a high proportion of patients. Host factors are of less importance than the inherent toxicity of the drug. Acetaminophen overdose, carbon tetrachloride hepatitis, or oral contraceptive cholestasis are examples.

Unpredictable hepatotoxins produce clinically apparent injury in less than 1% of patients exposed, seem unrelated to dose, and most often seem to resemble a hypersensitivity reaction. The evidence of hypersensitivity is circumstantial but compelling. Thus, eosinophilia, rash, a fixed one- to three-week latent period, and rapid response to rechallenge favor an immune-mediated mechanism. In this case the host response appears to be the critical determinant of hepatotoxicity rather than the inherent toxicity of the drug. This type of injury is exemplified by methyldopa (Aldomet) hepatitis and phenothiazine cholestasis.

How Do I Make the Diagnosis?

The diagnosis of drug-induced liver disease is based on the circumstantial ingestion of a drug and the expected clinical manifestations (Table 2). Therefore, it is mandatory that the physician always have a high index of suspicion and carefully question the patient about drugs. This often requires questioning and then rephrasing the question since patients often forget their medications or do not consider over-the-counter pharmaceuticals as medication. Therefore, in the cholestatic setting I may ask the patient specifically about phenothiazines and antibiotics. In the hepatitis setting, I may ask about Aldomet, isoniazid, and acetaminophen. A sufficient drug history is not obtained from a negative response to the simple question, "Do you take medications?"

If the patient is taking a potential offending drug, its use should be stopped immediately. There is a major rule in this situation: continued liver injury depends on continued drug use, or, conversely, stopping the drug will result in rapid improvement. Since many hepatic drug reactions are allergic in nature, the finding of rash, eosinophilia, or the characteristic one- to three-week sensitization interval is useful.

Finally, in the case of drug allergy, rechallenge with the drug will usually result in a rapid recurrence of symptoms and biochemical abnormalities. However, the latter maneuver should be reserved for cases in which the drug is absolutely essential and no replacement will suffice. Rechallenge is dangerous and rarely justified and it should never be attempted without informed consent. Consequently, drug-induced liver disease is usually diagnosed on clinical grounds without definitive proof. In many cases, however, the etiologic relationship is obvious, such as in the setting of acetaminophen overdose or intrahepatic cholestasis two weeks after starting erythromycin estolate, among others. In other circumstances, the association is not so obvious but should always be given the benefit of the doubt.

Table 2 **Diagnosis of Drug-Induced Liver Disease**

1. Have a high index of suspicion
2. Take a careful drug history
3. Stop the drug immediately
4. Assess clinical response to stopping drug
5. Search for signs of allergy
6. ? ? Rechallenge

Liver biopsy has very little role in the diagnosis of acute hepatic drug reactions since it tends to show either typical hepatitis or cholestasis. Certain intrinsic toxins such as acetaminophen and carbon tetrachloride produce a characteristic centrizonal coagulative necrosis without inflammation that is histologically distinct from viral hepatitis. However, the effect of most toxins, such as isoniazid, Aldomet, halothane, and others, cannot be distinguished from viral disease. Besides, since withdrawal of the drug leads to the rapid disappearance of liver disease, biopsy is rarely indicated.

Special Considerations

Acetaminophen Hepatotoxicity

Overdose of acetaminophen has been the most common form of suicide in Great Britain during the past decade. Recently, it has been increasing in the United States and all physicians need to be aware of this drug's effects. After ingesting 10 to 20 gm of acetaminophen, patients develop gastrointestinal upset and obtundation, which last for several hours, followed by an asymptomatic interval of one to two days. This is followed by acute hepatitis, which may be fulminant and cause death in several days. When a patient is seen in the emergency room during the first 12 hours, a blood level should be drawn and gastric lavage performed. If the blood level is greater than 150 to 200 μg/ml at four hours or 50 μg/ml at 12 hours, there is a significant risk of severe hepatitis. If the patient is seen within 24 hours of the ingestion, immediate therapy with N-acetylcysteine (Mucomyst, 20%) should be instituted by mouth or nasogastric tube. The initial dose is 140 mg/kg, followed every four hours by 70 mg/kg for three days. This agent is highly effective in preventing acetaminophen metabolites from attacking the liver.

Drug-Induced Chronic Liver Disease

Chronic active hepatitis leading to cirrhosis may occur as a result of continued administration of a drug to which the individual is sensitized (Table 3). Well-documented examples are Aldomet, isoniazid, nitrofurantoin, and dantrolene. Rare cases have been attributed to acetaminophen, aspirin, and halothane. It should be noted that all of these drugs produce hepatitis in a small proportion of users and clinically this is usually acute hepatitis. Fulminant

Histologic Type	Drug
Chronic active hepatitis	Oxyphenisatin
	Alpha-methyldopa
	Isoniazid
	Nitrofurantoin
	Dantrolene
Alcoholic-like hepatitis	Perhexilene
Alcoholic-like cirrhosis	Methotrexate
Biliary cirrhosis	Chlorpromazine
Budd-Chiari syndrome	Estrogens
	Alkaloids
Hepatic adenoma	Estrogens
Hepatocellular carcinoma	Androgens

hepatitis or chronic liver disease is more likely to develop in those patients who continue the drug because of lack of recognition of its association with the liver injury. If given long enough under this circumstance, progressive fibrosis and even cirrhosis can occur. However, when the drug is stopped, regardless of the stage, the activity (necrosis) rapidly disappears and transaminases return to normal. Steroid therapy is not needed.

Recently, a coronary vasodilator used extensively in Europe, perhexilene, has been associated with a chronic liver disease with features of alcoholic hepatitis. This observation raises the possibility of this type of reaction occurring with other drugs.

Dose-related hepatic fibrosis culminating in cirrhosis, but without significant ongoing liver necrosis, has been described in association with methotrexate. This drug appears to directly stimulate specialized sinusoidal lipocytes, called Ito cells, to produce collagen. The pattern of cirrhosis and fibrosis resembles that seen in the alcoholic, but there is no hyaline necrosis.

Biliary cirrhosis can occur in a small proportion of patients in whom an acute "allergic" cholestatic liver disease secondary to chlorpromazine develops. This intrahepatic cholestasis and biliary fibrosis can progress over a prolonged period of time after discontinuation of the drug. This situation is the only well-documented example of self-perpetuating liver disease initiated by a drug. The liver disease resembles primary biliary cirrhosis but the antimitochondrial antibody is not present.

Estrogens are of interest in producing several forms of chronic liver disease in addition to benign intrahepatic canalicular cholestasis: Budd-Chiari syndrome (hepatic vein thrombosis due to the hypercoagulopathy) and hepatic adenoma. The latter rarely undergoes malignant transformation but is clinically important because of symptoms and danger of rupture. Androgen therapy has been associated with the development of well-differentiated, hormone-sensitive, hepatocellular carcinoma (hepatoma), which may regress when therapy is stopped. Peliosis hepatitis is another rare, sometimes fatal, complication of these agents. This is a replacement of liver parenchyma by blood-filled cysts.

ALCOHOL AND THE LIVER

Alcohol is probably the most important cause of chronic liver disease in the United States. Alcohol should be viewed as a hepatotoxin; nutritional deficiency is no longer considered a key aspect in the pathophysiology of this liver disease. The dose and duration of alcohol consumption necessary to produce cirrhosis are not well defined. A minimum average figure is about one-half to one pint of whiskey per day for 15 to 20 years. There is some suggestion that women are more susceptible than men to the adverse effects of alcohol, since they develop alcoholic hepatitis and cirrhosis with a lower dose and shorter duration of drinking. Not everyone who drinks develops cirrhosis; in fact, probably fewer than one-half of heavy chronic alcohol abusers do so. The explanation for the susceptibility of some is uncertain. The dose of alcohol itself rather than the type of alcoholic beverage consumed (i.e., beer, wine, whiskey, etc.), determines whether the patient is at increased risk of developing liver disease.

Stages of Alcoholic Liver Disease

Fatty Liver

Alcoholic liver disease may be divided into three stages: fatty liver, alcoholic hepatitis, and cirrhosis (Fig. 1). Fat accumulation

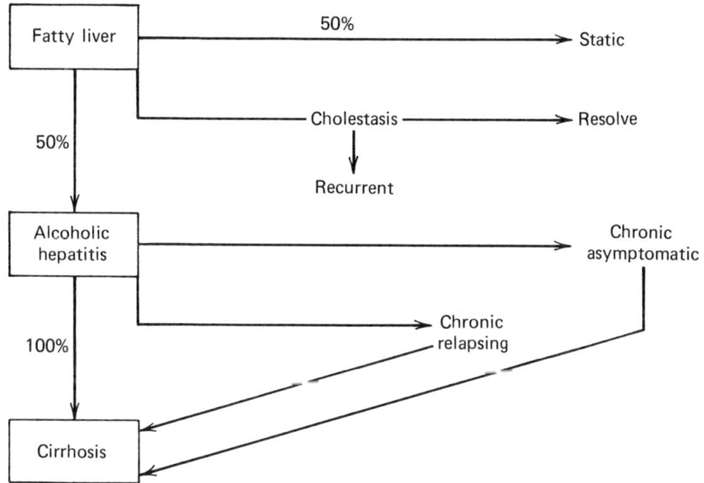

Figure 1 Natural history of liver disease in chronic alcoholics who do not abstain.

in the liver occurs very rapidly (in just a few days) in drinkers and usually persists in active alcoholics. The fatty liver represents a net result of the effects of alcohol on fat metabolism. There is no evidence that fat is bad for the liver or that it causes progressive liver disease in and of itself. Furthermore, there are a host of causes of fatty liver unrelated to alcohol that are not associated with progressive liver failure.

Fatty liver is usually asymptomatic and patients just have an enlarged liver. Liver function tests are normal or there may be a slight increase in the SGOT. Rarely, patients with fatty liver may have a cholestatic disease with jaundice, pruritus, and markedly increased alkaline phosphatase. Both the fatty liver and this cholestasis improve rapidly with abstinence. In contrast, the other forms of alcoholic liver disease do not improve rapidly.

Alcoholic Hepatitis

Clinical Spectrum Alcoholic hepatitis may be viewed on a histologic basis as liver necrosis, usually with alcoholic hyaline and polymorphonuclear leukocytes and associated fibrosis in the centrilobular region of the liver lobule. However, this histologic lesion is associated with a broad clinical spectrum, enumerated in **Table 4.** Alcoholic hepatitis with scarring accounts for the progression to cirrhosis. Once alcoholic hepatitis develops continued drinking will always lead to cirrhosis. Alcoholic hepatitis rarely presents before five to 10 years of heavy alcohol consumption, usually is associated with considerable fibrosis, and persists indefinitely in active drinkers while disappearing very slowly over months in abstainers. These features of chronicity lead one to conclude that alcoholic hepatitis is a chronic inflammatory condition that may or may not have associated clinical exacerbations.

On one end of the clinical spectrum of alcoholic hepatitis is the asymptomatic patient who clinically may have disease that resembles fatty liver and has hepatomegaly and mild SGOT elevation. This pattern of low-grade, smoldering hepatitis in an alcoholic probably accounts for the not infrequently seen cirrhotic who has never had clinically overt alcoholic hepatitis.

The most common or "garden-variety" form of alcoholic hepatitis presents with jaundice, tender hepatomegaly, fever, and leukocytosis. Although a cholestatic biochemical picture may be seen (and will be discussed later), usually a hepatocellular pattern is appreciated. These patients usually have no or minimal clotting disturbances and lack encephalopathy. They have a good short-term prognosis with a very low mortality during any index hospitalization.

On the severe end of the spectrum is a presentation of alcoholic hepatitis referred to by some as sclerosing hyaline necrosis. These patients have rapid onset, severe encephalopathy, and clotting disturbances, all superimposed on the typical features. The mortality

Table 4   Presentations of Alcoholic Liver Disease

Hepatocellular (alcoholic hepatitis)
    Asymptomatic (anicteric, hepatomegaly, $\uparrow$ SGOT)
      "Garden variety" alcoholic hepatitis (fever, jaundice, leukocytosis)
                    $< 5\%$ MORTALITY
    Sclerosing hyaline necrosis (ascites, jaundice, abnormal prothrombin time, encephalopathy)
                    $> 50\%$ MORTALITY
Cholestatic (jaundice, $\uparrow$ alkaline phosphatase, $\uparrow$ cholesterol, pruritus, fatty liver)
Combination

of this group during a hospitalization is nearly 50% (80% with spontaneous encephalopathy). The pathology is one of marked necrosis and fibrosis in the liver lobule.

Patients with alcoholic hepatitis may or may not be jaundiced. The prothrombin time is a reasonable prognostic test in that marked abnormality is associated with a higher mortality. The serum transaminases remain a uniquely valuable test in the alcoholic. Despite marked liver destruction, they are almost never more than mildly elevated. The SGOT is usually two to five times normal, rarely more. The SGPT is especially helpful in that it is usually within normal limits. Rarely, it may be increased, but always less than two-fold. Therefore, a moderate elevation of SGOT with a normal SGPT in a patient with obvious liver disease (such as with jaundice, ascites, clotting disturbances, etc.) points very strongly to alcoholic hepatitis. Empirically, this characteristic is the strongest reason to perform transaminase determinations in the setting of hepatobiliary disease, and it seems the only legitimate circumstance in which the relationship of SGOT to SGPT is of value.

Some patients with alcoholic hepatitis will have a cholestatic picture. Cholestasis may be from intrahepatic or extrahepatic causes (Table 5). Inadvertently operating on a patient with intrahepatic cholestasis for suspected biliary tract disease is associated with a very high anesthetic mortality (approximately 50%). On the other hand, chronic relapsing pancreatitis, another complication of alcoholism, can also lead to cholestasis. The common bile duct is anatomically adjacent to or embedded in the head of the pancreas. Thus, edema or scarring in the pancreas can extrinsically compress the common bile duct. In exacerbations of pancreatitis, this may produce transient obstructive jaundice. In addition, chronic stricturing of the common bile duct occurs in about 10% of patients with chronic pancreatitis. These patients usually have marked eleva-

Table 5 **Cholestasis in the Alcoholic**

Intrahepatic cholestasis—? toxic effect of alcohol

Extrahepatic obstruction
    Gallstone (one-third of cirrhotics have gallstones)
    Pancreatitis (transient or persistent common bile duct stenosis)
    Hepatoma invading biliary tree (rare)

Dilemma: fever, jaundice, leukocytosis, right upper quadrant pain
Clues to correct diagnosis: massive tender hepatomegaly
        ascites
        SGOT/SGPT, abnormal prothrombin time
Differential diagnosis: Acute viral hepatitis—serum transaminases
        HB_sAg
        Acute cholecystitis—localized tenderness
        mild jaundice
        + HIDA or PIPIDA scan
        Choledocholithiasis
        cholangiography
        Alcoholic pancreatitis
Difficult cases: liver biopsy or cholangiography

tion of serum alkaline phosphatase, and jaundice, cholangitis, or even secondary biliary cirrhosis may develop.

Cholestasis in the alcoholic often presents a real diagnostic dilemma, since the patient has jaundice, fever, leukocytosis, abdominal pain, and a variable cholestatic profile (Table 6). Aside from a history of high alcohol intake, the clues that the process is intrahepatic are the presence of massive tender hepatomegaly, ascites, an abnormal prothrombin time that does not correct with vitamin K, and the characteristic SGOT/SGPT ratio. However, the differential diagnosis is extensive, including: (1) acute viral hepatitis, which can be distinguished by a striking elevation in SGOT and SGPT and appropriate viral serology; (2) acute cholecystitis, which is characterized by localized right upper quadrant tenderness, very mild icterus, and cholescintigraphy showing no filling of the gallbladder; (3) choledocholithiasis, which is usually marked by biliary colic and cholangitis; and (4) alcoholic pancreatitis with common duct stenosis, which has already been discussed.

Cholestasis in the alcoholic should be approached in a similar fashion to that in the nonalcoholic. However, even if biliary obstruction is proved in the alcoholic by cholangiography we generally perform a liver biopsy. The purpose of the biopsy is to evaluate the liver complications of alcoholism, which help us to decide the operative risk. In other words, an alcoholic with cholangitis from calculus or pancreatitis obstructing the bile duct who also has alcoholic hepatitis will probably be treated conservatively and nonoperatively with antibiotics unless sepsis is uncontrollable. Resolution of active alcoholic hepatitis will markedly improve the operative risk.

Course   As noted previously patients with clinically overt alcoholic hepatitis tend to have a slow recovery clinically and a variable but significant short-term mortality. The subsequent course of survivors is determined predominantly by whether or not they continue to drink. Those who abstain will revert to histologically inactive, healed disease and possibly even to normal. Those who continue to drink will have subclinical alcoholic hepatitis, often punctuated by clinically overt exacerbations, and cirrhosis will develop within a few years on the average. Once cirrhosis has become fully developed, the alcoholic's drinking habits continue to play a key role in dictating the course. Abstinence will result in the slow reversion to inactive cirrhosis, whereas continued drinking will produce the superimposition of the spectrum of alcoholic hepatitis leading to a progressive downhill course. Since complications of cirrhosis in the alcoholic are covered elsewhere, brief consideration needs to be presented at this juncture. There are two major classes of complications: those related to hepatocellular failure and those related to the hemodynamic consequences of portal hypertension. The important point is that alcoholic liver disease tends to be associated with both types of complications concurrently. In addition, another serious complication is hepatocellular carcinoma, a complication of all forms of cirrhosis. This complication ultimately develops in roughly 5% to 10% of alcoholic cirrhotics, with greater likelihood in reformed drinkers who have quiescent cirrhosis. (For a discussion of cirrhosis, please see the previous chapter.)

Liver Biopsy in the Alcoholic

As noted previously, I perform a liver biopsy whenever contemplating operation in an alcoholic so as to gain insight into the severity of acute and chronic liver disease and the risk of surgery. However, if the biopsy is contraindicated by coagulation abnormalities or ascites, one can assume the liver disease is very serious. The decision regarding surgery in the face of significant liver disease is very difficult and must be individualized; unfortunately such a decision may be absolutely unavoidable.

Liver biopsy outside of this setting is less clearly indicated. I believe that any form of chronic liver disease should be assessed histologically as standard practice in order to exclude unexpected and potentially treatable conditions. Thus, biopsy of an alcoholic will, to one's surprise, occasionally reveal features of large-duct obstruction, granuloma, or chronic active hepatitis instead of alcoholic liver disease.

The histologic features that one calls alcoholic hepatitis are typical but not pathognomonic of an alcohol etiology. Thus, similar pathology has been described in nonalcoholic, obese, middle-aged female diabetics; in postjejunoileal bypass liver disease; and in association with certain drugs. However, the typical lesion in the alcoholic should be viewed as compelling evidence for alcoholic liver disease. It would be premature, however, to label patients who deny alcohol but have a suggestive lesion as alcoholics.

Treatment of Alcoholic Liver Disease

The therapy for alcoholic liver disease can be either short-term or long-term. Short-term therapy for alcoholic hepatitis is directed at withdrawal from alcohol, good nutrition, vitamins, and patience. It remains controversial as to whether steroids or propylthiouracil affect short-term survival. Probably, for the time being, neither should be used.

Long-term therapy is directed at psychosocial rehabilitation leading to abstinence. Stopping alcohol improves survival dramatically compared to continued imbibing. This is true even when cirrhosis is present and the patient has ascites, jaundice, or clotting disturbances. Because of the serious nature of bleeding from esophageal varices, it is more controversial if abstention helps survival in that setting. The reason why cirrhotics who abstain have improved survival is that cirrhosis is not an end-all. Continued drinking produces continued alcoholic hepatitis, which progressively worsens the cirrhosis and increases the likelihood of complications.

SELECTED READING

Lieber C: Pathogenesis and early diagnosis of alcoholic liver injury. *N Engl J Med* 298:888–893, 1978.

Maddrey WC, Boitnott JK: Drug-induced chronic liver disease. *Gastro-enterology* 72:1348–1353, 1977.

Mitchell JR, Tollows DJ: Metabolic activation of drugs to toxic substances. *Gastroenterology* 68:392–410, 1975.

Mitchell JR, Zimmerman HJ, Ishak KG, et al: Isoniazid liver injury: clinical spectrum, pathology, and probable pathogenesis. *Ann Intern Med* 84:181–192, 1976.

Prescott LF, Ballantyne A, Park J, et al: Treatment of paracetamol (acetaminophen) poisoning with N-acetylcysteine. *Lancet* 2:432–434, 1977.

Zimmerman HJ: Liver injury induced by chemicals and drugs, in Bockus HL: *Gastroenterology,* vol 3, ed 3. Philadelphia, WB Saunders Co, 1976, pp 299–341.

CLINICAL PROBLEMS

I. A 33-year-old woman complains of generalized pruritus and jaundice of several weeks' duration. She has no past history of any medical problems. She denies any exposure to hepatitis or medications except birth control pills. She has had no abdominal pain, weight loss, or fever. She specifically denies any intestinal symptoms other than light-colored stools and dark urine. Her physical examination is normal except for obvious jaundice and skin excoriations.

Preliminary laboratory data reveal a normal blood count (including the white cell differential), a slightly elevated SGPT, an alkaline phosphatase five times the upper limit of normal, and a bilirubin of 6.8 mg%.

1. What further diagnostic tests should be undertaken?
2. What type of drug-induced liver injury does she have?
3. How should she be managed?

II. A 35-year-old woman has been receiving chronic nitrofurantoin therapy for two years because of recurrent bouts of pyelonephritis. For the past two months, she has noted gradual fatigue, anorexia, weight loss, and, most recently, jaundice. She has had no abdominal pain, fever, or urinary tract symptoms. Review of her chart reveals that, for at least the past six months, the serum transaminases have been elevated. Physical examination demonstrates mild scleral icterus and a slightly enlarged liver.

Laboratory evaluation reveals elevated transaminases (eight times normal), bilirubin of 3.5 mg%, and a slightly abnormal alkaline phosphatase. The hepatitis B surface antigen is negative. There is no biliary tree dilatation demonstrated on ultrasound examination. Liver biopsy is undertaken.

1. What is the biopsy likely to demonstrate?
2. What other drugs produce a picture of chronic active hepatitis?
3. What other types of chronic liver disease can drugs produce?

III. A 46-year-old man who is a chronic alcoholic is admitted to the hospital with jaundice, fever, and tender hepatomegaly of two weeks' duration. Mild ascites is also present. Encephalopathy is absent. His admitting laboratory tests reveal leukocytosis (white blood cell count, 17,000/mm^3, with 72% polymorphonuclear leukocytes and 12% band forms); serum albumin, 3.4 gm%, SGOT, 107 IU (normal value, < 35 IU), an SGPT of 21 IU (normal value, < 40 IU); a bilirubin of 18.6 mg%; an alkaline phosphatase of 117 IU (normal, < 105 IU); and a normal prothrombin time.

1. What are the likely diagnoses?
2. What further evaluation should be done?
3. How should the patient be managed?

Discussion

I. 1. The likely problem is that the patient's disease is related to the birth control pills. Since the question of extrahepatic biliary obstruction is still open, an ultrasound examination should be ordered.

2. This represents a typical cholestatic pattern that can be produced by estrogen. This would also be a "predictable" reaction.

3. Clearly the birth control pills should be stopped. She should be instructed in the relationship between the drug and the symptoms, and advised not to take contraceptive steroids anymore. The patient should be followed until the symptoms resolve and the biochemical tests return to normal. If the jaundice persists, a cholangiogram should be obtained.

II. 1. The biochemical picture is consistent with hepatocellular necrosis. Presumably this hepatitis has been present for at least six months. Thus, it would not be surprising to find some form of chronic hepatitis. In view of the symptoms, chronic active hepatitis would be most likely. Cirrhosis may or may not also be present. Nitrofurantoin, when consumed chronically, is associated with this clinical and histologic picture in a small proportion of patients.

2. Most drugs that are hepatotoxic produce "acute" disease. A few drugs are known to lead to chronic active hepatitis. These include alpha-methyldopa, isoniazid, and dantrolene.

3. Several other drugs produce other forms of chronic liver disease. Chlorpromazine use may be associated with a clinical syndrome and histologic picture similar to that of primary biliary cirrhosis. Estrogens and androgens can produce benign and malignant primary hepatic tumors. Methotrexate can produce progressive fibrosis without much hepatonecrosis. Perhexilene has been associated with a picture similar to that of alcoholic hepatitis. Both estrogens and alkaloids can cause thrombosis of hepatic veins (Budd-Chiari syndrome).

III. 1. This is a fairly typical picture of alcoholic hepatitis. However, several other possibilities need to be considered. Any acute upper abdominal process in an alcoholic may present a similar picture. Thus, one must consider acute cholecystitis or cholangitis, perforated (and sealed over) peptic ulcer disease, liver abscess, pancreatitis, and even an acute complication of a liver tumor. Other nonabdominal causes of fever (specifically other sites of infection) must also be sought.

2. The biochemical picture is most compatible with alcoholic liver disease. Nonetheless, a serum amylase, hepatitis serology, radiographic study of the upper gastrointestinal tract,

and an abdominal ultrasound could be appropriately ordered. Blood culture, chest x-ray, and a urinalysis and culture should also be obtained. A diagnostic paracentesis should be performed.

3. If, after this evaluation is done, the patient is still thought to have uncomplicated alcoholic hepatitis, supportive measures are indicated. These include appropriate fluid and electrolyte management, vitamin and caloric replenishment, and, most importantly, alcohol abstinence. In the absence of encephalopathy or a coagulopathy, the prognosis for survival of the acute illness is good. The patient must be educated to the threat of continued drinking and a long-term alcoholic rehabilitation program should be begun.

Index